KT-564-624

Biomechanics: Problem Solving for Functional Activity

SUSAN L. ROBERTS, M.DIV., O.T.R.
SHARON A. FALKENBURG, M.S., O.T.R.

Illustrated by Avtar Dunaway

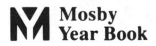

Mosby
Year Book

St. Louis   Baltimore   Boston   Chicago   London   Philadelphia   Sydney   Toronto

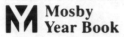
Mosby
Year Book

Dedicated to Publishing Excellence

Sponsoring Editor: David K. Marshall
Assistant Editor: Julie Tryboski
Associate Managing Editor, Manuscript Services: Deborah Thorp
Production Project Coordinator: Carol Reynolds
Proofroom Manager: Barbara Kelly

Copyright © 1992 by Mosby-Year Book, Inc.
A. C.V. Mosby imprint of Mosby-Year Book, Inc.

Mosby-Year Book, Inc.
11830 Westline Industrial Drive
St. Louis, MO 63146

All rights reserved. No part of this publication may be reproduced, stored in a retrieval system, or transmitted, in any form or by any means, electronic, mechanical, photocopying, recording, or otherwise, without prior written permission from the publisher. Printed in the United States of America. Permission to photocopy or reproduce solely for internal or personal use is permitted for libraries or other users registered with the Copyright Clearance Center, provided that the base fee of $4.00 per chapter plus $.10 per page is paid directly to the Copyright Clearance Center, 21 Congress Street, Salem, MA 01970. This consent does not extend to other kinds of copying, such as copying for general distribution, for advertising or promotional purposes, for creating new collected works, or for resale.

1 2 3 4 5 6 7 8 9 0 CL ML 96 95 94 93 92

Library of Congress Cataloging-in-Publication Data
Roberts, Susan L., 1951-
    Biomechanics : problem solving for functional activity / Susan L.
Roberts, Sharon A. Falkenburg.
        p.   cm.
    Includes bibliographical references and index.
    ISBN 0-8016-4047-4
    1. Biomechanics.   2. Human mechanics.   I. Falkenburg, Sharon A.
II. Title.
    [DNLM: 1. Biomechanics.   2. Models, Biological.   3. Movement.
4. Problem Solving.   WE 103 R647b]
QP303.R58   1991   91-22785
612.7'6—dc20   CIP
DNLM/DLC
for Library of Congress

HAMMERSMITH AND WEST
LONDON COLLEGE
LIBRARY

14 APR 1996

DAW B147125 £16.00
612.044
281569

281569

*I wish to dedicate this book to my former
kinesiology students at Eastern Kentucky
University, who taught me at least as much
as I taught them.*

S.L.R.

*I wish to dedicate this book to Doug and Barb,
the nurturers of my dreams; and to my family,
especially my parents, Eunice and Don, for
allowing me to discover and choose.*

S.A.F.

FOREWORD

The use of purposeful activity to prevent and restore dysfunction or to maintain function is a major therapeutic process of occupational therapy. Activities are selected for therapeutic intervention based on analysis of their inherent characteristics as well as the meaningfulness of a particular activity for a particular patient. Occupational therapists who treat persons with physical dysfunction analyze activities preparatory to using them as therapeutic media, to determine their potential effectiveness to prevent or correct a particular physical problem. Occupational therapists assess the demands of daily life tasks to determine whether persons with diseased joints or weak muscles can or should engage in particular activities with or without adaptations. Occupational therapists design tool and environmental adaptations to allow independence in life tasks. They design and construct orthoses to prevent or correct deformities or assist function. Occupational therapists also assess job demands to determine the fitness of a worker to return to a previous job or to determine the need for modifications of the workplace, the tools, or the routine in order to prevent work-related cumulative trauma. All these therapeutic interventions involve determination of the forces acting on the body or of those that the body must produce to engage in the task. They involve biomechanical principles that have heretofore been learned as "rules" such as "the location, in relation to the patient, of the objects used in an activity changes the muscles used and/or the forces required of the muscles" or "persons with arthritis should prevent damage to joints by use of the strongest/largest joints available for the job rather than weaker/smaller joints" or "a wrist splint extends two thirds the length of the forearm for proper leverage to maintain neutral wrist position" or "the pull of elastics in a traction splint should be at 90 degrees to the part to which it is attached" or "high repetitions of a particular motion, especially if resisted, increase the likelihood of developing cumulative trauma injury."

Beyond these "rules" of practice for specific treatment situations, occupational therapists need to have a thorough knowledge of biomechanical concepts to guide therapeutic decision making and professional judgment. For example, those who treat persons with rheumatoid arthritis need to understand the biomechanical basis for joint deformities that arise due to displacement of tendons secondary to joint swelling or destruction of supportive tissue so that they can explain the rationale of activity prescription and prohibition to the patient, the patient's family, and to professional colleagues. Those who treat persons with neurological dysfunction must realize that tasks performed in certain positions are more biomechanically demanding than others, and will stress the nervous system and affect responses.

With this book, Roberts and Falkenburg have made a major contribution to the advancement of occupational therapy by capturing into the practice of occupational therapy the physical and mathematical concepts that underlie the "rules of practice" and the mechanisms that underlie normal neuromusculoskeletal function. There are many biomechanical texts and journals, but they presuppose knowledge of mathematics and physics beyond the level of currently trained occupational therapists. Roberts and Falkenburg have stripped the mystery away from biomechanics and have enabled the reader with no more than high school level knowledge of mathematics and physics to understand and use biomechanical principles. By giving examples of the application of these principles to practice problems and by guiding the reader through the solution to the problems, the authors have enabled occupational therapists to learn to use biomechanical analysis as a regular tool of their profession. Whenever a person gains conceptual knowledge and the ability to apply it to special circumstances, he or she is free to be a creative problem solver, an important characteristic of professionals, rather than being bound to operate from a rulebook as would be more characteristic of technicians. Therapists so empowered will now be more able to seek creative solutions to problems presented in their practice by individual patients in individual circumstances.

Catherine A. Trombly, Sc.D., OTR, F.A.O.T.A.
Professor
Department of Occupational Therapy
Sargent College of Allied Health Professions
Boston University
Boston, Massachusetts

PREFACE

The material in this book was first presented to the "Human Motion and Activity" class at Eastern Kentucky University in the fall of 1986. Many of the students in that class confessed that one reason they had chosen careers in occupational therapy was because it "did not require any math." I understood their position very well. The lack of required coursework in math, chemistry, and physics had drawn me to occupational therapy as well. Later in my career I learned to value these courses and regret that I had not taken them in high school and college. When I finally decided to tackle them, I learned to my dismay that I had a serious learning disability in these areas and mastering them would take more time than I had available to me.

However, in 1986 I became responsible for teaching biomechanics to occupational therapy students at Eastern Kentucky University. At that time the Kentucky Occupational Therapy Association was working to get state licensure. There was strong opposition for licensure coming from academic physical therapists who maintained that occupational therapists had insufficient knowledge of biomechanics to perform such treatments as joint mobilization. One of the course objectives of "Human Motion and Activity" was to learn principles of biomechanics so that my course outlines would be presented as part of the licensure arguments.

During the summer recess I dutifully took home books on biomechanics and studied diligently, or tried to. Most of the summer I spent looking for *sines* and *cosines* until a math teacher finally explained that these were concepts, not locations. This revelation not only opened the door for biomechanics, but to a whole new perspective on occupational therapy.

Before learning biomechanics, I had designed splints and adaptive equipment intuitively, and gave explanations such as, "it fits the normal arch of the hand," or "it gives more power to weak muscles." After learning biomechanics, I still designed splints and adaptive equipment intuitively, but I could make drawings that clearly showed important dimensions of length and placement. I could justify the need for these pieces of equipment with explanations such as, "it displaces the force of the intrinsic muscles without losing any power," and "the lever arm doubles the force produced by weak muscles." The reasons for the equipment had not changed, but the vocabulary had, and this new vocabulary gave more credibility to what I was doing.

In addition, biomechanics opened up arenas in ergonomics and human factors engineering that seemed to be perfect for occupational therapists if they could speak the language. Adaptation of environments is increasingly important in the workplace, and ergonomics is a field that is opening up for occupational therapists. Adaptation to environments is even more important in fields such as aerospace, and occupational therapists need to begin to communicate their expertise in adaptation to those who work in aerospace human factors engineering. A fluency in the principles of biomechanics is one way that we can do this.

Most of the concepts presented here are not new. They are based in common sense and everyday experience. What is new is naming these concepts with numbers and vocabulary from the worlds of math and physics. Even those with a serious math disability can learn this vocabulary. There were students who entered my course and had never seen a variable (like x) in an equation. By the end of the semester they could draw diagrams that showed the interaction of gravitational and muscle forces that produced movement.

Many occupational therapists are scared of numbers and therefore scared of biomechanics. Numbers are simply a means of describing concepts. These concepts explain phenomena that can be useful for understanding human activity. Play with the math. Use it to see if concepts are understood. Do not be upset if your method of solving the problem is different than that contained in this book. If your answers are close, you are probably understanding the concepts. As occupational therapists know best, there is always more than one way to solve a problem.

Susan L. Roberts, M.Div., O.T.R.

ACKNOWLEDGMENTS _____

Many people were helpful in the writing of this book. Without their assistance and support the tasks of writing would have been much more difficult.

Avtar Dunaway, our illustrator, not only produced fine drawings, but had infinite patience to redo them as we changed our minds. Her insights about how biomechanics affects everyday activities were valuable for many of the problems found in the text.

Fran Heron read through the entire manuscript and offered editorial suggestions where needed.

Many of our colleagues discussed the book with us and gave us suggestions for illustrating and clarifying concepts contained in the text. Marge Campbell and Lynn Carlson read through the chapter on the lower extremity, and provided us with expertise from a physical therapist's perspective. Nancy Harris Ossman, Barbara Brown, Martha Flores, Judy Jorgensen, and Kay Benjamin discussed with us aspects of biomechanics that affect their practice of occupational therapy.

We received lots of encouragement from friends, family, and colleagues throughout the entire process. Cindy Carlson, Bob Minton, and the staff of the Center for Occupational Rehabilitation and Education of Tucson were enthusiastic and generous in their support of the entire endeavor, especially in the early stages. The occupational therapy staff of Tucson Medical Center provided time to work and encouragement when needed as the manuscript neared completion. Diane Deyoe provided much-needed support and working space when it was needed to put the final manuscript together. Staff members at NATLSCO read the parts of the final copy and gave us valuable feedback based on their areas of expertise.

Susan L. Roberts, M.Div., O.T.R.
Sharon A. Falkenburg, M.S., O.T.R.

CONTENTS _____

PART **I** _____

Overview

Chapter 1

Philosophy

What does philosophy have to do with occupational therapy and biomechanics? Philosophy is a way of organizing human experience. Personal experiences are organized into **assumptions** that become a **model** for understanding new experiences. Groups of people may incorporate models into a system that forms a **frame of reference** for their collective experience. Compatible frames of reference make up culturally accepted **philosophies** that affect individual perceptions of experience. Scientific **theories** develop within and occasionally challenge accepted philosophies.

Assumptions about how activity affects human life are grouped together to form **models** of occupational therapy practice. A number of these models are based on a frame of reference known as biomechanics.

BIOMECHANICS AS A FRAME OF REFERENCE

Biomechanics is a system of assumptions about forces affecting the human body. Mathematics is used to understand these effects. Basic principles of biomechanics can be applied to all human activities of self-care, work, or recreation.

Biomechanics developed from a mechanistic philosophy or worldview. This philosophy was conceived in the late Middle Ages and reached maturity during the Industrial Revolution.

Mechanistic philosophies separate mind from body. Individuals are viewed as a composition of interrelated components. Time is linear and evolutionary. The past is a focus that may be used as an example to try to manage events in the future. Relationships between people and objects are viewed as parts in a machine. If the machine is well managed and well maintained, it will function at peak efficiency. Conflict, trauma, and other difficulties are interpreted as breakdowns in the machine. People, communities, or objects at the center of these breakdowns are viewed as victims that may or may not be restored to working order. Those who choose to intervene with a mechanistic philosophy often use a managerial style in order to coordinate all of the isolated parts.

In the 15th century Galileo combined his observations of the world around him with mathematics. He is considered the father of modern science. Descartes, in the 17th century, outlined a mechanistic philosophy that separated mind from matter. Influenced by Descartes, Newton used Galileo's studies to construct a system of mechanics that became the foundation of classic physics. Newtonian physics was not seriously challenged until Einstein's work in the 20th century. Einstein's theories and the advent of nuclear technology caused major upheavals in both science and philosophy that resulted in a number of new theories and philosophies.

One of these theories involves the study of chaos as a mathematic construct. Scientists trying to understand phenomena as diverse as weather and cardiac rhythms have begun to devise mathematic assumptions for understanding what was previously unpredictable. The assumptions they have made indicate that seemingly insignificant changes at a particular moment in time will produce more global changes at a later time. It is as if a butterfly flapping its wings in China could produce rainstorms in Iowa.

The mathematics of chaos reflects and influences a newer transformative philosophy. In transformative philosophy the individual is never separated from the environment but is always part of a much larger and interdependent open system. Time is relative. New emerges from old, and both are changed. Relationships are part of dynamic, infinitely unique patterns and harmonies. Conflict, trauma, and difficulty are thought to be part of a larger pattern, perhaps serving as a catalyst for creative adaptation. People and communities who adapt and create new ways of being are viewed as survivors or artists who have found a dynamic and harmonious place within their system.

USING BIOMECHANICS AS A MODEL TO DEVELOP OCCUPATIONAL THERAPY PRACTICE

Biomechanics is based on a mechanistic worldview. Several occupational therapy models for evaluation and treatment are based on biomechanics. Models that come out of this frame of reference isolate body parts for further examination and analysis.

In 1918 psychologist Bird T. Baldwin organized an occupational therapy department at Walter Reed General Hospital in Washington, D.C. Baldwin began routine measurements of joint motion and muscle strength and used these data to develop a method of evaluation and treatment. Baldwin believed that voluntary activities, graded and adapted to specific muscles and joints, would result in a return of function. His model is called the **Reconstruction Model.**

In the first half of the century occupational therapist Marjorie Taylor used knowledge of anatomy, physiology, pathology, and kinesiology to develop activities designed for specific muscle and joint problems. She believed that treatment should be specific to the problem muscles and joints. Her model is called the **Orthopedic Model.**

In 1950 physicians Sidney Licht and William R. Dunton, Jr., wrote a textbook of occupational therapy. Licht outlined another model for occupational therapy evaluation and treatment in the belief that occupational therapists needed to become more scientific. To this end he developed many working definitions of occupational therapy practice that are still valuable. Licht's model is called the **Kinetic Model.**

These biomechanical models have provided occupational therapists with a way to (1) objectively outline and define musculoskeletal problems, (2) develop exercise and activity that restores and maintains function, (3) design and fabricate adaptive equipment to meet functional activity goals, and (4) objectively measure functional musculoskeletal progress in treatment.

Biomechanics can be used to research the effects of activity on the musculoskeletal system. It provides an approach that is most useful in hand clinics, centers for physical rehabilitation, work-hardening clinics, and industry. Because biomechanics is a reductionistic model used in a profession that stresses a holistic approach, it is often used in conjunction with other models of occupational therapy.

LIMITATIONS OF BIOMECHANICS AS A MODEL FOR OCCUPATIONAL THERAPY PRACTICE

In occupational therapy biomechanics is based primarily on the mechanics of the musculoskeletal system. Biomechanics does not concern itself with the rest of the person, that is, cognitive, emotional, and social aspects of function. There is little attempt to balance these components of individual function with the environment in which a person operates. Biomechanics has not led to a comprehensive framework for occupational therapy practice. It has often contributed to confusion between occupational and physical therapy because of the focus on exercise as an activity to improve and maintain musculoskeletal function.

USING BIOMECHANICS WITH OTHER OCCUPATIONAL THERAPY MODELS OF PRACTICE

Biomechanics provides an objective means for evaluating musculoskeletal function in activity. This is an important aspect of physical function and needs to be addressed as part of any occupational therapy evaluation. Biomechanics can be a lens through which to look at a specific part of function. However, this model needs to be blended and combined with others in order to be part of contemporary occupational therapy practice.

Occupational therapists are creating new models that more closely guide and describe what it is that they do best. A. Jean Ayres' model of sensory integration practice presupposes that small changes in the processing of sensory input will produce global adaptive responses in people's interaction with their environment. Lorna Jean King has elaborated on Ayres' work to develop a model of adaptive responses for understanding patterns of change and growth. Mary Reilly and Gary Kielhofner have used an open systems model for describing human activity. All of these models use a neurobehavioral frame of reference that does not assume that growth and change will be a linear process. Belief in the uniqueness of individual experience comes out a transformative rather than mechanistic philosophy.

Occupational therapists use biomechanics to design and modify adaptive equipment, to evaluate the safety of home and work environments, and to create therapeutic activities and exercise programs. Most occupational therapists try to be aware of how a piece of equipment, a modified workstation, or a trip to the mall will enable individuals to participate more fully in their community. Like the Chinese butterfly that sets off a weather pattern leading to rain in Iowa, occupational therapists expect their little bit to go a long way.

BIBLIOGRAPHY

Cannon K: Resources for a Constructive Ethic—the Black Woman's Literary Tradition. Course taught in Cambridge, Mass, Harvard Divinity School, 1984.
Fritjof C: *The Tao of Physics.* New York, Bantam Press, 1984.
Gleick J: *Chaos: Making a New Science.* New York, Viking Press, 1987.
Reed K: *Models of Practice in Occupational Therapy,* Baltimore, Williams & Wilkins, 1984.

Chapter 2

How to Use This Book

Biomechanics is a frame of reference that can be used to analyze human activity. To do so requires an understanding of mechanical physics as it applies to the human musculoskeletal system. Basic vocabulary for discussing the human body and physics is provided in Chapters 3 and 4. The physics needed for solving basic problems in biomechanics is covered in Chapters 5 through 8. Biomechanics used as a tool for analyzing human activity is the focus of Chapters 9 through 11.

Problems are presented throughout the book to enable readers to get experience with an application of biomechanics to human activity. Solving these problems requires an ability to make a diagram organizing the information, some basic mathematics, and a few tools, such as a goniometer. The book is structured in a logical progression. Information is learned in much the same order as would be followed in solving a clinical problem involving biomechanics.

USING LINE DRAWINGS TO ORGANIZE PROBLEMS IN BIOMECHANICS

Line drawings require no artistic skill but can give an accurate representation of biomechanics in a problem. These drawings can be used to communicate information to bioengineers, physicians, clients, and other people who may be involved in the treatment process. Biomechanics provides a framework for understanding how movement is taking place. The steps for organizing information into a line drawing are as follows:

1. Look at the parts of the body used in an activity. Observe the activity as a whole to determine where movement is taking place. Note whether there is more than one movement.
2. Identify which specific joints and active muscle groups play a major role in the activity. Some muscles and joints will be less important. Joints and muscles playing a major role may change with different phases of an activity. (Anatomic terms for specific movements are covered in Chapter 3.)

3. Decide which plane or planes of motion will provide for the best analysis. Since analysis will be done from a two-dimensional drawing, it is important to find out which plane gives the clearest view of the entire motion. Different phases of an activity may require different views. (Planes of motion and their axes are covered in Chapter 3.)

4. Draw a line diagram that includes all of the relevant information (see Fig 2–1):

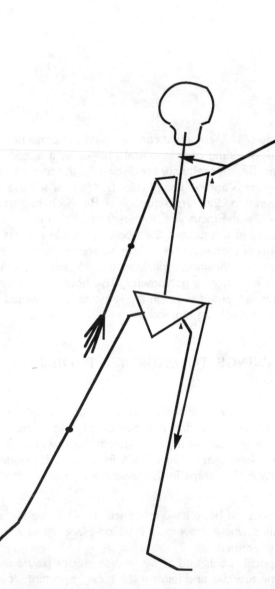

FIG 2–1.
Line drawings do not need to be works of art but should indicate the relationships of bones, joints, and active muscle groups.

    a. Skeletal segments—use bold lines to indicate the bones that are moving.

    b. Joints—use triangles to indicate the axis of movement that is taking place (a goniometer may be helpful to determine joint angles and can be used to draw these angles for a diagram).

    c. Muscles—use light lines from the muscle's point of origin to its point of insertion.

    d. Objects or tools—use circles, squares, or other simple geometric shapes that approximate the object's size.

5. Determine where and how gravity is acting on the human body and on tools or other objects. (Gravity is covered in Chapter 5.)

6. Determine what forces are operating to move specific body parts, objects, or tools. (Linear force, torque, and equilibrium are covered in Chapters 6, 7, and 8, respectively.)

USING MATHEMATICS TO SOLVE PROBLEMS IN BIOMECHANICS

Although this book does not propose to be a text in mathematics, math is the language of physics and engineering. Some knowledge of basic mathematic concepts is essential to solve problems in biomechanics. Schematic drawings can be used to communicate these problems and solutions to others. Understanding how math works in biomechanics will also help therapists identify relevant data needed to solve clinical problems, especially those that may require teamwork with bioengineers or orthotists.

In this text math is used primarily to demonstrate principles of biomechanics. Math problems are rounded off to two decimal places. Doing this means that mathematic answers are not up to bioengineering standards, which require more precise measurement and answers that give an average error of measurement. Such strict standards are not necessary in typical occupational therapy practice and lie beyond the mathematic level of this textbook. Nevertheless, occupational therapists can and do work with engineers whose knowledge and understanding of mechanics permits the precise mathematics necessary for designing complex adaptive equipment, orthotics, and ergonomic tools for industry.

The following section contains ten mathematic problems common to biomechanics. When the mathematic principles in these problems are understood, other problems in biomechanics can be readily solved.

Solutions to these problems are found at the end of the chapter. Explanations of how they are solved are found in Appendix A. Use the appendix as a resource when looking at other problems involving biomechanics. Problems solved in each chapter make use of mathematic calculation so that therapists can gain familiarity with the mathematics needed to analyze human activity. Numerical results are discussed and interpreted for use in the clinical setting.

WORKING WITH VARIABLES IN AN EQUATION

1. $8x = 48$
2. $0.3x + (0.25 \times 4) - 16 = 0$
3. $5(x - 4) + 10 = 45$
4. $12x - 6 - 2(4x + 8) = 0$
5. $x13 + \frac{1}{2} = \frac{3}{4}$

SIMPLE GEOMETRY

6. In the parallelogram *ABCD* in the figure below, side *a* is 5 cm, and side *b* is 8.5 cm. Angle *A* is 40 degrees. Line *e* divides the parallelogram into two equal triangles. Line *f* divides *ABC* into two right triangles. What are the values of the angles in each right triangle?

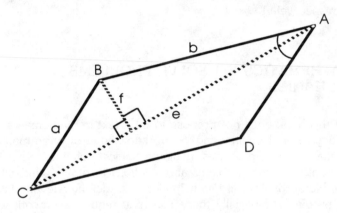

7. In the right triangle *ABC* in the figure below, side *a* is 4 cm, and side *b* is 3 cm long. How long is hypotenuse *c*?

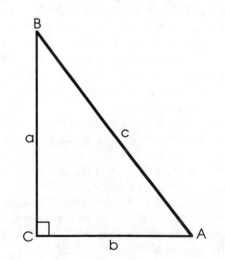

BASIC TRIGONOMETRY

8. In the right triangle *ABC* in the figure below, side *a* is 4 cm, and side *c* is 8 cm. How large is angle *A*?

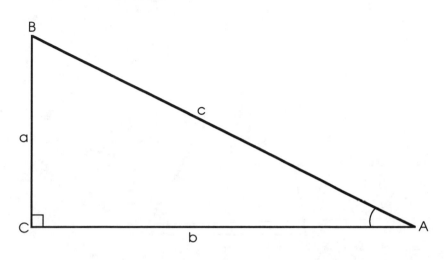

9. In the right triangle *ABC* in the figure below, the hypotenuse is 12 cm, and angle *A* is 15 degrees. How long are the sides?

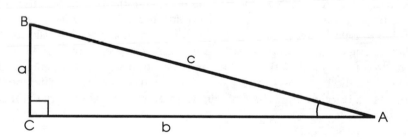

10. In the triangle *ABC* in the figure below, side *b* = 6.0 cm, side *c* = 9.0 cm, and angle *A* = 60 degrees. How long is side *a*?

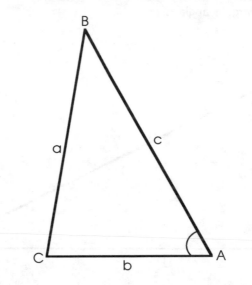

TOOLS FOR SOLVING PROBLEMS IN BIOMECHANICS

Biomechanics requires a few tools. The most important of these is the goniometer. It is used to measure joint angles. Knowing these angles provides a gauge for measuring muscle forces. A calculator is helpful for reaching mathematic solutions. A scientific calculator that computes sines and cosines is even more useful. A table of sines and cosines is included in Appendix B, so the use of a calculator is optional when working the problems in this text. Colored pens or pencils to differentiate muscles, bones, and forces in a schematic drawing are another aid to organization.

ANSWERS TO PROBLEMS
1. $x = 6$
2. $x = 50$
3. $x = 11$
4. $x = 5.5$
5. $x = \frac{3}{4}$
6. 20, 70, and 90 degrees
7. 5 cm
8. 30 degrees
9. 3.1 and 11.6 cm
10. 7.9 cm

PART II

Vocabulary: Basic Concepts

Chapter 3

The Human Body: Concepts From Medicine

The language of medicine is rich with words that describe unique physiologic conditions and minute areas of anatomic geography. These words are derived from Greek and Latin as well as a variety of other language roots. Although medical terms are often confusing to the uninitiated, the ability to say something in one word that would otherwise take several phrases is very useful. This chapter will cover terms that are commonly used to describe human movement.

GENERAL TERMS

Pinpointing specific areas of the human body is of utmost importance in medicine. In most instances the body is envisioned in **anatomic position,** that is, upright with the face, feet, and palms facing forward. When one body part is above another, it is referred to as **superior** or **superficial** to that part. Body parts are **inferior** or **deep** to body parts that are above them. Body parts closer to the front of the body are referred to as **anterior,** and those that are closer to the back are referred to as **posterior. Medial** body parts lie nearer the middle of the body, and **lateral** body parts lie nearer the right or left sides of the body. Arms and legs are referred to as **extremities,** and they connect to the trunk at their **proximal** ends. Fingers and toes are found at the **distal** ends.

THE NERVOUS SYSTEM

Biomechanics of the musculoskeletal system is the focus of this book. Understanding the role of the nervous system is essential to understanding the musculoskeletal system. It is briefly reviewed in this chapter.

The Central Nervous System

The **brain** and **spinal cord** make up the **central nervous system,** which controls all of the body's activities.

The Brain is divided into three major anatomic parts: cerebrum, cerebellum, and brainstem. The **cerebrum** receives sensory information and processes it to produce body responses, including movement. The cerebrum is divided into two **hemispheres.** Information from these hemispheres crosses from one side to the other via the **corpus callosum** and other pathways. The right hemisphere controls the left side of the body, and the left hemisphere controls the right side of the body. The **cortex** is the superficial layer of the cerebrum and processes information for all tasks requiring conscious thought. In a part of the cortex that runs from ear to ear there are two strips of cells lying side by side. These cells are primary processors of **sensory** information and primary directors of **motor** performance.

The cerebrum contains other important centers for processing sensory information and for organizing **subcortical** responses that do not require conscious thought. The cortex and corpus callosum surround the **limbic lobe** and **basal ganglia.** These contain collections of cells known as **nuclei** that coordinate complex motor responses to environmental stimulation.

The **brainstem** connects the cerebrum with the spinal cord. It contains a number of differentiated cellular structures. Two of them, the **thalamus** and **hypothalamus,** primarily regulate functions such as breathing, digestion, alertness, hormonal balance, and temperature control.

The **cerebellum** rises out of the brainstem but forms a special structure of its own. The cerebellum functions chiefly to regulate muscle **tone** and **equilibrium** or balance responses.

The spinal cord carries information to the brain from the body and to the body from the brain. Cells carrying specific kinds of information are grouped together to form pathways known as **tracts.**

The Peripheral Nervous System

Information is brought to and from the body via branches of nerve cells located in the brain and spinal cord or in special structures called **ganglia. Afferent** branches carry information from the body to the brain. **Efferent** branches carry information from the brain to muscles and glands. **Somatic** nerves carry information to and from muscles. **Visceral** nerves carry information to and from organs and glands.

Spinal nerves branch out from the spinal cord. In several locations spinal nerves are grouped to form a network known as a **plexus.** The **cervical plexus** located in the neck supplies structures in the neck and shoulder. The **brachial plexus** under the arm in the **axilla** supplies the upper extremity. **Lumbar** and **sacral plexuses** supply the lower extremity.

Cranial nerves branch out from the brain. There are 12 pairs of cranial nerves. All of these nerves except the tenth pair supply structures in the head and neck. The tenth pair of cranial nerves supplies organs and other structures in the trunk and abdomen.

The central nervous system controls organs and glands through a system of visceral efferent fibers and ganglia known as the **autonomic nervous system.** Visceral afferent fibers do not run through these ganglia and are not considered part of the autonomic system. The autonomic system is divided into two parts to balance bodily functions. The **parasympathetic** fibers and ganglia emerge from the brain and lower portion of the spinal cord **(craniosacral).** These fibers work to conserve and build up energy and have a calming affect on the body. The **sympathetic** fibers and ganglia emerge from the middle **(thoracolumbar)** portion of the spinal cord. Their function is to prepare for any environmental crisis, and they have an excitatory affect on the body.

Control of Movement

The nervous system controls movement in the body and limbs. Information reaches the central nervous system from sensory **receptors** in the skin, muscles, and related tissues. This information stimulates a variety of motor responses, depending on what part of the central nervous system the information reaches. Skeletal muscle fibers contain **muscle spindles.** These receptors are sensitive to changes in the length of muscle fibers. Responses to prolonged lengthening are called **tonic.** Responses to rapid changes in length are called **phasic. Golgi tendon organs** are receptors that protect muscles from tearing by causing them to relax when there is too much stretch on the tendons.

Responses to sensory receptors can occur without conscious thought. They follow subcortical pathways known as **reflexes.** Pathways that make a complete sensory-to-motor connection within the spinal cord are **spinal reflexes.** Spinal reflexes give protective responses to noxious stimuli or to stretching of the muscle spindle. Pathways that make connections in the brainstem are **brainstem reflexes.** Muscle responses to gravity acting on the body are regulated by brainstem reflexes. Movements of the head that affect the entire body are also regulated by brainstem reflexes.

More complex interconnections called **righting reactions** travel pathways to higher levels of the brainstem. These responses primarily involve positioning the head in relation to gravity. **Equilibrium reactions** require integrated connections between the cortex, basal ganglia, and cerebellum. They involve adjustments of the entire body to changes in its center of gravity.

THE MUSCULOSKELETAL SYSTEM

Bones

The skeletal system is made up of more than 200 bones. Although bones are rigid and generally considered to be permanent, bony tissue is dynamic and changes throughout life. The most obvious of these changes is the **ossification** of **cartilage** and **membrane** in early development. An infant skeleton has less bone than an adult skeleton. Centers of cartilaginous growth called **epiphyseal plates** allow bones to grow throughout childhood and into the early twenties. Bony tissue is laid down in response to stress from carrying weight and through movement or trauma. Bone continually remodels itself throughout life by absorbing existing bone and laying down new cells where they are needed.

Joints

Bones are connected to each other with joints. **Diarthrodial** joints have a fluid-filled space between the two or more bones. Bony surfaces are covered with smooth cartilage, and the whole joint is surrounded by a strong ligamentous capsule. Because of these characteristics, diarthrodial joints are the most mobile. In **synarthrodial** joints, bones are joined together with cartilage, fiber, or ligament. **Cartilaginous** and **ligamentous** joints allow some limited movement, but **fibrous** joints permit no movement.

Descriptions of Skeletal Movement

Joint movement is measured with a **goniometer.** The goniometer measures a full 360 degrees of movement. For measurement it is necessary that everyone look at movement in the same way; therefore, movement has been divided into three planes, each of which has a separate axis around which movement takes place.

Figure 3–1 shows a person divided by each of these three planes. The **sagittal plane** cuts the body into right and left sides. The **coronal plane** cuts the body into front and back, and the **horizontal plane** cuts the body into top and bottom. Each axis of movement passes perpendicularly through the plane. The plane revolves around its axis. The sagittal plane has a **frontal-horizontal** or **lateral axis.** The coronal plane has a **sagittal-horizontal** or **anteroposterior axis.** The horizontal plane has a **vertical axis.**

Movements are defined by the plane and axis where they occur. **Flexion** and **extension** take place in a sagittal plane around a lateral axis. **Abduction** and **adduction** take place in a coronal plane around an anteroposterior axis. **Rotation** takes place in a horizontal plane around a vertical axis. Rotation can be **medial** or **lateral** depending on its direction. Forearm rotation is described as **supination** when the palm is turned toward the front of the body and **pronation** when the palm is turned toward the back of the body.

Most active movements do not occur in these anatomic planes but are more often in an **oblique plane** around an **oblique axis.** A great many joints can and do move in all planes to form a cone-shaped movement known as **circumduction.**

Muscles are highly elastic tissues composed of fibers that can shorten to half their resting length or stretch up to 50% longer than their resting length to produce movement. Muscles are intimately connected to the skeletal system through tissue called **fascia.** Fascia makes up the **muscle sheaths** surrounding muscles and becomes the **tendons** that attach muscle to bone. Muscles have many different shapes based on the way they attach to bones via the fascia.

Muscle fiber movement occurs through a chemical process involving **oxygen** and

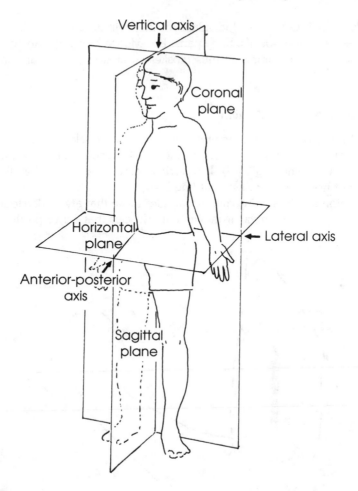

FIG 3–1.
The human body can be divided into three anatomic planes, each of which has an axis around which movement takes place.

adenosine triphosphate **(ATP).** The primary source of oxygen in muscle tissue is **myoglobin.** Like hemoglobin in the blood, myoglobin contains oxygen bonded to iron, and this produces its characteristic red color. Muscle fibers that contain high concentrations of myoglobin are **red.** Those with low concentrations of myoglobin are **white.** Muscles that move rapidly are called **fast-twitch,** whereas postural muscles must work more constantly and are called **slow-twitch.** Slow-twitch fibers depend on a steady supply of oxygen through myoglobin and the blood supply and are generally smaller and redder than fast-twitch fibers, which can produce ATP rapidly without oxygen for limited amounts of time. Muscles are believed to develop into fast-twitch or slow-twitch types because of the type of nerve that innervates them.

Muscle fibers lie parallel to one another. The shape of a muscle and its points of attachment to bone and fascia indicate its potential power for movement as well as which body parts it will move. Individual muscles will be discussed in the chapters that cover movement of specific body parts. Knowledge of human anatomy is essential to biomechanics. Diagrams of musculoskeletal anatomy are found in Appendix H.

Descriptions of Muscular Activity

Several types of **contractions** are common to all muscles. **Concentric** contractions cause muscles to shorten in length (Fig 3–2). **Eccentric** contractions occur as muscles are lengthening (Fig 3–3). **Isometric** contractions occur when there is muscle activity but no outward movement (Fig 3–4).

Every action involves many muscles besides those that are understood to be primarily responsible for a particular movement. Muscles that act to produce a specific

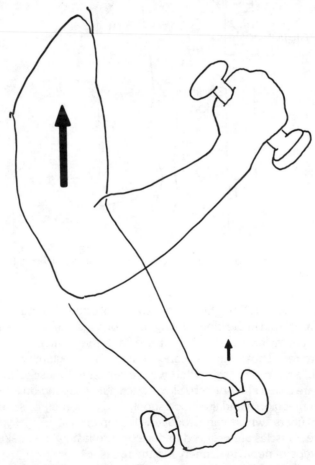

FIG 3–2.
A concentric contraction causes muscle fibers to shorten.

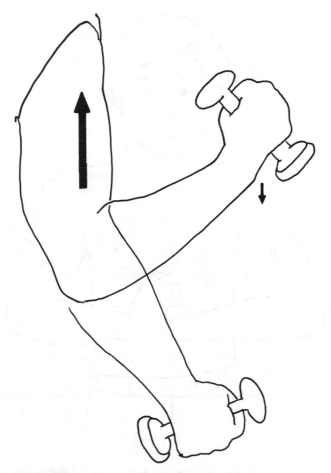

FIG 3–3.
An eccentric contraction allows muscle fibers to lengthen.

movement are called **movers** or **agonists.** Opposing muscles are called **antagonists.** Antagonists must relax to allow agonists to be movers. To protect joints antagonists brake movement at the end of a range of motion. When gravity is the primary force causing movement to take place, antagonists control movement through eccentric contraction.

Muscles that act together to produce specific movements are working in **synergy.** If a muscle performs more than one action, another muscle might act to **neutralize** the unwanted action and produce a different type of movement than the first muscle working alone. **Supporting** muscles hold the trunk and proximal parts of the limbs in advantageous positions. **Fixators** or **stabilizers** create a base for movement by holding bones steady. When agonists and antagonists contract simultaneously to stabilize a joint, it is known as **cocontraction.**

Movement of body parts is **active** when it is produced by muscle actions. **Pas-**

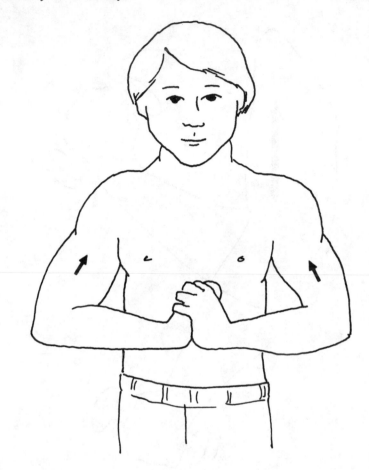

FIG 3–4.
Isometric contraction involves shortening of the muscle fibers without any movement taking place.

sive movement is produced by forces outside the body and involves no muscle activity. Slow active movement involves continuous muscle tension throughout a range of motion. **Ballistic** movements are initiated by rapid strong contractions but completed primarily through momentum. Ballistic movements are controlled through contraction of antagonistic muscles. They can be stopped passively by muscles, ligaments, and other joint tissues at the end of a range of motion or by meeting an outside obstacle or force. Ballistic movements that are passively controlled put joints at more risk for injury than those that are actively controlled.

BIBLIOGRAPHY

Fiorentino M: *Reflex Testing Methods for Evaluating CNS Development.* Springfield, Ill, Charles C Thomas Publishers, 1973.

Luttgens K, Wells K: *Kinesiology: Scientific Basis of Human Motion.* New York, WB Saunders Co, 1982.

Romanes GJ: *Cunningham's Textbook of Anatomy.* London, Oxford University Press, 1972.

Chapter 4 _____

The World: Concepts From Physics

In physics the world is described in mathematic terms that define relationships. These relationships help explain the past and predict the future. Biomechanics is based on the concepts of mechanical physics: the study of motion in gases, liquids, or solids. This chapter will focus on terms that apply to movement of the human musculoskeletal system.

GENERAL TERMS

When physicists talk about a **body,** they are referring to a collection of matter. A body may be incredibly small, like the protons and electrons that make up an atom, or very large like the sun. The human body is a collection of matter. Since "body" is a generic term, in physics it must have specific modifiers to avoid confusion.

TERMS OF MEASUREMENT

Space, time, and mass are all quantified in order to describe their relationship to one another. Different systems of measurement develop in different cultures. Most Americans use the English system, but the metric system is widely used in the scientific community. Metric will be the system used in this textbook. A complete conversion table of the English and metric systems is found in Appendix D.

Scalar Quantities

A **scalar** quantity is one that can be measured by an instrument or scale. Scalar quantities are static. They tend to stay in one place and allow themselves to be measured.

Measures of Space

Measurements of length, area, and volume are considered spatial measurements. In the metric system space is measured in **meters.** The English system measures space in **inches, feet,** and **yards. Length** is a linear, one-dimensional measure of distance (centimeters, meters, inches, miles). **Area** is a planar or two-dimensional measure of a flat surface (square meters or square feet). **Volume** is a cubic measurement of three dimensions (cubic meters, **liters,** cubic inches, **quarts,** or **gallons**).

Measure of Time

Time presents a fourth dimension. The basic unit of measurement for both the English and metric systems is the **second.**

Measures of Mass

Matter is composed of molecules made up of neutrons, protons, electrons, and whatever else physicists have found lately. **Mass** is a quantity of matter determined by the chemical composition of the substance and closeness of its molecules. For example, the hydrogen molecule has only 1 proton and electron pair, whereas larger molecules like carbon, nitrogen, and oxygen have 6, 7, and 8 proton-electron pairs. Potassium, calcium, and iron have 19, 20, and 26, respectively. Consult a periodic table of the elements to determine the number of proton-electron pairs in any of the 105 known elements.

The arrangement of these elements affects their mass. Molecules in solids are closely packed, liquid molecules move freely around each other, and gas molecules bounce around and keep their distance from everything else (think of them as tactually defensive). Water is in a class by itself. Body substances are mostly hydrogen, carbon, and oxygen compounds, but their slightly different chemical compositions determine their mass. Fat, for example, is less dense than bone or muscle, which have more calcium and iron in their composition.

In the metric system **mass** is measured in **grams.** In the English system it is measured in **slugs** (one slug is equal to 32 lb) (Fig 4–1).

Vectors

A **vector** indicates movement. It can only be measured for a specific moment of time because it is constantly changing. Vectors indicate both what can be measured and its direction of movement. Vectors are represented by arrows that show a starting point or point of application, the magnitude of what is measured, and its direction of movement.

Measures of Physical Movement

Speed is a measure of distance divided by time (65 mph). Add a starting point and a direction to make a vector quantity known as **displacement.** Figure 4–2,A shows 65 miles east on Route 66.

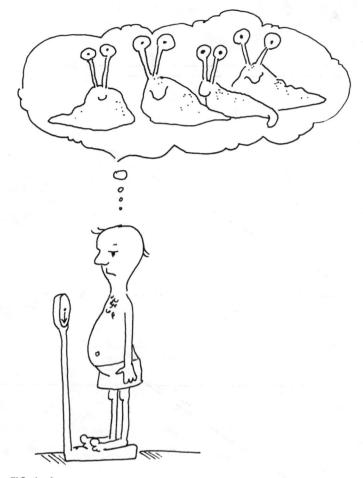

FIG 4-1.
One possible reason why the British measurement system did not flourish.

When displacement *(s)* is divided by time *(t)*, it becomes a vector quantity known as **velocity** *(v)*.

$$v = s/t$$

Figure 4–2,B shows 65 miles east on Route 66 in 60 minutes, which gives an average velocity of 65 mph.

Figure 4–2,C shows travel that begins in Winslow, Arizona; 65 miles east will be midway between exits 311 and 325 on Route 66 (now Interstate 40), and the first 7 miles go through construction for a total of 12 minutes. How much velocity is needed to cover the remaining 58 miles in 60 minutes? This change in velocity is a

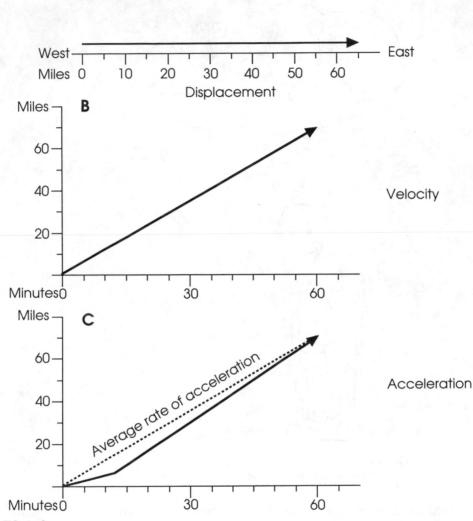

FIG 4–2.
Some common vectors indicating movement. Displacement is distance in a specific direction. Velocity is displacement occurring in a finite amount of time. Acceleration is change in velocity during a period of time.

vector quantity known as **acceleration.** To find an average rate of acceleration subtract the initial velocity *(u)* from the final velocity *(v)*, and divide the result by time *(t)*.

$$a = \frac{v - u}{t}$$

Velocity is always a measurement of displacement over time, so u = 7 miles/0.2 hr will be the time spent driving through construction, or 35 mph. The velocity of the remaining miles will be v = 58 miles/0.8 hr, or 72.5 mph. (Warning: the Arizona Department of Public Safety prohibits traveling at more than 65 mph on state highways.) The average rate of acceleration will be 37.5 mi/hr^2.

$$a = \frac{v - u}{t}$$

$$a = \frac{58 \text{ mi}/0.8 \text{ hr} - 7 \text{ mi}/0.2 \text{ hr}}{1 \text{ hr}}$$

$$a = \frac{72.5 \text{ mi/hr} - 35 \text{ mi/hr}}{1 \text{ hr}}$$

$$a = \frac{37.5 \text{ mi/hr}}{1 \text{ hr}}$$

$$a = 37.5 \text{ mi/hr}^2$$

Average acceleration is expressed in meters or feet by seconds squared, **m/sec^2**.

Measures of Weight

Weight measures both mass and the pull of gravity on that mass. Gravity always pulls toward the center of the earth, and this movement makes weight a vector quantity. Gravity is a constant factor, so as mass increases, weight will increase. In the English system weight is measured in **pounds.** In metric force and weight are measured in **newtons,** named after Sir Isaac Newton who first realized mass had direction when an apple landed on his head (Fig 4–3).

Measures of Force

In physics a force is defined as something that causes an object to be deformed or moved. Forces are measured in metric **newtons** or English **pounds.**

Normal forces are forces directed perpendicularly toward or away from a surface area. Normal forces that push two surfaces together are called **compressive forces** (Fig 4–4,A). Normal forces that pull two surfaces apart are called **tensile forces** (Fig 4–4,B). Forces that act parallel to the surfaces are called **shear** or **tangential forces** (Fig 4–5).

Gravity is a force. Muscle forces act with and against gravity. They also interact with normal forces called reaction forces. **Reaction forces** are opposing forces that are equal responses to gravity or other forces.

Measures of Stress

Stress is different from force. **Stress** is found in the material on which forces act. Tensile forces on the knee would produce tensile stress in the tissues of the knee joint. How much stress is present is determined by multiplying the amount of force by the specific quantity of tissue. Stress is measured in **pascal** (Pa) units, or newtons per meter squared (**n/m^2**).

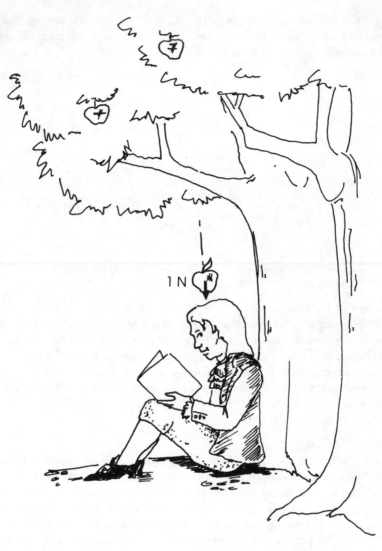

FIG 4–3.
As Newton discovered, gravity produces movement at a constant rate of acceleration. This means that weight can be indicated as a vector.

Measures of Friction

Friction is similar to stress. **Friction** (F) is determined by multiplying a normal force (N) times a coefficient (μ) that is unique to the material in question, $F = \mu N$. For instance, the coefficient of cartilage in a synovial joint is essentially zero, while the coefficient of a crutch tip on rough wood is about 0.70 to 0.75 (Fig 4–6). The closer the coefficient gets to 1.0, the more force will be needed to move this material across the surface in question.

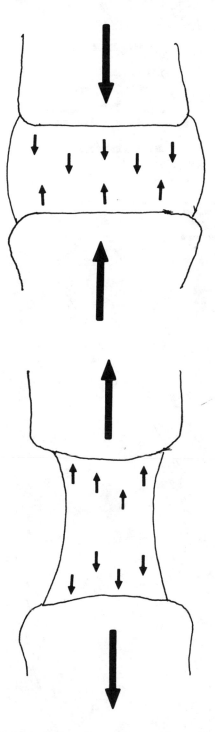

FIG 4-4.
Normal forces are perpendicular to body surfaces, either pushing surfaces together as compressive forces or pulling them apart as tensile forces. Stress occurs in the materials on which forces are acting.

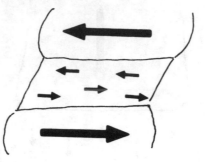

FIG 4–5.
Shear forces are parallel to body surfaces. They cause shear stress in the materials on which they act.

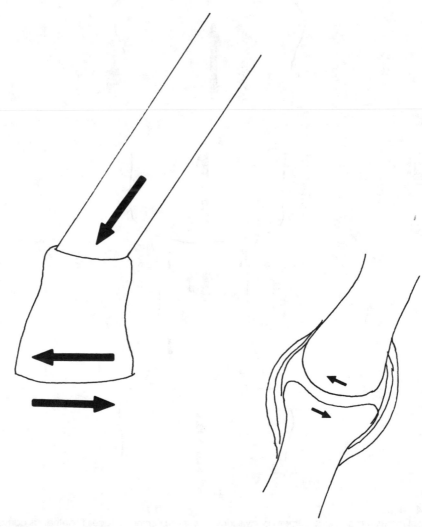

FIG 4–6.
Friction is determined by an object's substance. The friction between rubber and wood is much greater than that between cartilaginous surfaces in a normal synovial joint.

Measures of Work

Work is calculated by multiplying weight times distance times the number of repetitions. For example, to measure the amount of lifting work needed to do a job use the formula $L = mg \times h \times r$. Here, L represents lifting work; mg represents mass times gravity, or weight; h represents the height of objects lifted; and r represents the number of repetitions. To find the amount of hauling work done on a job use the formula $H = mg \times d \times r$. H represents hauling work, d is the distance traveled, and r is the number of repetitions.

TERMS OF RELATIONSHIP

Relationships can take place in many different dimensions. **Linear** relationships are one-dimensional and involve movement from one point to another along a line (usually a straight line). Two-dimensional relationships obviously involve more than one dimension but are conceived of as flat or operating in a single plane. More complex relationships have three or more dimensions. Although the human body is three-dimensional, most of the problems presented in this book will look only at two dimensions at a time.

Linear Relationships

In mechanical problems vectors are drawn with the base of the arrow at the point where movement begins or where a force is first applied. The arrow points in the direction of actual or potential movement. The length of the arrow indicates the quantity, or magnitude, of the movement or potential for movement.

Vectors with the same point of origin can be combined just like other numerical values and forms of measurement. These vectors, then, occur along the same **line of application.** The top of Figure 4–7 shows vectors with the same line of application added together because their arrows point in the same direction; the bottom shows vectors subtracted from each other because their arrows point in a different direction. The combination of vectors derived from these calculations is called a **resultant.**

Figure 4–8 shows how forces acting on a rigid body can be displaced along the

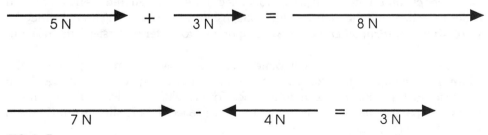

FIG 4–7.
Vectors acting on the same lines of application can be added or subtracted to get a resultant vector.

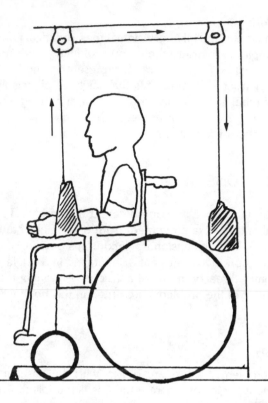

FIG 4–8.
Displacement of vectors. Vectors can be moved along the same line of application without changing their value.

line of application without changing its effect on that body. The mathematic theorem that explains this phenomenon is called the **displacement theorem.** The displacement theorem makes it possible to manipulate vectors to illustrate their resultants.

Two-Dimensional Relationships

If vectors acting on the same point come from different directions, they are called **concurrent.** Often multiple vectors need to be **resolved** into a single vector in order to understand the nature of the relationship. Likewise, a single vector may be resolved into **horizontal** and **vertical components** to better understand the relationship.

Figure 4–9,A shows two component vectors resolved by making a **parallelogram.** Each component makes up one side of the parallelogram, and the equal and opposite sides are drawn in with dotted lines. The resultant is a diagonal line running across the parallelogram. A mathematic construct called the **parallelogram theorem** explains why this is possible.

Figure 4–9,B shows a single vector broken down into two components. The vector becomes a diagonal line, and an imaginary rectangle of horizontal and vertical

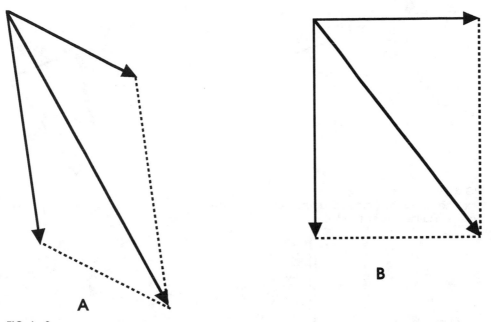

FIG 4–9.
Resolution of concurrent vectors. A diagonal vector can be resolved into horizontal and vertical components. Two vectors acting along different lines of application can be combined to make a parallelogram in order to find their resultant.

lines is drawn around it. Placing the horizontal and vertical components at right angles to each other makes it possible to use mathematic formulas to find a **resolution.**

Figure 4–10 shows how a **polygon** can be drawn to resolve more than two components or vectors operating in the same plane into a single vector. Each vector is drawn so that it connects to the previous one. Length, direction, and angle of orientation must be maintained. A vector line is drawn from the first vector to the last vector. The length and orientation of this vector will give the result of all the contributing vectors.

Forces are measured by using formulas of linear relationship. Detailed methods for determining forces are covered in Chapter 6.

Circular Relationships

When movement takes place around a fixed point (like a joint), different rules apply to the relationships. The fixed point is called an **axis.** The relationship of a vector to an axis is defined as the **radius** of a circle. As the vector moves around the circle, its radial relationship to the axis changes point by point. A force traveling around an axis is called a **moment,** and its radius is a **moment arm.** A moment is the product of a force times its distance from the axis. Circular relationships always gain or lose **momentum** based on the distance of the vector from the axis of the circle (Fig 4–11).

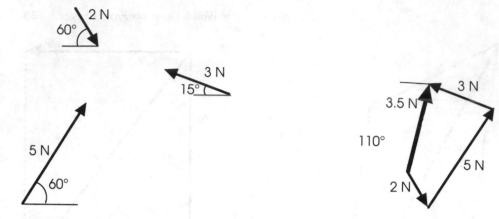

FIG 4–10.
More than two vectors acting at different angles to each other can be combined into a polygon in order to find the resultant vector.

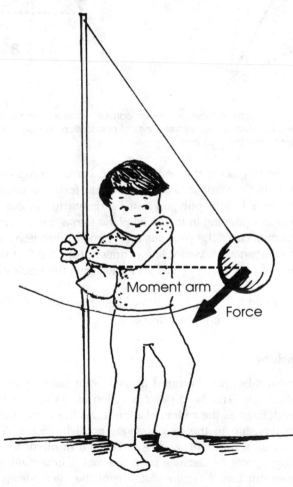

Moment arm

Force

FIG 4–11.
A vector that represents rotary forces will have a moment arm that represents the radius of its circular path at a given moment. Movement in a circle gains or loses momentum.

Torque is the relationship of a force traveling around a fixed point to that point. Torque is determined by multiplying a force times its distance from a fixed point.

Torque = force × moment arm

Human movement takes place around a joint. Methods for determining torque are covered in Chapter 7.

A **lever** is a rigid body (like a bone) traveling around an axis. Its length, therefore, is fixed and can be measured by using scalar measurements. Levers are moved by forces, and forces are measured by using vectors. The length of the lever from its axis to its terminus is called a **lever arm** (Fig 4–12). Sometimes the lever arm and

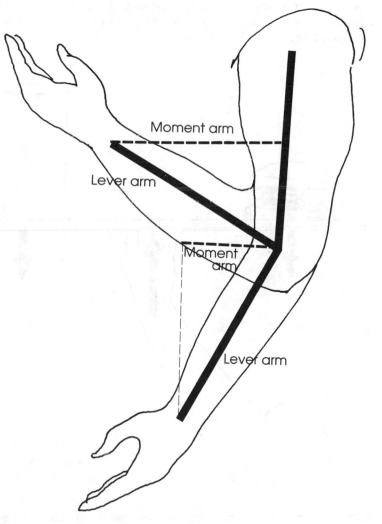

FIG 4–12.
A lever is a rigid body that moves around a fixed axis. The lever arm will remain the same throughout the movement, but the moment arm for the lever may change as the lever moves.

the moment arm are of equal length, but often they are different. Types of levers and calculations involving levers are covered in Chapter 8.

Balanced Relationships

Although most bodies are constantly moving and changing, they do have periods of stability called **equilibrium.** In physics equilibrium is governed by two conditions.

The **first equilibrium condition** looks at how linear or **translatory equilibrium** is achieved (Fig 4–13). In order for a rigid body to remain stable all vertical and horizontal forces acting on it must add up to zero ($\Sigma F = 0$).

To achieve this state with mathematics, horizontal forces are designated as **x.** Positive values are assigned to all forces directed to the right and negative values to all forces directed to the left ($\Sigma F_x = 0$). Vertical forces are designated as **y.** Positive

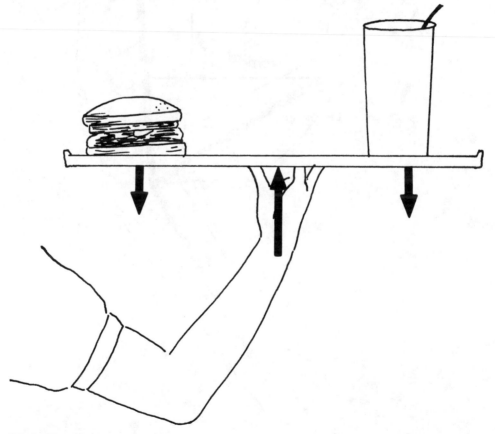

FIG 4–13.
The first equilibrium condition states that vertical and horizontal forces must be equal for a rigid body to remain stable.

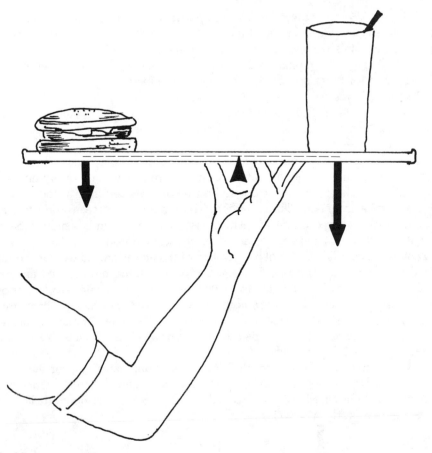

FIG 4–14.
The second equilibrium condition states that rotary movements must be equal for a rigid body to remain stable.

values are assigned to all upward forces and negative values to all downward forces ($\Sigma F_y = 0$). This type of equilibrium affects forces and is also known as **force equilibrium.**

The **second equilibrium condition** looks at how circular or **rotatory equilibrium** is achieved (Fig 4–14). All movement in one direction must equal all movement in the opposite direction ($\Sigma M = 0$). Clockwise movements are assigned positive values, and counterclockwise movements are assigned negative values. Since forces traveling in a circle are called moments, this type of equilibrium is known as **moment equilibrium.**

RULES OF RELATIONSHIP

Mechanical physics is based largely on the work of Sir Isaac Newton in the late 1600s. Newton's speculations about the universe changed the way Europeans perceived the world around them. **Newtonian physics** went unchallenged until the discovery of electromagnetic energy at the end of the 19th century. It was further challenged by Einstein's work at the beginning of the 20th century. Einstein's theories caused a change of perception in the world of science that has only begun to shift the perception for those outside the scientific community.

Classic physics based on Newton's mechanical models included three fundamental laws of motion. These laws are so much a part of western culture that stating them seems almost unnecessary. It is difficult to understand what a revelation they were four centuries ago.

Newton's first law of motion, the **law of inertia,** says that a body will continue in a state of rest or in a straight line of uniform motion unless acted on by an external force. All matter has inertia. Unless acted on by an outside force, a body either remains at rest or in uniform linear motion. The amount of force needed to start or stop movement is directly related to the mass of the body in question. Chapter 6 looks at how this law affects forces acting on the human body in activity.

Newton's second law of motion, the **law of acceleration,** states that the rate of change in momentum is proportional to and in the same direction as an applied force. The amount of force needed to move a heavy object will move a lighter object more quickly. It takes the same amount of force to stop a heavy object moving slowly as it does to stop a lighter object moving quickly. Stated in mathematic terms, force = mass × acceleration. Chapter 7 looks at how this law affects rotatory movement of the human body in activities.

Newton's third law of motion, the **law of reaction,** states that for every action there is an equal and opposite reaction. The law of reaction creates balance in relationships. It is how equilibrium is achieved. Chapter 8 looks at how equilibrium affects the human body in activities.

BIBLIOGRAPHY

Fritjof C: *The Tao of Physics.* New York, Bantam Press, 1984.

Luttgens K, Wells K: *Kinesiology: Scientific Basis of Human Motion.* New York, WB Saunders Co, 1982.

Wiktorin CH, Nordin M: *Introduction to Problem Solving in Biomechanics.* Philadelphia, Lea & Febiger, 1986.

PART III

Grammar

Chapter 5 _____

Gravity: A Constant Force

In the 15th century, Galileo did a series of experiments that involved rolling objects down ramps. From these experiments he developed **laws of uniform acceleration.** These laws can be written as mathematic equations. Newton used these formulas to develop his three laws of motion. These laws explain how the spinning of planetary bodies affects all movement. The Earth's rotation produces a force called gravity. Gravity provides a constant force on matter, which is commonly understood as weight. Weight is mass multiplied by gravity.

MASS, WEIGHT, AND THE AVERAGE RATE OF ACCELERATION FOR GRAVITY

In Figure 5–1 there is a tall building where each floor is spaced 4.9 m (or 16 ft) apart. If a bowling ball and a billiard ball are dropped off at various floors the following phenomena would be observed. When the balls drop from the first floor they will reach the ground in 1 second. When they drop from the fourth floor they will reach the ground in 2 seconds. When they are dropped from the ninth floor they will reach the ground in 3 seconds. It will take 4 seconds to reach the ground from the 16th floor.

Note that the balls always land simultaneously and that the rate of acceleration follows a certain pattern. The rate of acceleration is proportional to the square root of the distance traveled. The average rate of acceleration, caused by the earth's rotation, is 9.8 m/sec^2 (or 32 ft/sec^2). This can be rounded off to 10 m/sec^2, a constant, which is multiplied by the mass of any object to get its weight. In the metric system weight is measured in newtons; 1 N equals 9.8 kg.

PROBLEM 5.1: CALCULATING WEIGHT FOR A BASKET OF LAUNDRY
Figure 5–2 shows a basket of laundry with a mass of 10 kg. What is its weight (that is, the force of gravity acting on the basket of laundry)?

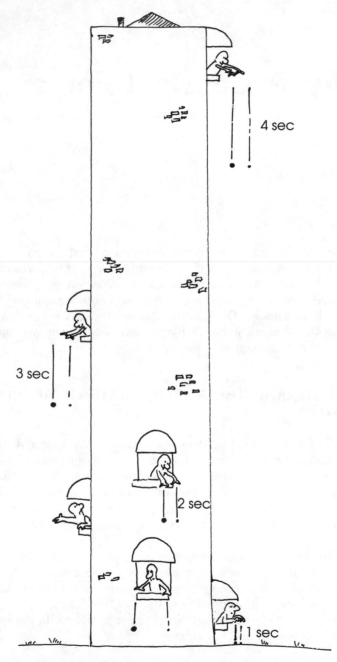

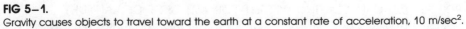

FIG 5–1.
Gravity causes objects to travel toward the earth at a constant rate of acceleration, 10 m/sec².

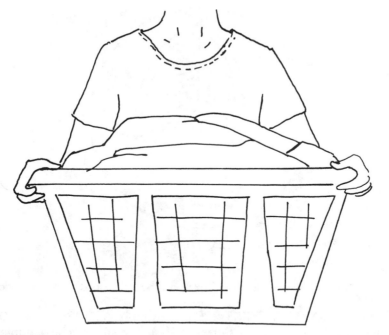

FIG 5–2.
A laundry basket has a mass of 10 kg. Draw in the vector representing its weight.

REPRESENTING GRAVITY IN A DIAGRAM

The force of gravity that acts on a body's center of gravity always moves toward the center of the earth. In symmetrical bodies like balls and cubes the center of gravity is easy to find since it is located in the exact center of the object. Material bodies are three-dimensional, so the center of gravity will be in the exact center of all three planes. Figure 5–3 has an orange cut in half, then into quarters, and then into eighths to show these three planes. The center of gravity will be at the point where the axes of all three planes meet.

Objects like people and tools are not symmetrical, but their center of gravity is found in much the same way. In the human body these three planes are called sagittal, coronal, and horizontal planes. A person's center of gravity will be the point where the axes of all three planes meet.

Any analysis of activity must account for the force of gravity acting on the person and on the tools or other objects involved. When diagraming an activity indicate vectors representing the force of gravity by drawing the following:

- The center of gravity (the point where the three axes meet)
- The direction of gravity (always perpendicular to the ground)
- The magnitude of the gravitational force (proportional to the mass of the body itself)

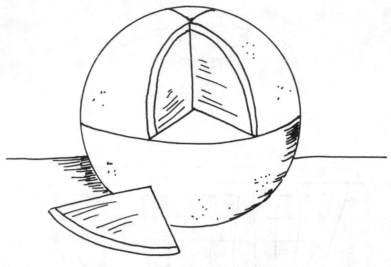

FIG 5–3.
An object's center of gravity will be at the point where the vertical and horizontal planes meet.

PROBLEM 5.2: ESTIMATING THE FORCE OF GRAVITY ACTING ON A SPOON

The spoon in Figure 5–4 has a mass of 40 g. The spoon is held in three different positions. How will the force of gravity acting on the spoon be drawn in each
different position? Will the center of gravity and its action on the spoon change as
the position of the spoon changes?

PROBLEM 5.3: ESTIMATING THE FORCE OF GRAVITY ACTING ON SPOONS OF
DIFFERENT WEIGHTS

In Figure 5–5 a spoon with a built-up handle has a mass of 60 g, and a regular
spoon has a mass of 40 g. How will the force of gravity acting on each spoon
be indicated in the diagram? Does weight affect the center of gravity for the
spoons?

WORKING WITH GRAVITY IN THE HUMAN BODY

The human body is almost constantly in motion. When standing still the center
of gravity is found in the abdominal cavity, about 6 in. above the pubis symphysis.
As the person's position changes, so does the center of gravity.

Centers of gravity can be calculated for each segment of the human body. This
is known as the **segmental method.** To use the segmental method a photograph or
a diagram is superimposed on a graph to plot centers of gravity for each body segment.

Appendix C contains each body segment's percentile weight and the location of
its center of gravity. These data are used to mark the center of gravity for each body

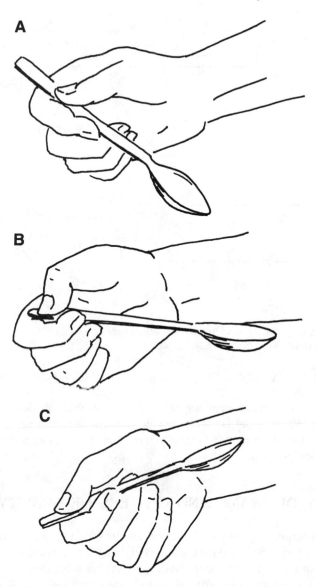

FIG 5–4.
This spoon weighs 40 g (0.4 kg). Draw a vector representing the force of gravity in positions **A–C**.

segment on a graph. The proportion of weight for that segment is multiplied by x- and y-coordinates for the segment's center of gravity. Add these products together to get a separate total for both x- and y-coordinates. These totals are the coordinates for the entire body's center of gravity. Table 5–1 is a blank form for making these calculations.

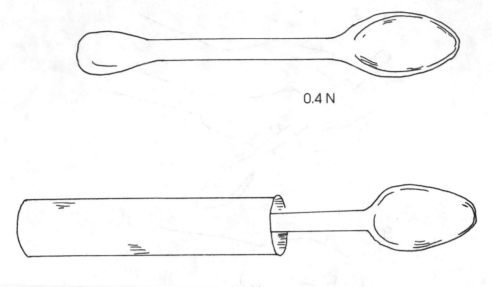

0.4 N

0.6 N

FIG 5−5.
This spoon weighs 40 g (0.4 kg), and this built-up handle spoon weighs 60 g. Draw a vector representing the force of gravity in both of these spoons.

PROBLEM 5.4: CALCULATING THE CENTER OF GRAVITY FOR A PERSON REACHING OVERHEAD
  In Figure 5−6 a person weighing 60 kg stands on the right leg to reach into an overhead shelf. Where is her center of gravity located? Is the center of gravity different than it would be if the person was simply standing? What factors make the center of gravity change position?

FREE BODY DIAGRAMS AND CENTERS OF GRAVITY

  Segmental center of gravity is also important when analyzing the forces that may be operating on a specific body part, such as in designing orthotic or adaptive equipment. When human body segments are diagramed this way, they are known as **free body diagrams.** Vectors can be drawn to indicate individual muscles, other forces, and the force of gravity acting on that specific joint segment. The percentage of total body mass for each body segment has already been determined through research. These values are found in Appendix C.

PROBLEM 5.5: CALCULATING GRAVITY OPERATING ON THE FOREARM
  Using the data from Problem 5.3 and your own arm, draw a forearm with a spoon (Fig 5−7). Which has greater gravitational force, the forearm or the spoons? How heavy would a spoon need to be to affect function of the forearm?

TABLE 5–1.

Blank Form for Calculating the Center of Gravity in the Human Body

Body Segment	% of Body Wt.	x + or − Value	Products	y + or − Value	Products
Head and Trunk					
R. Upper Arm					
R. Forearm					
R. Hand					
L. Upper Arm					
L. Forearm					
L. Hand					
R. Thigh					
R. Lower Leg					
R. Foot					
L. Thigh					
L. Lower Leg					
L. Foot					
Product Total					

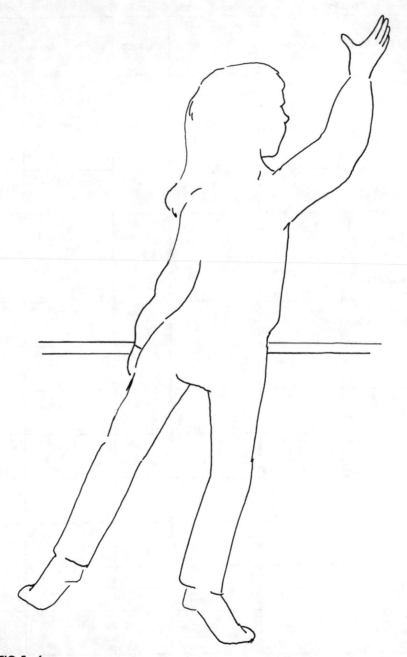

FIG 5—6.
A person weighing 60 kg stands on the right leg to reach into an overhead cabinet.

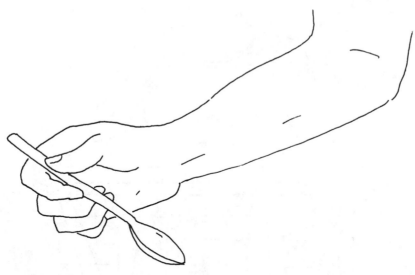

FIG 5–7.
Draw separate vectors indicating the weight of the spoon and the forearm.

SOLUTIONS TO PROBLEMS

SOLUTION TO PROBLEM 5.1: CALCULATING WEIGHT FOR A BASKET OF LAUNDRY

The mass of the laundry basket is 10 kg. Multiply this times the average rate of acceleration (gravity) to get the weight of the laundry basket. Figure 5–8 shows the weight of the basket drawn as a vector.

$$10 \text{ kg} \times 10 \text{ m/sec}^2 = \text{weight of laundry basket}$$
$$10 \text{ kg} \times 10 \text{ m/sec}^2 = 100 \text{ N}$$

SOLUTION TO PROBLEM 5.2: ESTIMATING THE FORCE OF GRAVITY ACTING ON A SPOON

To find the center of gravity for the spoon balance it on a finger (Fig 5–9). The point where the spoon balances is its center of gravity. Indicate this center with a dot on the drawing. Calculate the magnitude of the force by multiplying its mass times 10 m/sec^2.

$$0.04 \text{ kg} \times 10 \text{ m/sec}^2 = 0.4 \text{ N}$$

This can be drawn as an arrow of a specific length (for example, 0.4 N = 1 cm). In Figure 5–10,A–C the arrows point directly downward regardless of the angle of the spoon itself. The center of gravity stays the same no matter how an object is positioned. Gravity always pulls toward the center of the earth. The arrow's length must remain the same in each diagram because it indicates the actual weight of the spoon itself.

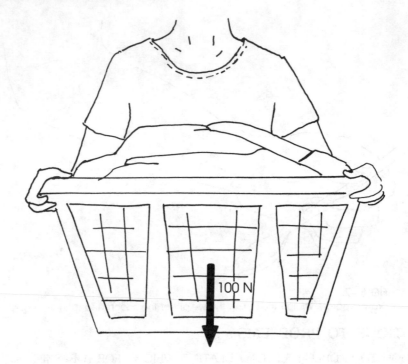

1 cm = 5 N

FIG 5-8.
A vector representing 100 N points directly downward from the center of this laundry basket.

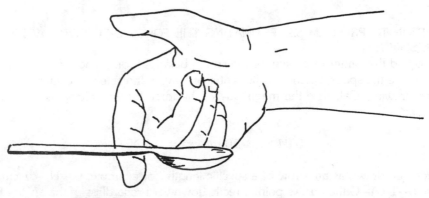

FIG 5-9.
Balance a spoon on one finger to find its center of gravity.

A

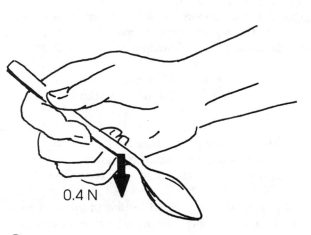

B

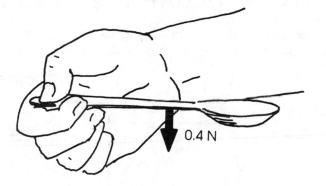

C

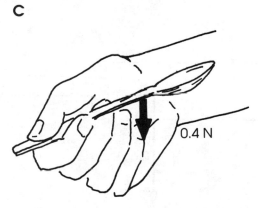

FIG 5–10.
Regardless of the spoon's position the vector representing gravity will always point directly downward.

SOLUTION TO PROBLEM 5.3: ESTIMATING THE FORCE OF GRAVITY ACTING
ON SPOONS OF DIFFERENT WEIGHTS
     Draw a diagram of each spoon. To find the center of gravity for each spoon,
balance it on a finger. The center of gravity may differ by several centimeters. Calculate the magnitude of the force by multiplying its mass times 10 m/sec^2.

$$0.04 \text{ kg} \times 10 \text{ m/sec}^2 = 0.4 \text{ N}$$
$$0.06 \text{ kg} \times 10 \text{ m/sec}^2 = 0.6 \text{ N}$$

Gravity for the built-up handle spoon has a force of 0.2 N greater than the gravity of
the regular spoon. This is indicated in Figure 5–11 by a slightly longer arrow in the
diagram. Keep vectors to scale, and indicate what the scale is somewhere on the
diagram. Gravity vectors point directly downward regardless of the angle of the object itself.
     The center of gravity will be affected by the distribution of weight. Individual
spoons need to be balanced to find their unique center of gravity.

SOLUTION TO PROBLEM 5.4: CALCULATING THE CENTER OF GRAVITY FOR A
PERSON REACHING OVERHEAD
     To find the center of gravity a graph is superimposed over a diagram of the per-
son reaching into an overhead cabinet (Fig 5–12). The x- and y-coordinates for

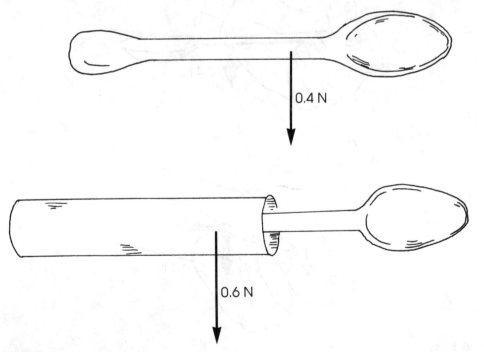

0.4 N

0.6 N

FIG 5–11.
The extra weight of the built-up handle shifts the spoon's center of gravity away from the bowl of
the spoon.

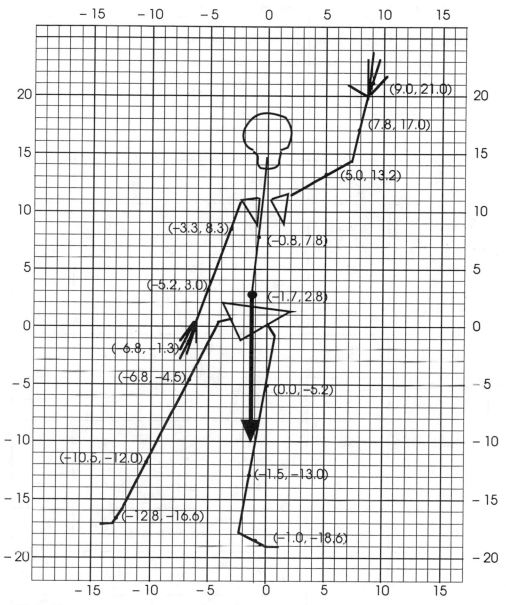

FIG 5–12.
Reaching into a cabinet changes the body's center of gravity in response to the proportion of body weight and its distance from the body's midline. In this case the center of gravity has shifted upward. If this person was leaning far enough forward, the body's center of gravity could be outside the body.

TABLE 5–2.

Calculations for the Finding Center of Gravity in Problem 5.4

Body Segment	% of Body Wt.	x + or − Value	Products	y + or − Value	Products
Head and Trunk	.565	−0.8	−0.45	7.8	4.41
R. Upper Arm	.027	5.0	0.14	13.2	0.36
R. Forearm	.015	7.8	0.12	17.0	0.13
R. Hand	.006	9.0	0.05	21.0	0.22
L. Upper Arm	.027	−3.3	−0.09	8.3	0.12
L. Forearm	.015	−5.2	−0.08	3.0	0.05
L. Hand	.006	−6.8	−0.04	−1.3	0.01
R. Thigh	.097	0.0	0.00	−5.2	−0.50
R. Lower Leg	.045	−1.5	−0.07	−13.0	−0.59
R. Foot	.014	−1.0	−0.01	−18.6	−0.26
L. Thigh	.097	−6.8	−0.66	−4.5	−0.44
L. Lower Leg	.045	−10.5	−0.47	−12.0	−0.54
L. Foot	.014	−12.8	−0.18	−16.6	−0.23
Product Total*			−1.75		2.85

*x coordinate = −1.75; y coordinate = 2.85.

each body segment's center of gravity are entered into Table 5–1 to calculate the center of gravity. Each coordinate is multiplied by the percentage of weight for that body segment. Adding the products of the segmental x- and y-coordinates gives the product totals that are used for the x- and y-coordinates for the entire body's center of gravity. Table 5–2 contains these calculations. Figure 5–12 shows how the product totals are plotted as the body's center of gravity.

The human body's center of gravity is shifted upward by the added length and weight of the arm reaching overhead. Since the human body's center of gravity is the summation of all of its segments, the center of gravity will shift in the direction where most body mass is located.

SOLUTION TO PROBLEM 5.5: CALCULATING GRAVITY OPERATING ON THE FOREARM

Use Appendix C to determine the center of gravity of your forearm, and mark this with a dot. Measure the total distance from the olecranon process to the styloid process. Multiply this distance times 0.43 or 0.57.

0.43 × length of forearm = distance from olecranon to center of gravity

0.57 × length of forearm = distance from styloid process to center of gravity

Multiply your total body weight times 0.021 (for the forearm and hand). Remember to use kilograms. This will give you the mass of your forearm. Multiply by 10 m/sec^2 to get the force of gravity operating on your forearm. Remember to keep the measurement scale the same when drawing in vectors representing the forearm and the tools (i.e., the spoons).

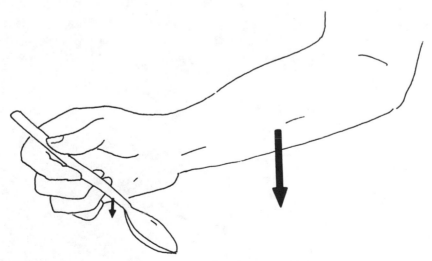

FIG 5–13.
The vector representing the weight of the forearm is greater than the vector representing the weight of the spoon.

The spoons have a gravitational force that is less than that of the forearm (Fig 5–13). When eating the weight of the forearm will be more important than the weight of the spoon. If the weight of the spoon or another object were greater than the weight of the forearm, the focus of the problem would shift to the weight of that tool, and the forearm weight might be considered negligible.

BIBLIOGRAPHY

Fritjof C: *The Tao of Physics.* New York, Bantam Press, 1984.

Luttgens K, Wells K: *Kinesiology: Scientific Basis of Human Motion.* New York, WB Saunders Co, 1982.

Nordin M, Frankel VH: *Basic Biomechanics of the Musculoskeletal System.* Philadelphia, Lea & Febiger, 1989.

Wiktorin CH, Nordin M: *Introduction to Problem Solving in Biomechanics.* Philadelphia, Lea & Febiger, 1986.

ANSWERS TO PROBLEMS

5.1: 100 N

5.2: 0.4 N arrow points downward regardless of the spoon angle

5.3: 0.6 N arrow will be proportionally longer than the 0.4-N arrow

5.4: x-Coordinate = -1.75

y-Coordinate = 2.85

5.5: The weight of spoons is negligible when compared with the weight of the forearm

Chapter 6

Problems of Linear Motion: Force

Newton's first law of motion, the law of inertia, states that all matter has inertia. Unless acted on by an outside force a body remains either at rest or in uniform linear motion. The amount of force needed to start or stop movement is directly related to the mass of the body in question. Force acting on mass is the focus of this chapter.

Figure 6–1,A–C shows a child with a ball. The child can kick or hit the ball. She can catch or stop the ball. She can sit on the ball. This covers all aspects of linear motion, which is also called **force**. Force can be used to start or stop motion, and force can be used to change the shape of an object.

FORCES ACTING ON THE HUMAN BODY

The same principles of inertia work on and in the human body. External forces as well as internal forces such as muscles cause movement. Forces also stop movement and cause human tissues to change shape.

Normal Forces

Normal forces push joint surfaces together or pull them apart. In Figure 6–2 the person leaning on a table pushes the surfaces of the glenohumeral joint together. In Figure 6–3 hanging motionless from an overhead bar pulls these same joint surfaces apart. Anatomic structures respond to these forces by altering their shape. **Compressive forces** push tissues together and cause anatomic structures to get shorter and

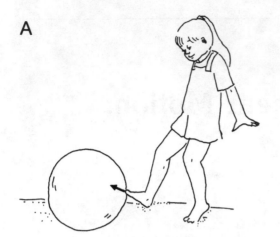

A

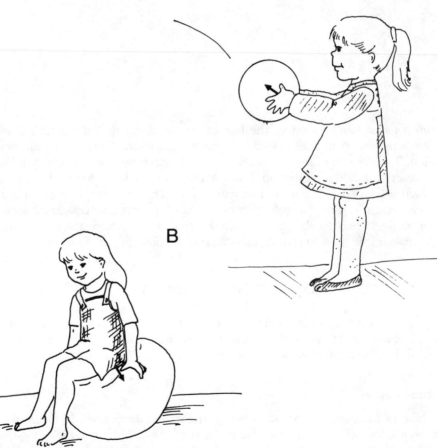

B

C

FIG 6–1.
Force can accelerate and decelerate motion or deform materials.

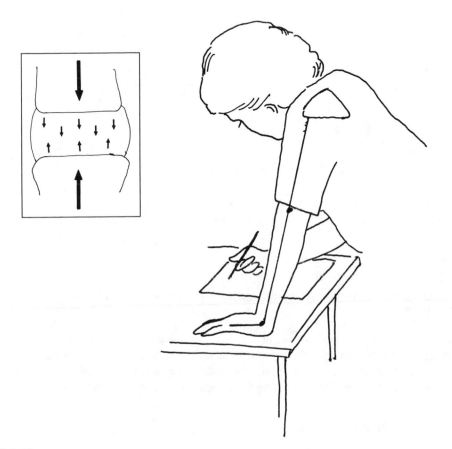

FIG 6—2.
Leaning on a table causes compressive forces to operate at the elbow and shoulder, with corresponding compressive stress in joint tissues.

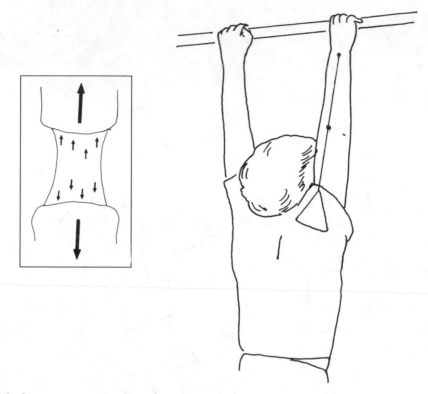

FIG 6–3.
Hanging on a bar causes tensile forces to operate at the elbow and shoulder, with corresponding tensile stress in joint tissues.

wider. **Tensile forces** pull tissues apart and cause anatomic structures to get longer and narrower. Anatomic structures usually return to their original shape once the forces acting on them have stopped. The ability to return to original shape is known as **elasticity.** If this ability is exceeded, the result is injury to human tissues.

Shear or Tangential Forces

Forces can also operate on the surface of a joint or parallel to the cross section of a joint. When the arm is raised above the head, the humerus produces a **shear** force on the glenoid fossa. Because they touch the surface of the structure, shear forces are also called **tangential** forces.

Stress

When a force is applied to a material substance like a joint capsule, it causes stress inside that material. Stress is measured in units of area: metric **pascals (Pa)** or newtons per meter squared (N/m^2). When stress inside human tissue exceeds the tissue's elasticity, breakdown of the tissue results in injury.

DRAWING FORCES IN A DIAGRAM

Since forces have magnitude and a direction of movement, they are vector quantities. They are measured in pounds or newtons. Vectors that represent forces are carefully drawn with arrows to show three things:

- The point where the force is first applied (the base of the arrow)
- The direction of the force (the orientation of the arrow)
- The magnitude of the force (the length of the arrow)

Muscle forces act along the length of the muscle in the direction of the tendons. Muscles pull from their point of origin, or insertion, toward maximum stabilization. As the point of stabilization changes, so does the direction of the force. In Figure 6–4 the biceps pulls a hand-held weight toward the shoulder, which is stabilized by scapular muscles. In Figure 6–5 the biceps pulls the body toward a bar held in the hands.

The magnitude of muscle force is determined by the number of fibers that are activated. The arrow representing the force is drawn longer to indicate increased force. When solving problems, graphic units of length will equal specific units of force.

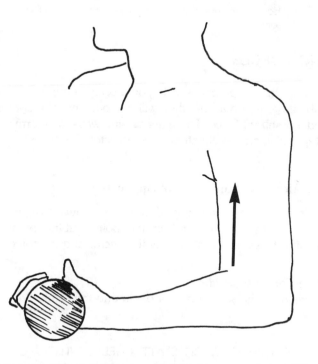

FIG 6–4.
When lifting a weight the shoulder is stabilized, causing the biceps muscle to pull the forearm closer to the body.

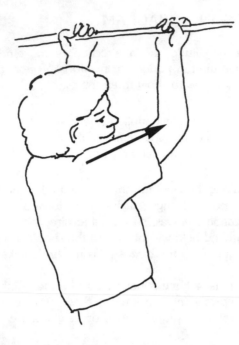

FIG 6–5.
When pulling up on a bar the wrist and hand are stabilized, causing the biceps muscle to bring the body closer to the forearm.

COMBINING FORCES

Suppose more than one force is acting on a body at the same time. These forces must be combined to find out how they will act together. The combination of these forces is called a **resultant force.** There are several ways to determine the magnitude of a vector depending on the directions of the vectors.

Forces Acting Along the Same Line of Application

Forces acting along the same line of application always originate from a single point. They may act at some distance from that point, but that point will always lie in a straight line with the same orientation as the vector and the force it represents.

Combining Forces by Addition

When forces have the same point of origin and the same direction, they can be added together.

PROBLEM 6.1: COMBINING WEIGHTS ATTACHED TO THE WRIST

In Figure 6–6 a person is exercising the biceps muscle by using a 5-kg wrist weight, which will produce a force of 50 N (mass × gravity = 5 kg × 10 m/sec^2). If

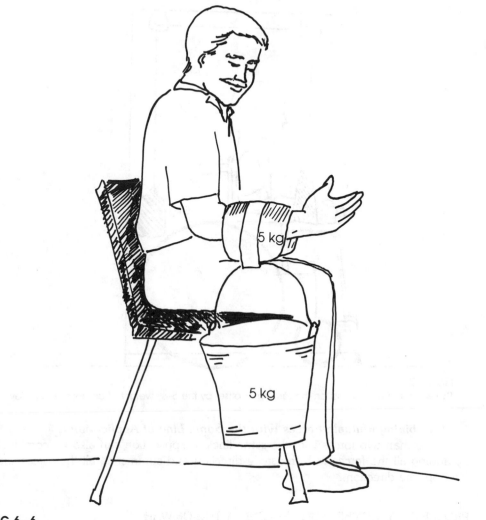

FIG 6–6.
A 5-kg bucket of sand is added to a 5-kg wrist weight to increase the amount of weight that is lifted.

a bucket of sand weighing 5 kg is attached to the wrist weight, what will the resultant force be?

Combining Forces by Subtraction
When forces have the same point of application and an opposite direction, they can be subtracted from each other.

PROBLEM 6.2: COMBINING WEIGHTS BY USING A PULLEY SYSTEM
In Figure 6–7 a person in an overhead pulley cast has a cast weighing 6 kg. If a 5-kg weight is attached to the same point on the forearm, how much weight is actually being lifted?

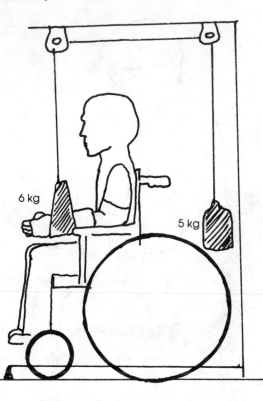

FIG 6–7.
The weight of a 6-kg cast on the forearm is offset by the 5-kg weight of an overhead pulley.

Combining Multiple Forces With the Same Line of Application

More than two forces with the same lines of application can also be combined by adding all the forces with the same direction and subtracting all the forces with the opposite direction.

PROBLEM 6.3: COMBINING FORCES IN A TUG-OF-WAR

In Figure 6–8 five children tugging on a rope have different pulling power. On the right side John pulls with a force of 400 N, Keesha with 300 N, Mary with 100 N; on the left side Miguel pulls with 200 N and Mai Li with 500 N. Which side will win the tug-of-war?

Forces Coming From Different Directions in the Same Plane

Forces acting on the same point but coming from different directions are called **concurrent** forces. To find the resultant of concurrent forces two methods are used: the parallelogram method and the polygon method.

In the body, the direction of force parallels muscle fibers and tendons. Some

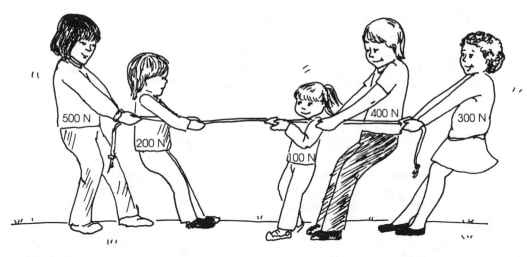

FIG 6–8.
Five children play tug-of-war. Which side will win?

muscles have fibers that go in different directions. These forces can be combined by mathematics to give a **resultant force.** For example, since the pectoralis major muscle has a fan shape, its direction of movement will be a resultant of the active muscle fibers operating in it.

Using a Parallelogram to Determine a Resultant Force

The parallelogram method relies on the **parallelogram theorem.** This states that if two forces are acting on the same point, their resultant can be measured as the diagonal of a parallelogram constructed with those forces as its sides. In Figure 6–9 each concurrent force represents a side of a parallelogram, and the resultant is represented by a diagonal line down the center of the parallelogram. Once the parallelogram is drawn, the problem can be solved by measurement, the Pythagorean theorem, or trigonometry.

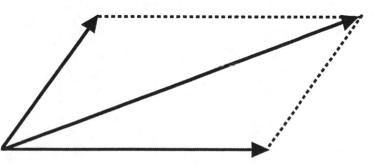

FIG 6–9.
A parallelogram diagram can be used to find the resultant of forces acting in two different directions.

PROBLEM 6.4: ONE OR TWO PEOPLE PUSHING A CRATE

In Figure 6–10 two workers must move a 1 m × 1 m × 1.5 m crate filled with metal parts as one of their daily tasks. When two workers push the crate, one worker pushes with a force of 125 N and the other with a force of 225 N. If only one worker pushes the crate how much force will be required? Would it be safe for one worker to push the crate alone?

Using a Polygon to Determine the Resultant of More Than Two Forces

This method is helpful when more than two forces are acting on a rigid body. Arrows that represent the forces are drawn base to tip. The lengths of these arrows are scaled in proportion to the magnitudes of the forces. The orientation of the arrows corresponds to the direction of the forces.

PROBLEM 6.5: A GROUP OF FIVE PEOPLE PLAYING WITH A LARGE-DIAMETER BALL

In Figure 6–11 five people push a large-diameter "Earth" ball. Ron pushes east with 300 N of force. Jack pushes 45° northeast with 150 N of force. Sam pushes north with 450 N. Fred pushes 45° northwest with 225 N of force. Jacob pushes west with 75 N of force. Which direction will the ball roll and with how much force?

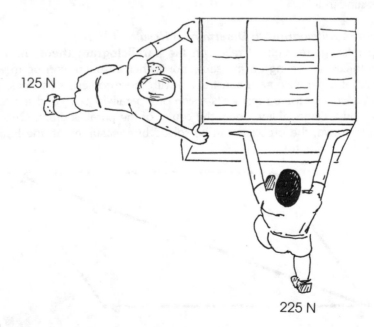

125 N

225 N

FIG 6–10.
Two people pushing a crate use 125 and 225 N of force. How much force would be needed by one person pushing the same cart?

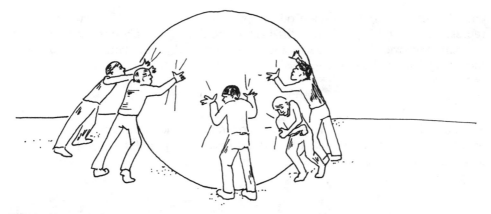

FIG 6–11.
Five people playing with a large-diameter ball all push with different amounts of force to move the ball.

SOLUTIONS TO PROBLEMS

SOLUTION TO PROBLEM 6.1: COMBINING WEIGHTS ATTACHED TO THE WRIST

Figure 6–12 shows a graphic representation of this problem. If the vectors are drawn to scale (for example, 50 N = 1 cm), the resultant would measure 5 cm, the combined length of both vectors.

$$50 \text{ N} + 50 \text{ N} = 100 \text{ N}$$

SOLUTION TO PROBLEM 6.2: COMBINING WEIGHTS BY USING A PULLEY SYSTEM

Make use of the **displacement theorem** to solve this problem. *The point of application of a force acting on a rigid body can be displaced along the line of application without changing its effect on the body.* The amount of force is not changed by

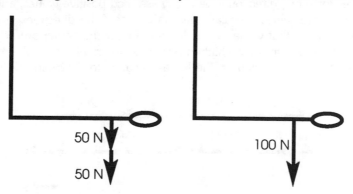

FIG 6–12.
A 5-kg bucket of sand is added to a 5-kg wrist weight to increase the amount of weight that is lifted to 10 kg, or 100 N of force.

changing its point of application on the pulley line. Figure 6–13 shows a graphic representation of this problem. If the vectors are drawn to scale (for example, 20 N = 1 cm) and placed next to each other, the downward vector would be longer than the upward vector by 0.5 cm.

$$60 \text{ N} - 50 \text{ N} = 10 \text{ N}$$

The person is lifting 10 kg. This type of apparatus would allow a person to use his available muscle strength even if he did not have enough to lift the cast without assistance. Ten newtons would approximate the weight of the forearm without the weight of the cast.

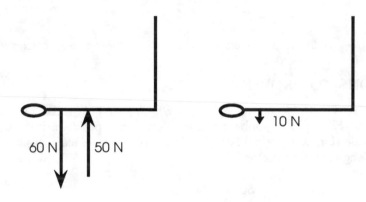

FIG 6–13.
The weight of a 6-kg cast on the forearm is offset by the 5-kg weight of an overhead pulley so that only 1 kg, or 10 N is actually lifted.

SOLUTION TO PROBLEM 6.3: COMBINING FORCES IN A TUG-OF-WAR

In setting up problems where forces act along the same line of application but in different directions, one direction is generally assigned positive values, and the other is assigned negative values. Typically this is done as if the directions were *x* and *y* values on a graph so that values to the left and below the center are negative. Following this pattern, assign those children pulling on the right side of the rope as positive and those children pulling on the left as negative to determine which side has

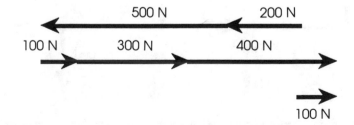

FIG 6–14.
The three children on the right have a combined force of 100 N more than the combined force of the children on the left.

more force. Figure 6–14 shows a graphic representation of this problem. If vectors are drawn to scale (for example, 200 N = 1 cm) and lined up next to each other, the vector to the right would be 0.5 cm longer than the combined vector to the right.

$$-500 \text{ N} - 200\text{N} + 100 \text{ N} + 300 \text{ N} + 400 \text{ N} = 100 \text{ N}$$

SOLUTION TO PROBLEM 6.4: ONE OR TWO PEOPLE PUSHING A CRATE

Figure 6–15 shows a graphic representation of this problem. If the vectors are drawn in accurately, the diagonal line can be measured to find the resultant. Use a scale to convert centimeters to newtons. Each side of the parallelogram represents one of the workers. The vectors intersect at 90°. One vector represents 125 N and the other 225 N. The diagonal line will represent the amount of force needed by one worker to push the crate.

For a mathematic solution use the Pythagorean theorem.

$$a^2 + b^2 = c^2$$
$$125^2 + 225^2 = c^2$$
$$15{,}625 + 50{,}625 = 66{,}250$$
$$c^2 = 66{,}250$$
$$c = 257 \text{ N}$$

Appendix F contains a table of acceptable standards for average workers.

A force of 257 N is within acceptable limits for the average worker. It would not jeopardize the safety of an individual worker to push the cart alone.

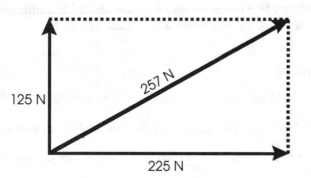

FIG 6–15.
Two people pushing a cart use 125 N and 225 N of force. One person pushing the same cart would need to use 257 N of force.

SOLUTION TO PROBLEM 6.5: A GROUP OF FIVE PEOPLE PLAYING WITH A LARGE-DIAMETER BALL

Figure 6–16 shows a graphic representation of this problem. To solve the problem vectors must be drawn accurately and to scale (for example, 1 cm = 50 N). The vectors are placed end to end. The resultant connects the last vector with the first

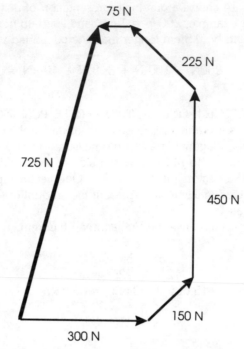

75 N

225 N

725 N

450 N

300 N   150 N

FIG 6–16.
Five people move a large ball northwest with a force of 725 N.

vector. Using the scale that was given the resultant would measure 14.5 cm, which gives a value of 725 N. This vector should point about 75° northwest.

The ball would roll 75° northwest with a force of 725 N.

BIBLIOGRAPHY

Luttgens K, Wells K: *Kinesiology: Scientific Basis of Human Motion,* New York, WB Saunders Co, 1982.
Nordin M, Frankel VH: *Basic Biomechanics of the Musculoskeletal System.* Philadelphia, Lea & Febiger, 1989.
Wiktorin CH, Nordin M: *Introduction to Problem Solving in Biomechanics.* Philadelphia, Lea & Febiger, 1986.

ANSWERS TO PROBLEMS
    6.1: 100 N
    6.2: 10 N
    6.3: 100 N to the left
    6.4: 257 N
    6.5: 75° northwest with a force of 725 N

Chapter 7 _____

Problems of Rotary Motion: Torque

Newton's second law of motion, the law of acceleration, describes the relationship between force, matter, and acceleration: force is equal to mass times the average amount of distance covered in a unit of time. This means that the amount of force needed to move a heavy object will move a lighter object more quickly. It takes the same amount of force to stop a heavy object moving slowly as it does to stop a lighter object moving rapidly. To measure these forces we need to know both their mass and their rate of acceleration:

Force = mass × acceleration (F = ma)

Figure 7–1,A and B shows a ball attached to a pole by a rope that limits its range of movement to the length of the rope. The speed of the ball's travel around the pole is regulated by the amount of force used to hit the ball and the composition of the ball itself. As the speed of the ball increases, less force is needed to move it. A heavy ball traveling at the same speed as a lighter ball will hit against our hands harder when we stop it because it has more force. These are the basic relationships of rotary motion, which is commonly called **torque.**

TORQUE, LEVERS, AND MOMENT ARMS

Two kinds of torque operate on the human body: internal and external. External torque is produced by forces operating outside of the body. Internal torque is produced by muscles, tendons, and other soft tissues operating inside the body.

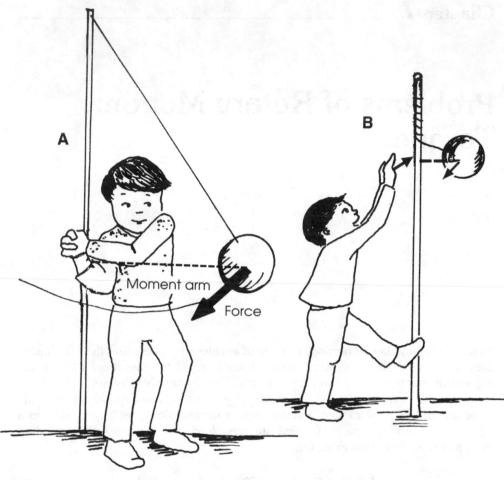

FIG 7–1.
A, the amount of force needed for circular movement depends on the mass of the object that is moved and its distance from the axis of movement. **B,** when the mass of an object is multiplied by its distance from an axis of movement, that relationship is called torque.

Inside the human body almost all movement involves torque. Torque is produced by **levers.** Levers are any rigid body that rotates around a fixed point. In the human body the most frequently considered levers are bones. Bones move around joints that form an axis for rotation. In the forearm the biceps produces a linear force that pulls the radius bone around the humerus. The biceps and radius work together to produce torque.

Rotation makes an arc or circle. A goniometer, which measures degrees in an arc, is used to assess joint motion. Since the size of a circle is determined by its radius, it is important to find the radius of specific arcs of motion in order to assess torque. This radius is called the **moment arm** or **torque arm.**

Figure 7–2 shows a moment arm. It is the line that runs perpendicularly from

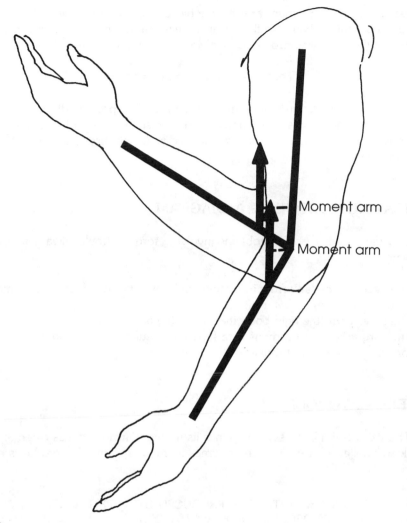

FIG 7–2.
A lever arm is the rigid body that moves around an axis, while a moment arm is the radius from the line of force to the axis of motion.

the line of force to the axis of rotation. It is called a moment arm because it only exists for a moment. The lever arm is the bone that is in movement. The moment arm changes throughout the arc of rotation.

The lever arm is the distance between the center of the joint and the insertion of the biceps. A line from the axis of motion to the biceps tendon will form the moment arm. This distance will change as muscle fibers contract and lengthen. The change can be felt by placing the thumb on the medial epicondyle of the humerus (which is approximately the center of the joint) and the fingers on the biceps tendon. With the forearm held in supination, the distance between the thumb and fingers is a good approximation of the moment arm for the biceps. As the elbow flexes and extends, there is a noticeable change in the distance between the thumb and fingers.

A formula for solving problems involving rotary motion is as follows:

$$\textbf{Torque = force} \times \textbf{moment arm}$$

Torque is measured in newton-meters (Nm) or foot-pounds (ft-lb). As the lever arm moves around its axis, the moment arm representing the radius of a circle may change its length. The amount of force needed is directly proportional to the length of the moment arm.

INDICATING TORQUE IN A DIAGRAM

Drawings used to solve problems involving torque should always indicate the following:

- The vector force (an arrow indicating application point, direction, and magnitude of the force)
- The **lever arm** (the rigid body that is moving around an axis)
- The **torque arm** or **moment arm** (a perpendicular line running from the vector force to the axis of movement)

EXTERNAL TORQUE

The weight of a body segment times its moment arm produces external torque. Any load applied to a body segment times its moment arm also produces external torque.

PROBLEM 7.1: EXTERNAL TORQUE PRODUCED BY A 5-KG BARBELL HELD AT 30, 60, 90, AND 120 DEGREES OF ELBOW FLEXION
In Figure 7–3 a client lifts a 5-kg barbell weight from a seated position. The client's forearm measures 30 cm (0.3 m) from the elbow joint to the palmar creases where the barbell rests. What is the amount of external torque produced by the barbell when the elbow is at 30°, 60°, 90°, and 120° of motion? Is the external torque the same throughout the range of motion? If it changes, how does it change and why?

INTERNAL TORQUE

Internal torque is the force produced around a joint by muscles, tendons, and other soft tissues. It is measured by the force of muscle contraction times the length of its moment arm. The moment arm for internal torque is drawn perpendicular to the line of the muscle's pull. Individual muscle force depends both on the size of the muscle and its location in relation to the center of motion in the joint. With movement, the relationship of muscle to joint changes, so the internal torque increases and decreases throughout a range of motion. The maximum isometric torque at specific joint angles can be plotted on a graph. It is useful to know where in the range of motion a muscle will have its greatest strength.

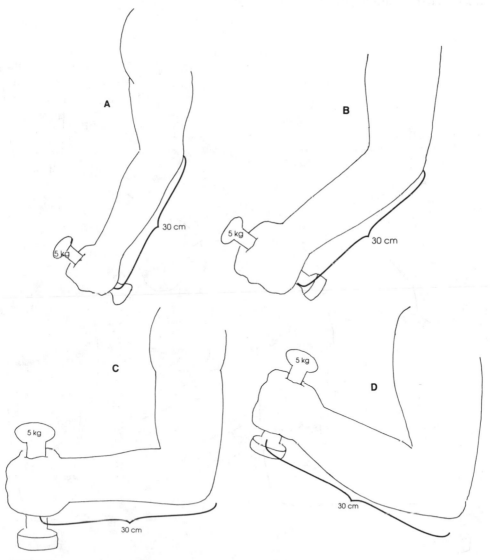

FIG 7–3.
External torque produced by a 5-kg barbell changes as the elbow moves from 30° **(A)**, 60° **(B)**, 90° **(C)**, and 120° **(D)** of flexion.

PROBLEM 7.2: INTERNAL TORQUE PRODUCED BY THE BICEPS AT 30°, 60°, 90°, AND 120° OF FLEXION

In Figure 7–4 a client lifts a 5-kg barbell weight from a seated position. The biceps tendon lies 4 cm from the radioulnar joint. For this problem we assume that the force of the biceps is 375 N at 30° and 90°, and 433 N at 60 and 120 degrees. What is the amount of internal torque produced at 30°, 60°, 90°, and 120° of flexion? Is the amount of internal torque the same throughout the operation? If it changes, how does it change and why?

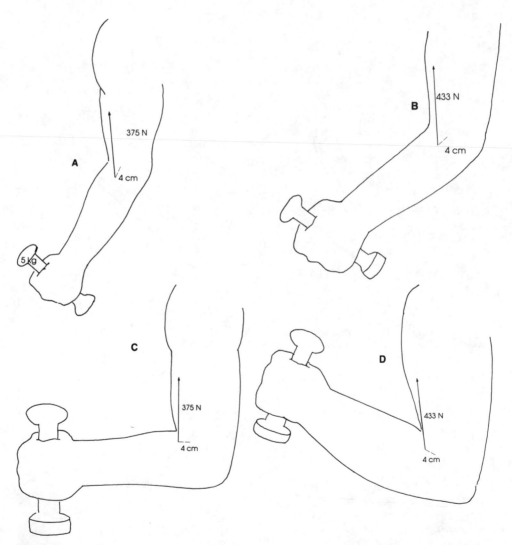

FIG 7–4.
Internal torque produced by the biceps when lifting a 5-kg barbell changes as the elbow moves from 30° **(A)**, 60° **(B)**, 90° **(C)**, and 120° **(D)** of flexion.

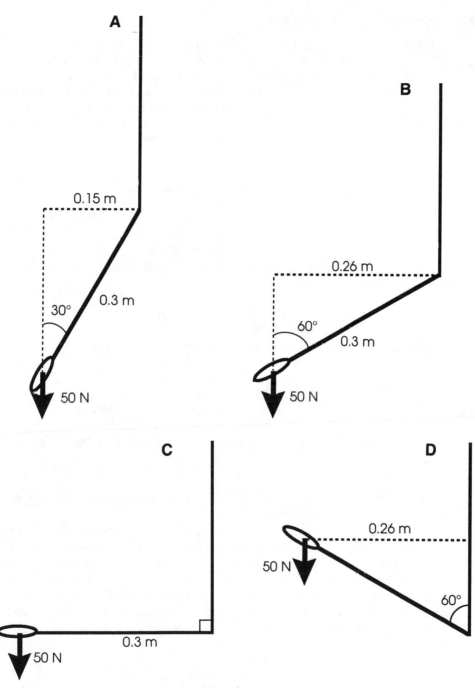

FIG 7–5.
External torque changes as the line of force moves closer and farther from the axis of movement in the elbow joint.

SOLUTIONS TO PROBLEMS

SOLUTION TO PROBLEM 7.1: EXTERNAL TORQUE PRODUCED BY A 5-KG
BARBELL HELD AT 30, 60, 90, AND 120 DEGREES OF ELBOW FLEXION
   Figure 7−5 shows the four elbow placements. The lines that represent the forearm and the force of the barbell are made to scale and identical for each drawing.
The length of the moment arm can be estimated by measuring with a ruler and scaling it, but for a more accurate length of the moment arm use sines. The forearm is
the hypotenuse in a right triangle, and side a is the moment arm.

$$\sin A = a/c$$
$$\sin 30 \text{ degrees} = a/0.3 \text{ m}$$
$$0.50 = a/0.3 \text{ m}$$
$$a = 0.50 \times 0.3 \text{ m}$$
$$a = 0.15 \text{ m}$$

   Multiply the length of the moment arm by the force of the barbell to get the
torque produced by the barbell.

$$50 \text{ N} \times 0.15 \text{ m} = 7.5 \text{ Nm}$$

Repeat this process to solve the rest of the problem.

$$60° = 13 \text{ Nm}$$
$$90° = 15 \text{ Nm}$$
$$120° = 13 \text{ Nm}$$

   External torque will change throughout the range of motion as the length of the
moment arm changes.

SOLUTION TO PROBLEM 7.2: INTERNAL TORQUE PRODUCED BY THE BICEPS
AT 30, 60, 90, AND 120 DEGREES OF FLEXION
   Figure 7−6 shows four figures representing the four ranges of motion. The lines
that represent the distance to the biceps tendon and the force of the biceps are made
to scale for each drawing. The biceps pulls directly upward and parallel to the humerus. The length of the moment arm can be estimated by measuring with a ruler
and scaling it, but for a more accurate length of the moment arm use sines. The distance from the elbow joint to the biceps tendon is the hypotenuse of a right triangle,
and side a is the moment arm.

$$\sin A = a/c$$
$$\sin 30° = a/0.04 \text{ m}$$
$$0.50 = a/0.04 \text{ m}$$
$$a = 0.50 \times 0.04 \text{ m}$$
$$a = 0.02 \text{ m}$$

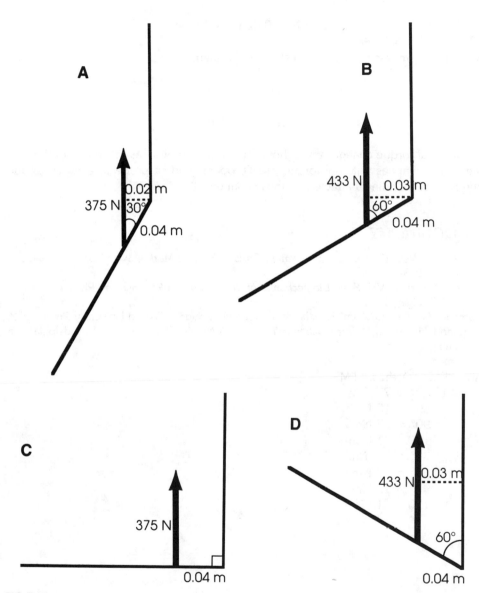

FIG 7–6.
Internal torque changes as the line of force produced by the biceps moves closer and farther from the axis of motion in the elbow joint.

Multiply the length of the moment arm by the force of the biceps to get the torque produced by the biceps.

$$375 \text{ N} \times 0.02 \text{ m} = 7.5 \text{ Nm}$$

Repeat this process to solve the rest of the problem.

$$60° = 13 \text{ Nm}$$
$$90° = 15 \text{ Nm}$$
$$120° = 13 \text{ Nm}$$

Internal torque changes throughout the range of motion as the length of the moment arm changes. Internal torque usually operates in response to external torque and is correspondingly affected by those changes.

BIBLIOGRAPHY

Luttgens K, Wells K: *Kinesiology: Scientific Basis of Human Motion.* New York, WB Saunders Co, 1982.
Nordin M, Frankel VH: *Basic Biomechanics of the Musculoskeletal System.* Philadelphia, Lea & Febiger, 1989.
Romanes GJ: *Cunningham's Textbook of Anatomy.* London, Oxford University Press, 1972.
Wiktorin CH, Nordin M: *Introduction to Problem Solving in Biomechanics.* Philadelphia, Lea & Febiger, 1986.

ANSWERS TO PROBLEMS
    7.1: 30° = 7.5 Nm
          60° = 13 Nm
          90° = 15 Nm
         120° = 13 Nm
    7.2: 30° = 7.5 Nm
          60° = 13 Nm
          90° = 15 Nm
         120° = 13 Nm

Chapter 8 _____

Problems of Moment and Force Equilibrium

Newton's third law of motion, the law of reaction, states that for every action, there is an equal and opposite reaction. Knowing this allows us to determine both magnitude and direction of forces.

In the human body muscles maintain equilibrium by contracting and relaxing. Internal and external torque create corresponding reaction forces in bones, muscles, joints, and other soft tissues. These forces are **compressive** if they push tissues closer together or **tensile** if they pull tissues apart (see Chapter 6).

FORCE EQUILIBRIUM OR TRANSLATORY EQUILIBRIUM: THE FIRST EQUILIBRIUM CONDITION

A simple way of stating this is what goes up must also come down.

A mathematic way of stating this is in order for a rigid body to remain stable (that is, in equilibrium), all forces acting on it must add up to zero ($\Sigma F = 0$). That is, all vertical forces must equal zero ($\Sigma F_y = 0$), and all horizontal forces must equal zero ($\Sigma F_x = 0$). To achieve this mathematic state, assign positive values to all upward forces and negative values to all downward forces. Likewise, assign positive values to all forces directed to the right and negative values to all forces directed to the left.

PROBLEM 8.1: A FOOD SERVER HOLDS A TRAY OF FOOD

In Figure 8–1 a food server carries a tray weighing 0.35 kg. It contains a soft drink weighing 0.5 kg and a sandwich weighing 0.3 kg. How much force is needed to hold up this tray of food?

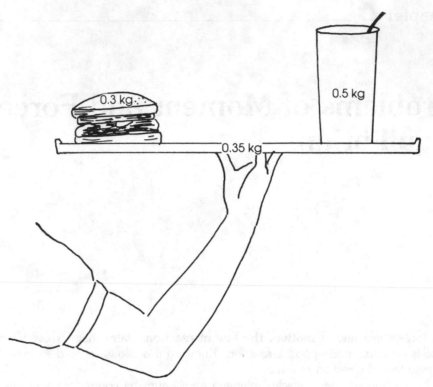

FIG 8–1.
A force equal to the weight of its mass is needed to hold up this tray of food.

MOMENT EQUILIBRIUM OR ROTARY EQUILIBRIUM: THE SECOND EQUILIBRIUM CONDITION

Simply stated, clockwise torque is met by counterclockwise torque.

To solve these kinds of problems assign positive values to clockwise movements and negative values to counter clockwise movements. Add them together to get zero ($\Sigma M = 0$).

PROBLEM 8.2: A FOOD SERVER BALANCES FOOD PLACED ON A TRAY

In Figure 8–2 a food server carefully places each item a certain distance from the center of the tray (where it will be supported). If a soft drink weighing 0.5 kg is placed 6 cm from the center of the tray, how far must a sandwich weighing 0.3 kg be placed from the center of the tray?

CLASSIFICATION OF LEVERS

A **lever** is a rigid body acted upon at two different points by opposing forces. Levers are used to overcome a resisting force or to increase the amount of force im-

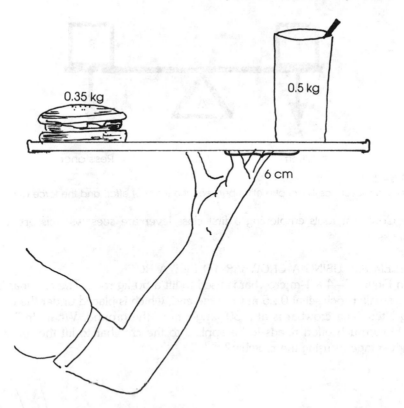

FIG 8–2.
In order to balance this tray of food on one hand the torque produced by the drink must equal the torque produced by the sandwich.

parted to a resisting force. Many tools make use of levers. Lever-type tools allow us either to do something with less effort or to increase the speed or force of an object we are moving.

The force that is imparted through a lever takes the form of movement. Levers are grouped into three categories based on the relationship of their axes of rotation and the placement of opposing forces. These opposing forces are labeled **effort** and **resistance.** Use Newton's law of reaction to set this up as a mathematic formula:

Effort × effort moment arm = resistance × resistance moment arm
$$E \times EMA = R \times RMA$$

This formula can be simplified to: $\Sigma M = 0$.

First-Class Levers

First class levers have their axis of movement placed so that it lies between the effort force and the resistance force (Fig 8–3). This type of a lever favors equilib-

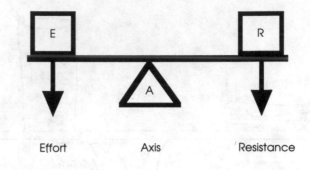

Effort   Axis   Resistance

FIG 8–3.

A first-class lever has its axis of motion between the force of effort and the force of resistance.

rium. Common tools employing a first class lever are seesaws, scissors, crowbars, and jacks.

PROBLEM 8.3: USING A CROWBAR TO LIFT A ROCK

In Figure 8–4 a 1-m crowbar is used to lift a 50-kg rock. The crowbar is placed over a smaller rock set at 0.25 m from the end, which is placed under the rock that is being lifted. The crowbar is at a 30° angle from the ground. What kind of lever is this? How much effort needs to be applied to the crowbar to lift the rock? What is the advantage of using the crowbar?

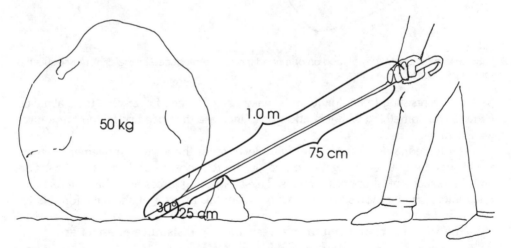

FIG 8–4.

A 1-m crowbar is placed so that its axis is 25 cm from a 50-kg rock and 75 cm from the end of the handle. The crowbar is angled 30° from the ground. How much effort is needed to lift the rock?

Second-Class Levers

In second-class levers, the resistance force lies between the force of effort and the axis of movement (Fig 8–5). This type of lever favors the force of effort because effort always has a longer moment arm. Common tools using a second class lever are wheelbarrows and nutcrackers.

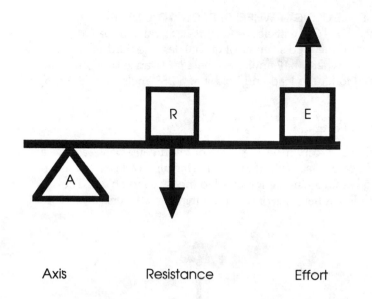

Axis   Resistance   Effort

FIG 8–5.
In a second-class lever the force of resistance lies between the axis of movement and the force of effort.

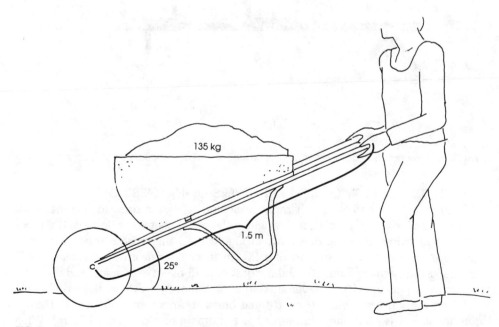

FIG 8–6.
A wheelbarrow has an axis of movement 1.5 m from where the handles are held. Its 135-kg load lies one third of the distance from its axis. The handles are 25° from the ground. How much effort is needed to lift this load?

PROBLEM 8.4: USING A WHEELBARROW TO CARRY A WEIGHT

In Figure 8–6 a wheelbarrow is used to carry a load of 135 kg. What kind of lever is this? If the load's center of gravity lies one third of the way between the axis and the point where the handles are held (a distance of 1.5 m), how much effort will be required to lift the load and hold it at a 25° angle from the ground?

Third-Class Levers

Third-class levers have the force of effort lying between the axis of movement and the force of resistance (Fig 8–7). This type of lever favors speed and distance because great force can be imparted to the resisting object. Tools used as extensions of the arm like a hammer or a bat are third-class levers.

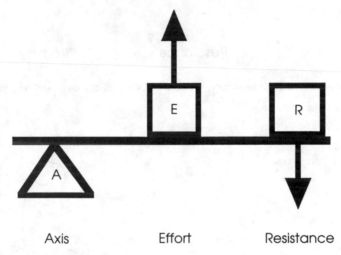

Axis   Effort   Resistance

FIG 8–7.
A third-class lever has its force of effort lying between the axis and the force of resistance.

PROBLEM 8.5: USING TWO DIFFERENT STYLES OF HAMMERING

In Figures 8–8 and 8–9 a hammer weighing 0.6 kg is used to hammer nails into a board placed on a workbench at elbow height. This task is done with an axis of motion at either the wrist or elbow. In Figure 8–8 the wrist is used as an axis point, and the hand becomes part of a 20-cm lever lifted from approximately 45° from the workbench. In Figure 8–9 the elbow is used as an axis point, and the forearm becomes part of a 45-cm lever lifted to approximately 45° from the workbench.

When the wrist is used, the effort force has a moment arm of 2 cm (0.02 m). When the elbow is used, the effort force has a moment arm of 3 cm (0.03 m). What types of levers are these? How much effort is needed to raise the hammer when the wrist is the axis of motion? How much effort is needed to raise the hammer when the elbow is the axis of motion? What would be the advantage to using either the wrist or the elbow as the primary axis of movement in a hammering task?

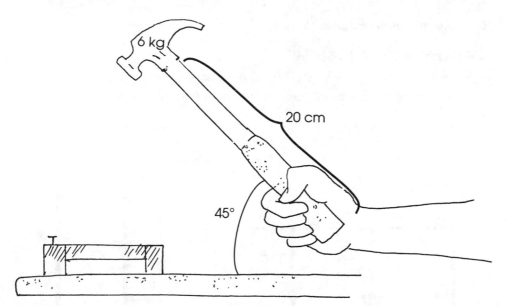

FIG 8–8.
A 6-kg hammer is held 45° from the surface to be hammered. The hammer's center of gravity is 20 cm from its axis of motion in the wrist. The muscles used to lift the hammer lie 2 cm from the axis of motion in the wrist.

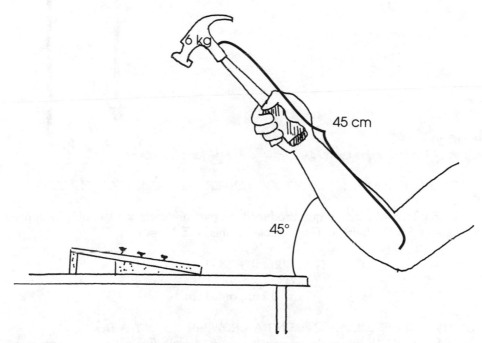

FIG 8–9.
A 6-kg hammer is held 45° from the surface to be hammered. The hammer's center of gravity is 45 cm from its axis of motion in the elbow. The muscles used to lift the hammer lie 3 cm from the axis of motion in the elbow.

SOLUTIONS TO PROBLEMS

SOLUTION TO PROBLEM 8.1: A FOOD SERVER HOLDS A TRAY OF FOOD

In Figure 8–10 downward forces must equal upward forces. The formula for this is: $\Sigma F = 0$.

$$3.5\text{ N} + 5\text{ N} + 3\text{ N} + x = 0$$
$$x = -11.5\text{ N directed upward}$$

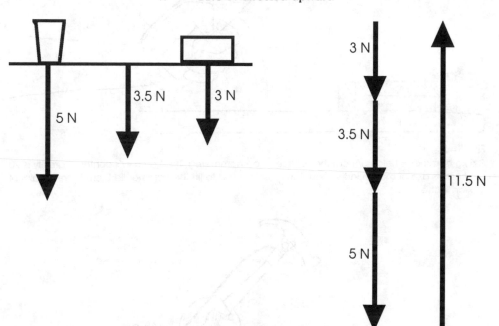

FIG 8–10.
A force of 11.5 N is needed to hold up the weight of the food and the tray.

SOLUTION TO PROBLEM 8.2: A FOOD SERVER BALANCES FOOD PLACED ON A TRAY

In Figure 8–11 the torque produced by the sandwich must equal the torque produced by the soft drink. The formula for this is: $\Sigma M = 0$.

$$(5\text{ N} \times 0.06\text{ m}) + (3\text{ N} \times x) = 0$$
$$3\text{ N} \times x = 0.3\text{ Nm}$$
$$x = 0.1\text{ m, or 10 cm}$$

SOLUTION TO PROBLEM 8.3: USING A CROWBAR TO LIFT A ROCK

In Figure 8–12 the crowbar/lever is drawn to scale (for example, 1 cm = 0.1 m). The smaller rock/axis lies a fourth of the distance from the end of the lever. The lever is a hypotenuse with a 30° angle to the base of a right triangle. A vector representing the rock is drawn to scale (for example, 1 cm = 100 N). A right triangle is

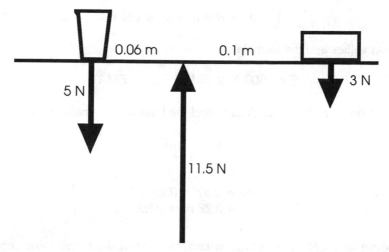

FIG 8–11.
The sandwich must be placed 10 cm from the center of the tray in order to balance the torque produced by the soft drink.

drawn with the resistance force as side a_1. The effort force is a_2. This is a first-class lever because the axis of movement lies between the effort force and the resistance force. See Problem 9.1 for an example of a first-class lever operating in the human body.

To determine the amount of force needed to lift the rock the formula $\Sigma M = 0$ is used.

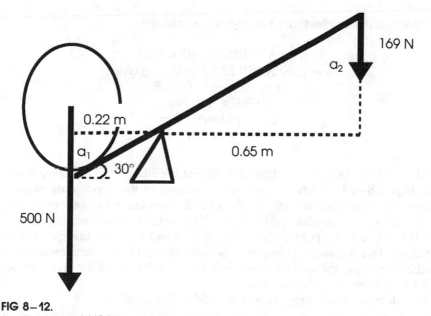

FIG 8–12.
An effort force of 169 N is needed to counteract the torque produced by this 50-kg rock.

$$0 = (R \times RMA) - (E \times EMA)$$

Put known values into the formula.

$$0 = (500 \text{ N} \times RMA) - (E \times EMA)$$

To determine RMA use cosines to find the base of the smaller right triangle b_1.

$$\cos A = b_1/c_1$$
$$\cos 30° = b_1/0.25 \text{ m}$$
$$0.87 = b_1/0.25 \text{ m}$$
$$b_1 = 0.87 \times 0.25 \text{ m}$$
$$b_1 = 0.22 \text{ m} = RMA$$

To determine EMA use cosines to find the base of the triangle and subtract b_1 from the result.

$$\cos A = b/c$$
$$\cos 30° = b/1 \text{ m}$$
$$0.87 = b/1 \text{ m}$$
$$b = 0.87 \text{ m}$$
$$b_2 = b - b_1$$
$$b_2 = 0.87 \text{ m} - 0.22 \text{ m}$$
$$b_2 = 0.65 \text{ m} = EMA$$

Substitute these values into the original formula.

$$0 = (R \times RMA) - (E \times EMA)$$
$$0 = (500 \text{ N} \times 0.22 \text{ m}) - (E \times 0.65 \text{ m})$$
$$0 = 110 \text{ Nm} - 0.65 E$$
$$0.65 E = 110 \text{ Nm}$$
$$E = 110 \text{ Nm}/0.65 \text{ m}$$
$$E = 169 \text{ N}$$

SOLUTION TO PROBLEM 8.4: USING A WHEELBARROW TO CARRY A WEIGHT

In Figure 8–13 the wheelbarrow/lever is drawn as the hypotenuse of two right triangles. The wheel/axis is angle A (25°) of both triangles. A vector representing the load is side a_1 of a smaller right triangle. The vector representing the effort force forms side a of a larger right triangle. The bases b and b_1 of the triangle are the moment arms. This is a second-class lever because the force of resistance lies between the effort force and the axis of movement. See Problem 11.3 for an example of a second-class lever in the human body.

To determine effort force the formula $\Sigma M = 0$ is used.

$$0 = (R \times RMA) - (E \times EMA)$$

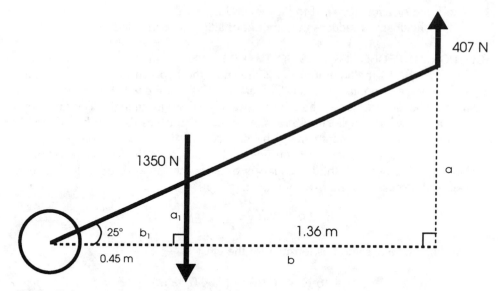

FIG 8-13.
A force of 450 N is needed to counteract the torque produced by this 135-kg load carried in a wheelbarrow.

Put known values into this formula.

$$0 = (1{,}350 \text{ N} \times RMA) - (E \times EMA)$$

Use cosines to determine *RMA* and *EMA*.

$$\cos A = b/c$$
$$\cos 25° = b/1.5 \text{ m}$$
$$0.91 = b/1.5 \text{ m}$$
$$b = 0.91 \times 1.5 \text{ m}$$
$$b = 1.36 \text{ m} = EMA$$

$$\cos A = b_1/c_1$$
$$\cos 25° = b_1/0.5 \text{ m}$$
$$0.91 = b_1/0.5 \text{ m}$$
$$b_1 = 0.91 \times 0.5 \text{ m}$$
$$b_1 = 0.45 \text{ m} = RMA$$

Substitute these values into the original formula.

$$0 = (R \times RMA) - (E \times EMA)$$
$$0 = (1{,}350 \text{ N} \times 0.45 \text{ m}) - (E \times 1.36 \text{ m})$$
$$0 = 607.5 \text{ Nm} - 1.36 \text{ Em}$$
$$E = 553.5 \text{ Nm}/1.36 \text{ m}$$
$$E = 407 \text{ N}$$

The force of effort required to lift the load is one third the weight of the entire load. The wheelbarrow reduces the amount of lifting effort needed by two thirds.

SOLUTION TO PROBLEM 8.5: USING TWO DIFFERENT STYLES OF HAMMERING

In Figure 8–14 the hammer/lever is drawn as the hypotenuse, c_1, of a right triangle. The angle opposite the axis will be angle A_1 (45° at the wrist). In Figure 8–15 the hammer/lever is drawn as the hypotenuse, C_2, of a right triangle. The angle opposite the axis will be angle A_2 (45° at the elbow). The bases, b_1 and b_2, of the triangles represent the moment arms. The direction of the effort vectors are determined by muscles. (Specific muscle groups will be covered in the following section of the book.) These are both third-class levers because the forces of effort lie between the resistance forces and the axes of movement.

$$0 = R \times RMA - E \times EMA$$

Put known values into this formula for the wrist.

$$0 = (6 \text{ N} \times RMA) - (E \times 0.02 \text{ m})$$

Use cosines to determine *RMA*.

$$\cos A = b_1/c_1$$
$$\cos 45° = b_1/0.2 \text{ m}$$
$$0.71 = b_1/0.2 \text{ m}$$
$$b_1 = 0.71 \times 0.2 \text{ m}$$
$$b_1 = 0.14 \text{ m} = RMA$$

Put this value into the formula for the wrist.

$$0 = (6 \text{ N} \times 0.14 \text{ m}) - (E \times 0.02 \text{ m})$$
$$0 = 0.85 \text{ Nm} - 0.02 \text{ Em}$$
$$E = 0.85 \text{ Nm}/0.02 \text{ m}$$
$$E = 43 \text{ N with the wrist as the axis}$$

For the elbow as axis,

$$0 = (6 \text{ N} \times RMA) - (E \times 0.03 \text{ m})$$

Use cosines to determine *RMA*.

$$\cos A = b_1/c_1$$
$$\cos 45° = b_1/0.45 \text{ m}$$
$$0.71 = b_1/0.45 \text{ m}$$
$$b_1 = 0.71 \times 0.45 \text{ m}$$
$$b_1 = 0.32 \text{ m} = RMA$$

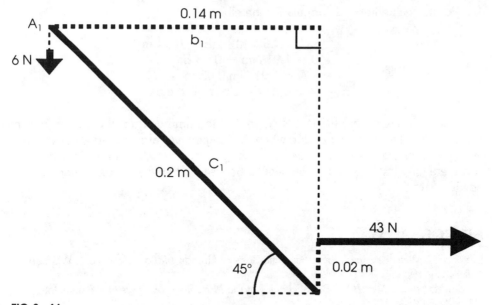

FIG 8–14.
Muscles must produce 42 N of force to use this hammer with the wrist as an axis of motion.

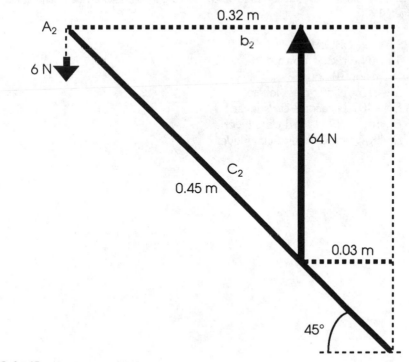

FIG 8–15.
Muscles must produce 64 N of force to use this hammer with the elbow as an axis of motion.

Put this value into the formula for the elbow.

$$0 = (6\ \text{N} \times 0.32\ \text{m}) - (E \times 0.03\ \text{m})$$
$$0 = 1.91\ \text{Nm} - 0.03\ Em$$
$$E = 1.91\ \text{Nm}/0.03\ \text{m}$$
$$E = 64\ \text{N with the elbow as the axis}$$

It takes a little more effort (22 N) to lift the hammer from the elbow, but the hammer doubles its impact torque when the longer lever arm is used. The wrist provides a better axis of motion for hammering when strength and endurance are a consideration, but elbow motion would be used whenever extra hitting force is needed.

BIBLIOGRAPHY

Luttgens K, Wells K: *Kinesiology: Scientific Basis of Human Motion.* New York, WB Saunders Co, 1982.

Nordin M, Frankel VH: *Basic Biomechanics of the Musculoskeletal System.* Philadelphia, Lea & Febiger, 1989.

Romanes GJ: *Cunningham's Textbook of Anatomy.* London, Oxford University Press, 1972.

Wiktorin CH, Nordin M: *Introduction to Problem Solving in Biomechanics.* Philadelphia, Lea & Febiger, 1986.

ANSWERS TO PROBLEMS
    8.1: 11.5 N directed upward
    8.2: 0.1 m or 10 cm
    8.3: $E = 169$ N first-class lever
    8.4: $E = 407$ N second-class lever
    8.5: E wrist $= 43$ N third-class lever
        E elbow $= 64$ N third-class lever

PART IV

Application: Biomechanics in the Human Body

Chapter 9

Head and Trunk

The head and trunk house all the organs that support life. Because these organs are made up of delicate tissues, the head and trunk must be able to protect these structures as well as move them. The skull, spine, rib cage, and pelvis are rigid bodies that protect delicate organs. Skin, tendons, ligaments, cartilage, and fascia provide additional protection. These structures are elastic and allow movement to take place. Muscles move as well as protect the structures they surround. Movement of the head and trunk takes place primarily at the neck, lower part of the back, and hips.

BASIC PROTECTIVE STRUCTURES OF THE SKULL AND SPINE

The skull and spine house the human body's most important structure, the central nervous system. The central nervous system is made up of the brain and spinal cord. The brain processes information from the senses and directs the body's internal and external activity. The spinal cord carries information to and from the brain and the rest of the body. The nerve cells that make up the brain and spinal cord are very delicate. If they are damaged, the body cannot repair or replace them. The bones and connective tissue surrounding the nerve cells provide maximum support and protection.

The ribs and pelvis house organs that are necessary for the continuation of life, most notably the heart, lungs, and reproductive organs. Support and protection for the digestive and eliminative organs is primarily provided by muscles attached to the rib cage, lumbar spine, and pelvis. These organs do have the ability to repair and replace themselves so that the structures around them can devote more effort to movement than protection.

The Skull

The skull is made up of 23 bones connected primarily with fibrous, suture-type joints. The jaw joins the skull at a synovial joint called the **temporomandibular joint,** which allows movement for eating and communication. Most muscles in the head perform the essential activities of eating and communication; however there are small muscles that control eye movement and blinking the eyelids.

The Vertebrae

With the exception of the first two vertebrae, all of the spinal vertebrae attach to each other on the horizontal plane via a cartilaginous joint called an **intervertebral disc.** This disc is made up of cartilaginous tissue attached to the vertebral body of the spine. In its center is a jelly-like substance known as the **nucleus pulposus.** The structure of the vertebrae and their intervening discs forms a strong, flexible column capable of absorbing a great deal of shock. There are many deep muscles of the back that attach to the skull, vertebrae, ribs, and pelvis. These deep muscles maintain the strength and integrity of the spinal column as well as provide for movement. Other superficial muscles that attach to the extremities and the vertebrae help maintain integrity of the spinal column while moving the limbs.

The spine continues into the buttocks where it is joined to the pelvis at the synovial **lumbosacral joint.** The pelvis is made up of the hip bones and sacrum. Each hip bone is made up of three smaller bones joined by fibrous suture joints. Anteriorly, the hip bones are joined together by a cartilaginous joint. Posteriorly, they are joined to the spine by a synovial joint. With the exception of the temporomandibular joint and the lumbosacral joint, movement between the bones of the skull and pelvis is extremely limited and occurs only with growth. In women there is potential for movement between pelvic bones since movement via softening and relaxation of ligaments occurs during pregnancy.

The Thoracic Region

The 12 thoracic vertebrae of the upper part of the back are unique because they have two facets on each side of the vertebral body. This is where the ribs attach and the spinous processes slope downward. The rib cage is made up of 7 pairs of **true ribs** that are joined to the thoracic vertebrae by synovial joints and to the sternum by cartilaginous and synovial joints. There are also 5 pairs of **false ribs** that are connected only to the thoracic spine. The thoracic vertebrae attach to one another with facets at a 60-degree angle to the vertebral body. The rib cage protects the heart and lungs by limiting movement of the thoracic spine in flexion or extension. The 12 units of the thoracic spine become fixed in flexion **(kyphosis)** during childhood. This kyphosis may increase with age and various disease processes. Some rotation and lateral flexion of the thoracic spine is possible, but this is limited both by spinal joint facets and the **intercostal** muscles between the ribs.

The Sacral Region

In the buttocks the spine continues as the **sacrum** and **coccyx.** The sacrum is joined to the pelvis at the synovial **lumbosacral joint.** This allows for positioning of the pelvis in relation to the lumbar spine. Anteriorly the hip bones are joined together by a cartilaginous joint, the **pubic symphysis.** Posteriorly they are joined to the sacrum by a synovial joint called the **sacroiliac joint.** Caudally the sacrum is joined to the coccyx by a cartilaginous joint. Muscles of the spine, abdomen, and extremities can adjust the relationship of the pelvis to the spine.

BASIC STRUCTURES OF MOVEMENT

The Cervical Region

The head must have a wide range of motion so that sensory organs such as eyes, ears, nose, and mouth can be positioned for optimal gathering of information. For this reason the cervical vertebrae form the most mobile section of the spine. Collectively the cervical spine has about 145° of flexion and extension, 180° of rotation, and 90° of lateral flexion. This spinal section is made up of seven cervical vertebrae that have protective bony openings for the vertebral arteries on either side.

The first cervical vertebra is called the **atlas.** The atlas is a ringlike structure that attaches to the skull via bilateral synovial joints. The skull can flex and extend a total of 10° to 15° and laterally flex about 4 degrees to either side on the atlas.

The second cervical vertebrae is called the **axis.** It has a toothlike protuberance known as the **dens** on which the atlas can rotate about 47 degrees. The synovial joint of the atlas and axis allows for a total of 10 degrees of flexion and extension but no lateral flexion.

The remaining five vertebrae attach with synovial joints at a 45° angle to the horizontal plane. They can rotate about 9 degrees to either side, flex 8 degrees, extend 5 degrees, and laterally flex about 10° to either side. Raising the head in infancy causes the intervertebral discs to develop so that they are thicker on the ventral surfaces and thinner on the dorsal ones. This gives the cervical vertebrae a **lordotic** curve, which provides additional ability to absorb shocks.

Neck movement is provided by a number of small muscles that span the cervical vertebrae. Many originate on the skull and have fibers inserted on the thoracic vertebrae and ribs. The muscles on the back of the neck are interlaced with the small and deep muscles of the lower portion of the spine and are called the **erector spinae.** The most prominent of the anterior neck muscles is the **sternomastoid,** which runs from below the ear to the center of the chest and attaches on top of the sternum. This muscle is visible as a "V" shape on the front of the neck. It pulls the head forward and helps to turn it from side to side.

PROBLEM 9.1: FORCES OPERATING ON THE NECK WHILE WORKING AT A VIDEO DISPLAY TERMINAL

Several computer operators in a small company complain of neck pain and upper back tightness during a normal working day, which includes 6 hours of work at the computer terminal. These operators' body weight runs from 60 to 65 kg. The weight of their heads is estimated at 5 kg. Figure 9–1,A and B shows operators with their heads in erect posture and at 45 degrees of flexion.

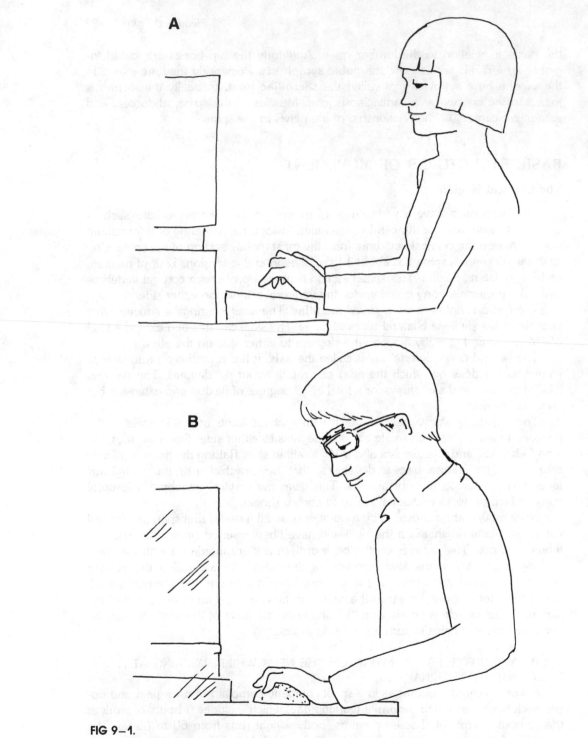

FIG 9–1.
A, a computer operator sits with the head erect. **B,** a computer operator sits with the head at 45° of flexion to the C5 vertebrae.

For this problem assume that the axis of movement occurs at the C5 vertebrae located about 3 cm above the palpable spine of the seventh cervical vertebra. The center of gravity for the head is at the portion of the temple closest to the temporo-mandibular joint. When the head is erect, the distance from the axis of motion to the center of gravity of the head is 2 cm. When the head is flexed, the distance from the axis of motion to the center of gravity of the head is 10 cm (Fig 9–1,B). The distance of the erector spinae to the axis of motion is 4 cm when the head is erect and 5 cm when it is flexed to 45°.

9.1A

What is the force of the erector spinae when the head is erect? What is the reaction force on the C5 disc?

9.1B

What is the force of the erector spinae when the head is flexed at 15 degrees? What is the reaction force on the C5 disc?

DISCUSSION

Movement of the head on the neck operates as what class of lever? How does this affect muscle forces acting on the head and spine? Do the muscle forces and reaction forces explain the computer operator's complaints of neck pain and upper back stiffness? What might be done to make the operator more comfortable? What other activities might be affected by a similar motion?

The Lumbar Region

The lower part of the back is made up of five lumbar vertebrae. These vertebrae attach to each other with facets at a 90° angle. This 90° angle severely limits rotation of the individual lumbar vertebrae. In the lumbar spine the intervertebral discs are wedge shaped, with the ventral surface thicker than the dorsal surface. The wedge shape of the disc gives the lumbar spine its characteristic **lordosis.** This concave curve takes shape as a child learns to sit and walk. It serves to keep the center of gravity of the head in line with the pelvis. The lumbar vertebrae each have the ability to flex about 9°, which gives the entire lumbar spine about 45° of flexion.

The **erector spinae** is a large complex muscle that arises from the sacrum and runs up the spine, fanning out as it attaches up the spine, to form a series of smaller muscles. These interlace with the neck muscles that run down from the head. The erector spinae are joined by smaller deeper muscles that run between vertebrae. These muscles together with the ligaments between vertebrae are responsible for both back extension and flexion, when flexion involves eccentric contraction.

PROBLEM 9.2: FORCE OF THE ERECTOR SPINAE LIFTING TWO DIFFERENT-SIZED BOXES

Workers in Figure 9–2 must lift 25- and 46-cm boxes to shoulder height. Both type of boxes weigh 18 kg. For this problem it is assumed that the erector spinae will counteract the force of the boxes. The force of these muscles operates at a distance

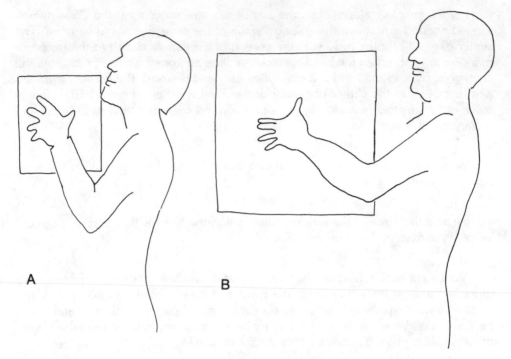

FIG 9–2.
A, a worker carries a 25-cm box held 20 cm from the axis of motion at the L5 vertebra. **B,** a worker carries a 46-cm box 40 cm from the axis of motion at the L5 vertebra.

of 5 cm from the axis of movement at the L5 disc. Workers weighing 65 to 75 kg have an upper body weight of about 40 kg. With the box lifted to shoulder height the center of gravity is 2 cm dorsal to the axis of movement in the L5 disc. The 25-cm box is held so that its center of gravity is 20 cm from the axis of motion. The 46-cm box is held so that its center of gravity is 40 cm from the axis of motion.

9.2A
What is force of the erector spinae muscles needed to lift the 25-cm box? What are the reaction forces on the L5 disc?

9.2B
What is the force of the erector spinae muscles needed to lift the 46-cm box? What are the reaction forces on the L5 disc?

Discussion
How does the size of the box change the strength needed for lifting? Does the difference in box size affect the loads on the disc? How could a work environment be adapted by using this knowledge?

PROBLEM 9.3: LOADS ON THE L5 DISC WHEN STANDING OR LEANING OVER A SINK

In Figure 9–3 a person stands and leans over a sink to perform self-care activities. For the purposes of this problem assume that both arms are held in a bilaterally symmetrical posture.

When standing, the angle of the L5 disc is at 30° to the floor, the center of gravity of the head and trunk falls 17 cm from the axis of motion in the L5 disc, and the center of gravity of the arms falls 20 cm from the L5 disc. When bending over, the L5 disc is at a 70° angle to the floor, the center of gravity of the head and trunk is 31 cm from the L5 disc, and the center of gravity of the arms is 52 cm away from the L5 disc. The person weighs 60 kg.

The erector spinae, which counteracts the force of gravity acting on the head, trunk, and arms, is located 5 cm from the axis of motion in the L5 disc. Its fibers pull at an angle of 90° to the surface of the vertebral body.

9.3A

What is the force of the erector spinae needed to counteract the weight of the head, trunk, and arms when standing or bending over?

9.3B

What are the compressive and shear forces operating on the L5 disc when standing or bending over the sink?

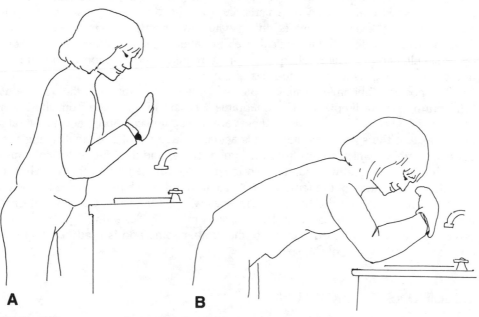

FIG 9–3.
A, a person is standing at a sink with the L5 vertebra at a 30-degree angle to the floor. The elbows are 20 cm from the axis of motion at L5. **B,** a person is bent over a sink with the L5 vertebra at a 70° angle to floor. The elbows are 52 cm from the axis of motion at L5.

Discussion

How much more muscle force is required when bending over the sink? Which position has more compressive and shear force operating on the disc? What would happen to the forces operating on the disc if the muscle strength of the erector spinae were not enough to handle the weight of the head, trunk, and arms? How could this activity be adapted to reduce the effort needed by the erector spinae and the loads imposed on the L5 disc?

The Abdominal Region

The internal contents are protected by three layers of muscle that attach to the rib cage, spine, and pelvis on the anterior wall of the abdomen. These muscles are also responsible for most trunk control and movement. The innermost layer is called the **transversus abdominis,** and its fibers run horizontally. This layer primarily provides support to the internal contents, but it is also involved in some lateral flexion and rotation of the trunk. The middle layers are called the **internal obliques,** and they run upward from the iliac crest to the lower three ribs at about a 45° angle. The topmost layers are called the **external obliques,** and they run downward from the lower eight ribs to the iliac crest and abdominal fascia. The fibers fan outward with an anterior angle of about 45°. These three layers of muscles are connected by fascia and remain continuous throughout the rib cage, with muscle fibers of all three layers running between each rib. In addition to these three layers there is another muscle, the **rectus abdominis,** which runs vertically from the pubis symphysis to the sternum. The rectus flexes the trunk against gravity and resists extension against gravity. The obliques provide both lateral flexion and rotation. In general these two motions occur simultaneously. Full rotation of the spine requires coordination of the internal and external obliques on opposite sides of the body.

The posterior abdominal wall is protected by two major muscles, the **quadratus lumborum** and the **iliopsoas.** The quadratus lies next to the spine from the lower ribs to the iliac crest of the pelvis. Its fibers are mostly vertical, and it acts to laterally flex or extend the spine. The iliopsoas is actually made up of two smaller muscles, the **psoas major,** which comes from the lumbar spine, and the **iliacus,** which comes from the pelvis. These two muscles join together to form a tendon that attaches to the inferior trochanter of the femur. The iliopsoas bends the hips and pulls the pelvis forward. When lying on the back, the iliopsoas will pull the trunk up to sitting once the shoulders are off the ground. The iliopsoas primarily flexes the hip, but it also serves to maintain the lordotic curve of the lumbar spine and is used in sitting balance and lateral flexion of the spine.

SOLUTIONS TO PROBLEMS

SOLUTION TO PROBLEM 9.1: FORCES OPERATING ON THE NECK WHILE WORKING AT A VIDEO DISPLAY TERMINAL

9.1a: When the Head Is Erect

In Figure 9–4 the force of the erector spinae muscles is calculated by using the formula for the second equilibrium condition, $\Sigma M = 0$ ($0 = EMA - RMA$). In this

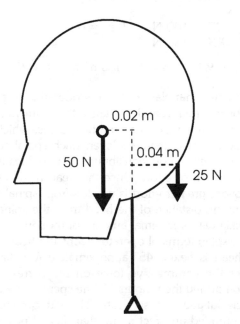

FIG 9–4.
When a computer operator sits with the head erect, the force of the erector spinae muscles needed to maintain this posture is 25 N. The reaction force on the C5 disc is 75 N directed upward.

problem E is the force of the erector spinae, and R is the force of gravity acting on the head.

$$0 = (E \times 0.04\text{m}) - (50\text{ N } [5\text{ kg} \times 10\text{ m/sec}^2] \times 0.02\text{ m})$$
$$0 = 0.04\ Em - 1\text{ Nm}$$
$$E = 1\text{ Nm} \div 0.04\text{ m}$$
$$E = 25\text{ N}$$

The reaction force on the C5 disc is calculated by using the first equilibrium condition, $\Sigma F = 0$. Since both gravity and the erector spinae muscles pull downward, the reaction force on the disc must be an equal upward force. Downward forces are negative.

$$RF - 25\text{ N} - 50\text{ N} = 0$$
$$RF = 25\text{ N} + 50\text{ N}$$
$$RF = 75\text{ N}$$

9.1B: When the Head is Flexed to 45 Degrees
In Figure 9–5 the force of the erector spinae is calculated as follows:

$$0 = (E \times 0.05\text{ m}) - (50\text{ N} \times 0.1\text{ m})$$
$$E = 5\text{ Nm} \div 0.05\text{ m}$$
$$E = 100\text{ N}$$

$$RF - 100 \text{ N} - 50 \text{ N} = 0$$
$$RF = 150 \text{ N}$$

Discussion of Problem 9.1: Forces Operating on the Neck While Working at a Video Display Terminal

In order to determine what class of lever is operating it is necessary to find the relationships of the forces of effort and resistance to the fulcrum or axis of motion. In this case the axis of motion lies between the two forces, which makes the action of the head on the neck that of a first-class lever. Each spinal segment acts as a first-class lever. This arrangement favors equilibrium and enables an erect posture to be maintained with a minimum of effort. Once the head moves out of alignment with the spinal axis of motion, greater effort is needed from spinal muscles. This effort is in direct proportion to the distance of the head from the spinal axis of motion. The effort force rises quickly with a minimal amount of motion.

While the video display terminal operator keeps the head erect, minimal effort is needed. Once the head is flexed 45° approximately four times as much effort is needed. This doubles the compressive force on the corresponding disc. Frequent repetition of this action during the 6 hours of time spent at the computer terminal will likely result in muscle fatigue and soreness. The video display terminal could be placed so that it encouraged an erect rather than flexed posture to relieve some of this muscle fatigue. The worker could also take frequent breaks and exercise the neck so that the forces of neck flexion are not so constant.

Observation of posture is important when considering factors of fatigue and discomfort in activities. If the head is out of alignment, activity will be more difficult, and

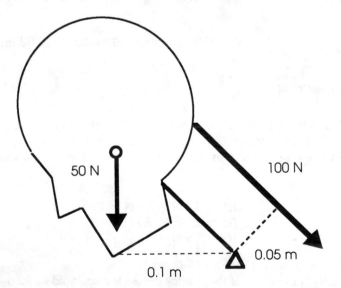

FIG 9–5.
When a computer operator sits with the head at a 45° angle, the force of the erector spinae muscles needed to maintain this posture is 125 N. The reaction force on the C5 disc is 175 N directed upward.

people will fatigue more easily. Figure 9–6 shows a client who has difficulty getting a utensil to his mouth. He flexes his head forward to meet the spoon. In so doing he uses more effort than would be needed with better posture. This extra fatigue and discomfort might cause him to stop feeding himself even though he is still hungry.

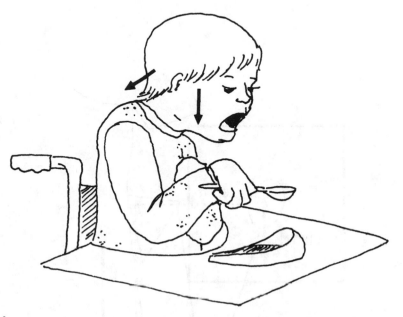

FIG 9–6.
Eating with the head angled forward may require more endurance than can be sustained throughout an entire mealtime.

SOLUTION TO PROBLEM 9.2: FORCE OF THE ERECTOR SPINAE LIFTING TWO DIFFERENT-SIZED BOXES

For this problem notice that the weight of the body falls dorsal to the axis of motion and decreases the amount of effort needed by the erector spinae to lift the boxes.

9.2A: A 25-CM BOX

In Figure 9–7 the force of the erector spinae muscles is calculated by using the formula for the second equilibrium condition, $\Sigma M = 0$. In this problem E is the force of the erector spinae and R is the force of gravity acting on the box. B is a third moment that represents gravity acting on the body. The problem will be set up like this: $0 = (R \times RMA) - (B \times BMA) - (E \times EMA)$

$$0 = (180\ N \times 0.2\ m) - (400\ N \times 0.02\ m) - (E \times 0.05\ m)$$
$$0 = 36\ Nm - 8\ Nm - 0.05\ Em$$
$$0.05\ E = 28\ Nm$$
$$E = 560\ N$$

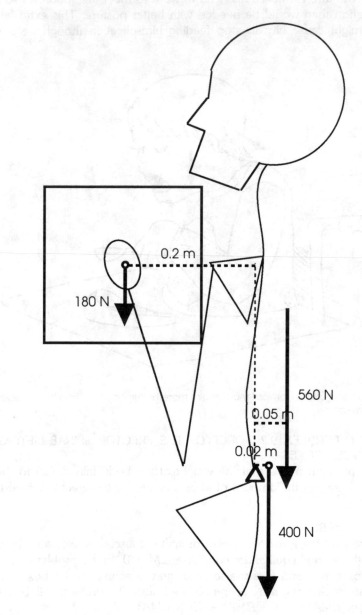

FIG 9–7.
A worker must use 560 N of force to hold a 25-cm box 20 cm from the axis of motion at L5. Carrying the box in this position will cause a reaction force of 1,140 N on the L5 disc.

The reaction force on the L5 disc is calculated by using the first equilibrium condition, $\Sigma F = 0$. Since the force of gravity on the box and the body as well as the erector spinae muscles pulls downward, the reaction force on the disc must be an equal upward force.

$$0 = RF - 180 \text{ N} - 400 \text{ N} - 560 \text{ N}$$
$$RF = 180 \text{ N} + 400 \text{ N} + 560 \text{ N}$$
$$RF = 1,140 \text{ N}$$

9.2B: A 46-CM BOX

In Figure 9–8 the force of the erector spinae is calculated as follows:

$$0 = (180 \text{ N} \times 0.4 \text{ m}) - (400 \text{ N} \times 0.02 \text{ m}) - (E \times 0.05 \text{ m})$$
$$0 = 72 \text{ Nm} - 8 \text{ Nm} - 0.05 \, E \text{ m}$$
$$0.05 \, Em = 64 \text{ Nm}$$
$$E = 1,280 \text{ N}$$

$$0 = RF - 180 \text{ N} - 400 \text{ N} - 1,280 \text{ N}$$
$$RF = 180 \text{ N} + 400 \text{ N} + 1280 \text{ N}$$
$$RF = 1860 \text{ N}$$

DISCUSSION OF PROBLEM 9.2: FORCE OF THE ERECTOR SPINAE LIFTING TWO DIFFERENT-SIZED BOXES

As the size of the box increases, its center of gravity moves farther away from the axis of motion in the L5 disc, thereby increasing its moment arm. The longer moment arm means that twice as much force must be used to lift the larger box even though its weight remains the same as the smaller box. The load on the disc is also increased significantly as the size of the larger box increases.

Using the smallest possible size of box for the objects that must be lifted would reduce the magnitude of the moment arm and decrease the amount of effort needed to do the job. Figure 9–9 shows how a long narrow box might decrease the effort needed from the erector spinae but would increase the amount of effort needed from the shoulder muscles.

As muscles fatigue, people may try to compensate by using rapid jerking motions to shift the load's center of gravity as close to the axis of motion as possible. One way of doing this is to arch the back, which shifts the body's center of gravity farther back and lengthens its moment arm. Ligaments running along the anterior portion of the vertebrae protect the spine from over arching movements, but hyperextension increases the load on the smaller facet joints. If at all possible, loads should be packaged and handled so that the center of gravity remains close to the body at all times.

SOLUTION TO PROBLEM 9.3: LOADS ON THE L5 DISC WHEN STANDING OR LEANING OVER A SINK

For this problem notice that the weight of the head, trunk, and arms falls anterior to the axis of motion and will be assigned positive values while counteractive force of the erector spinae will be assigned negative values. Percent weights of respective body parts can be found in Appendix C, "Body Segment Parameters."

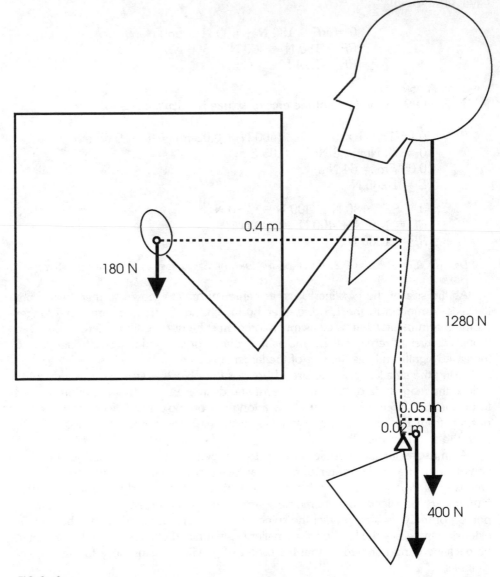

FIG 9–8.
A worker must use 1,280 N of force to hold a 46-cm box 40 cm from the axis of motion at L5. Carrying the box in this position will cause a reaction force of 1,860 N on the L5 disc.

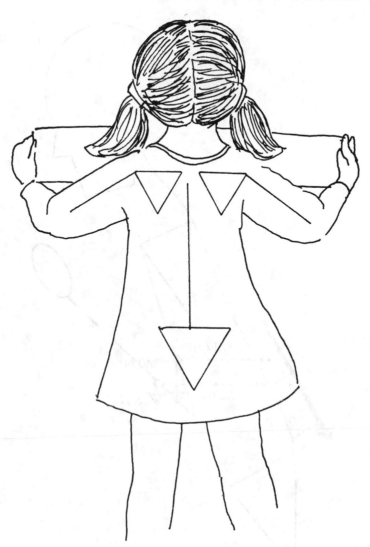

FIG 9–9.
Carrying a long narrow box may decrease loads on the vertebrae but will increase loads on the shoulders.

9.3A: FORCE OF THE ERECTOR SPINAE

In Figures 9–10 and 9–11 the force of the erector spinae muscles is calculated by using the formula for the second equilibrium condition, $\Sigma M = 0$. In this problem E is the force of the erector spinae, and R is the force of gravity acting on the body.

$$0 = (340 \text{ N} \times 0.17 \text{ m [head and trunk]}) + (60 \text{ N} \times 0.2 \text{ m [arms]})$$
$$- (E \times 0.05 \text{ m})$$
$$0 = 57.8 \text{ Nm} - 12 \text{ Nm} - 0.05 \, E \text{ m}$$
$$0.05 \, Em = 69.8 \text{ Nm}$$
$$E = 1{,}396 \text{ N standing upright}$$

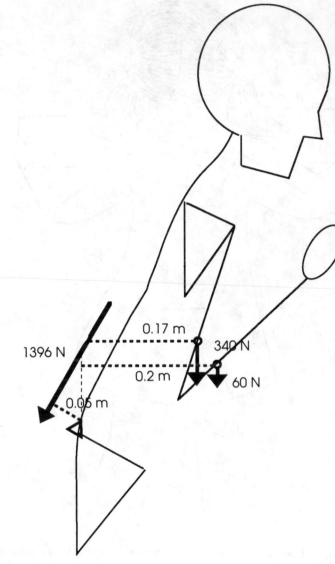

FIG 9–10.
A person must use 1,396 N of force from the erector spinae to maintain this standing posture at a sink. This posture causes 1,742 N of compressive force and 200 N of shear force on the L5 disc.

$$0 = (340 \text{ N} \times 0.31 \text{ m}) + (60 \text{ N} \times 0.52 \text{ m}) - (E \times 0.05 \text{ m})$$
$$0 = 105.4 \text{ Nm} - 31.2 \text{ Nm} - 0.05 \, Em$$
$$0.05 \, Em = 136.6 \text{ Nm}$$
$$E = 2{,}732 \text{ N bending over}$$

9.3B Compressive and Shear Forces Operating on the L5 Disc

In Figure 9–12 the compressive and shear forces can be calculated with graphics and with mathematics.

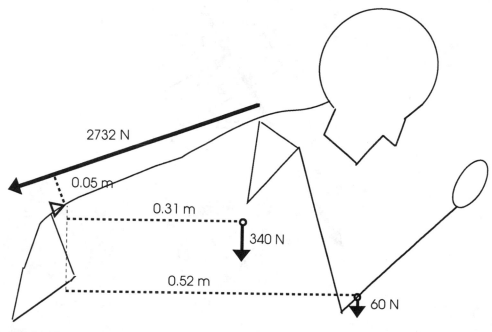

FIG 9–11.
A person must use 2,732 N of force from the erector spinae to maintain this bending posture at a sink. This posture causes 2,869 N of compressive force and 376 N of shear force on the L5 disc.

Graphic Solution.—The L5 discs are drawn at 30° and 70° to the horizontal plane. The weight of the body, which is known to be 400 newtons, lies 90° to the horizontal plane. This line forms the hypotenuse of a right triangle that has the disc surface as its base. The right triangle has an angle that corresponds to the angle of the disc on the horizontal plane, that is, 30° or 70°. The line C_w, which lies perpendicular to the base of the triangle, represents the compressive forces operating on the disc surface from the weight of the body. The line S, which connects these two lines, lies along the base of the disc surface and represents the shear forces operating on the disc. If the diagram is drawn to scale, then these lines can be measured to give estimates of the compressive and shear forces operating on the disc. Remember that the compressive weight of the body must be added to the compressive force of the erector spinae in order to get the total compressive force acting on the disc.

Mathematic Solution.—There is a right triangle with a hypotenuse of 400 N and one angle of 30° or 70°. The compressive force (C_w) of the weight of the body lies adjacent to this angle, and the shear force (S) lies opposite the known angle. Use sines to determine the sides of the opposite angles and cosines to determine the sides of the adjacent angles.

$$S = 400 \text{ N} \sin 30°$$
$$S = 200 \text{ N standing}$$

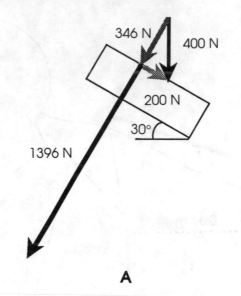

A

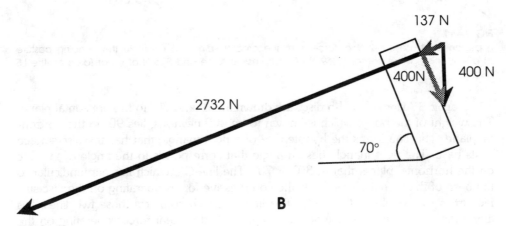

B

FIG 9–12.
Parallelograms give a graphic solution when finding compressive and shear forces operating on a disc.

$$S = 400 \text{ N sin } 30°$$
$$S = 200 \text{ N standing}$$

$$C_w = 400 \text{ N cos } 30°$$
$$C_w = 346 \text{ N}$$
$$C = 1,396 \text{ N} + 346 \text{ N}$$
$$C = 1,742 \text{ N standing}$$

$$C_w = 400 \text{ N cos } 70°$$
$$C_w = 137 \text{ N}$$
$$C = 2{,}732 \text{ N} + 137 \text{ N}$$
$$C = 2{,}869 \text{ N bending}$$

DISCUSSION OF PROBLEM 9.3: LOADS ON THE L5 DISC WHEN STANDING OR LEANING OVER A SINK

The erector spinae work twice as hard when bending over a sink as when standing next to a sink. Most of the compressive forces on the disc are caused by muscle force. The compressive forces on the disc, caused by the weight of the body, are actually less when bending over than they are when standing up. Shear force is nearly doubled when bending over, but it only accounts for about 13% of all the forces acting on the disc.

The spinal segments operate as first-class levers, with the erector spinae balancing out the weight of the body. If the erector spinae muscles were unable to handle

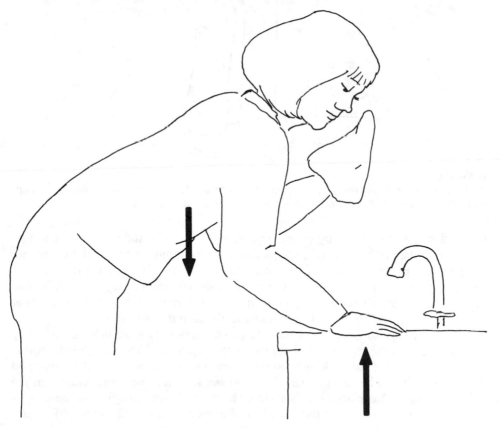

FIG 9–13.
Supporting the body with one arm while raising a washcloth to the face can decrease the forces operating in the lower part of the back while bending over a sink.

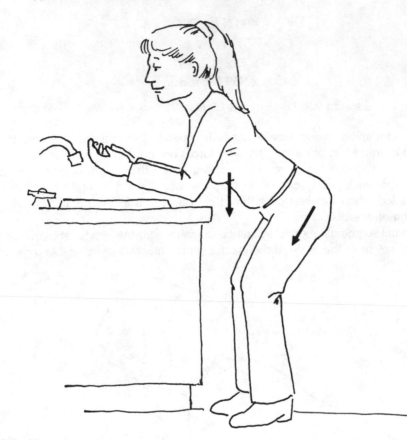

FIG 9–14.
Bending at the knees and keeping the lower portion of the back straight can decrease forces operating in the lower part of the back while bending over a sink.

the load imposed on them by bending over, this balance would be lost. The weight of the body still produces a compressive force on the anterior portion of the disc, but the posterior portion experiences a tensile force. The tensile force is the difference between the strength of the erector spinae and the forward-bending moment created by the weight of the body. This combination of compressive, tensile, and shear forces causes a twisting type of stress likely to damage disc tissue.

Most sinks are so low that it is necessary to bend over to effectively do such daily tasks as washing the face or brushing the teeth. Figure 9–13 shows stressful forces on the lower part of the back reduced when some of the body's weight is supported by one arm during bending. Figure 9–14 shows stressful forces reduced when the knees are bent. This places the face closer to the sink, and less lumbar bending is required. If the lower part of the back is held in extension during bending, force for maintaining the posture will be shared by the gluteal muscles.

BIBLIOGRAPHY

Caillet R: *Low Back Pain Syndrome.* Philadelphia, FA Davis Co, 1988.

Luttgens K, Wells K: *Kinesiology: Scientific Basis of Human Motion.* New York, WB Saunders Co, 1982.

Nordin M, Frankel VH: *Basic Biomechanics of the Musculoskeletal System.* Philadelphia, Lea & Febiger, 1989.

Romanes GJ: *Cunningham's Textbook of Anatomy.* London, Oxford University Press, 1972.

Wiktorin CH, Nordin M: *Introduction to Problem Solving in Biomechanics.* Philadelphia, Lea & Febiger, 1986.

ANSWERS TO PROBLEMS

- 9.1A: Force of erector spinae muscles = 25 N
  Reaction forces on C5 = 75 N directed upward
- 9.1B: Force of erector spinae muscles = 125 N
  Reaction forces on C5 = 175 N directed upward
- 9.2A: Force of the erector spinae = 560 N
  Reaction forces on the L5 disc = 1,140 N directed upward
- 9.2B: Force of the erector spinae = 1,280 N
  Reaction forces on the L5 disc = 1,860 N directed upward
- 9.3A: Standing upright = 1,396 N
  Bending over = 2,732 N
- 9.3B: Compressive forces:
    - Standing upright = 1,742 N
    - Bending over = 2,869 N
  Shear forces:
    - Standing upright = 200 N
    - Bending over = 376 N

Chapter **10** _____

The Upper Extremity

Through the ages people have used tools extensively to adapt to their environment. Most tools are used with a combination of reaching and grasping. The arms can be stabilized to permit fingers and thumbs to make fine manipulations of materials. The ability of the thumb to touch each fingertip has made technology possible. The hands are guided primarily by touch and sight, but they also work in conjunction with hearing.

The arm attaches to the body at the shoulder. The shoulder allows enough motion that the hand can be positioned the length of the arm in a 360-degree arc. The elbow brings the hand closer to the body for better visual contact. The elbow also acts to increase the amount of force that can be imparted to the hand through the levers of the arm and forearm. The wrist provides refined positioning and stability so that the fingers and thumb work to best advantage. The small joints of the hand allow the thumb and fingers to adapt to almost any shape. The small joints of the thumb and fingers move so that objects can be held tightly or loosely or released at will.

REACH

Reach is the ability of the arm to move the hand away from the body. In Figure 10–1 a person uses the upper extremity to extend the hand a distance about half the length of the body. This same person uses the trunk and lower extremities to reach a distance that is almost the length of the entire body. The shoulder, elbow, and forearm are structured to permit a maximum amount of movement.

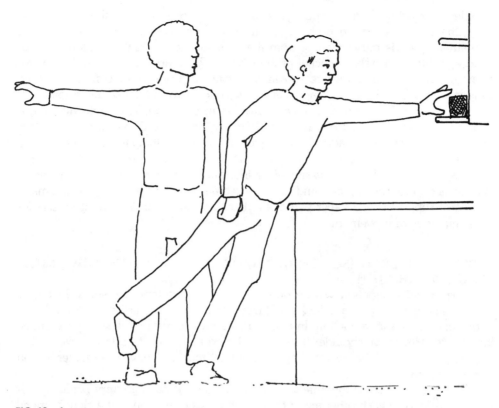

FIG 10—1.
Reaching distance is half the total body length. If a person leans to the side, the reaching distance increases to almost the entire body's length.

The Shoulder Region

Only one small skeletal attachment, the synovial **sternoclavicular joint,** connects the arm to the trunk. Otherwise the attachment of the shoulder to the trunk is muscular. The **clavicle** and **scapula** connect through the synovial **acromioclavicular joint** and a number of ligaments, of which the **coracoclavicular** ligament is the strongest. The clavicle and scapula are bases of attachment for muscles that provide stability for the shoulder. The **trapezius, rhomboids,** and **levator scapulae** connect the scapula to the spine. The **serratus anterior, subclavius,** and **pectoralis minor** connect the scapula to the rib cage. This arrangement holds the scapula to the trunk like a hinge so that the scapula generally stays close to the rib cage at its medial border. It pivots on this border and swings away from the trunk on the lateral border to provide extra range of motion for the arm. These muscles also work together to position the scapula so that movement of the arm above shoulder level is possible.

The shoulder joint has a complex muscle arrangement to compensate for the minimal stability provided by its modified ball-and-socket joint. Many of the shoulder muscles originating on the scapula cross to the anterior portion of the **humerus** to bring the arm close to the body. The **supraspinatus, infraspinatus, teres minor,** and **subscapularis** muscles come from the scapula: they hold the head of the **humerus** in the small dishlike socket of the scapula. They are also responsible for rotating the shoulder joint and are known collectively as the **rotator cuff.** The **deltoid** muscle comes from both the scapula and clavicle to surround the shoulder joint. It is primarily responsible for raising the arm away from the body. The **pectoralis major** is a large fan-shaped muscle that comes from the clavicle and the rib cage. It twists as it inserts, which gives it added strength for climbing and lifting types of movement. It is assisted by the **coracobrachialis.** On the back, the **latissimus dorsi** is another fan-shaped muscle that also twists before inserting on the humerus. The latissimus originates on thoracic, lumbar, and sacral vertebrae as well as the pelvis. It is a major source of support to the lower part of the back as well as an important muscle for climbing kinds of movement.

PROBLEM 10.1: DESIGNING ADAPTIVE EQUIPMENT FOR CLIENTS WITH LIMITED SHOULDER STRENGTH

Specialized equipment will be designed for two quadriplegic clients. In Figure 10–2 muscle testing of a 60-kg C5 quadriplegic reveals "fair" muscle grades in shoulder flexion and abduction. In Figure 10–3 muscle testing reveals "poor" muscle grades, with active shoulder flexion to 70° and abduction to 50°. A switch is being designed that can be operated by a movement midway between shoulder flexion and abduction.

The muscle fibers of the anterior and middle deltoid lie at an approximately 30-degree angle from each other and 2 cm from the axis of motion in the glenohumeral joint. With the arm outstretched the center of gravity for the entire upper extremity will fall approximately at the elbow, which is 30 cm from the shoulder joint in both these individuals.

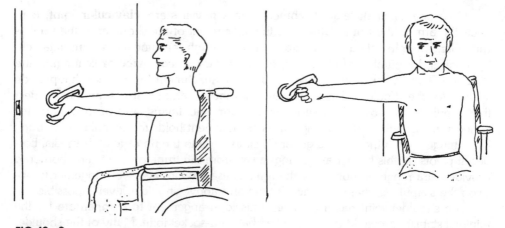

FIG 10–2.
Fair muscle grades for the anterior and middle deltoid are taken with the shoulder at 90°.

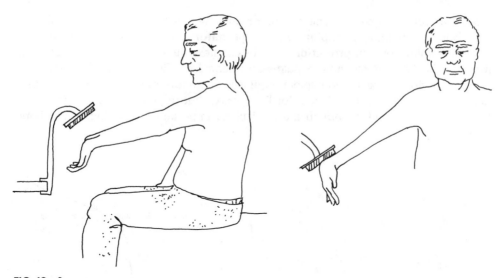

FIG 10—3.
This client has poor muscle grades. The anterior deltoid can lift the outstretched arm to only 70° of shoulder flexion. The middle deltoid can only lift the arm to 50° of abduction.

10.1A

What amount of force is available to the client with "fair" anterior and middle deltoid muscle grades?

10.1B

What amount of force is available to the client with "poor" anterior and middle deltoid muscle grades?

10.1C

What amount of force is available in "fair" and "poor" ranges when anterior and middle deltoid fibers are combined in the midrange?

DISCUSSION 10.1

Is there any advantage to be gained by using a range midway between shoulder flexion and abduction? How can manual muscle testing and goniometry be used as a noninvasive method of determining muscle forces available for daily activities?

The Elbow and Forearm

The elbow is made up of three bones that share a common joint capsule. The **ulna** and **radius** join the humerus in a hinge joint. The **biceps** and **brachialis** and **brachioradialis** muscles generally bring the hands closer to the face, and the **triceps** muscles pull the hands away from the face. Because the long head of the biceps attaches to the scapula, it also assists in flexing the shoulder during lifting tasks where the elbow is already bent.

The radius pivots at the humerus, which makes it possible for the hand to be rotated about 180 degrees. The **supinator** and the biceps, which attach to the radius, bring the palm up in **supination.** The **pronator teres** and **pronator quadratus** bring the palm down in **pronation.** The biceps flexes the elbow and supinates the hand for lifting tasks requiring a palms-up orientation. Since many lifting tasks require both elbow flexion and supination, this is an important combination. The pronator teres assists in elbow flexion for lifting tasks that require a palms-down orientation. Pronation and supination are particularly important in positioning the hand for grasping.

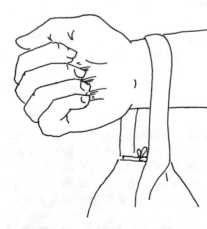

FIG 10–4.
A 5-kg handbag is carried at the wrist.

PROBLEM 10.2: FORCES OPERATING ON THE ELBOW JOINT WHEN A LOAD IS APPLIED TO THE FOREARM

In Figure 10–4 a person weighing 60 kg places a 5-kg handbag on her wrist 30 cm from the center of rotation at the elbow joint. The elbow is flexed 90 degrees and supinated. The force produced by the biceps muscle, which is assumed to be the only active muscle, has a moment arm of 0.04 m and a line of application parallel to the long axis of the humerus. In Figure 10–5 the same purse is moved closer to the elbow, 10 cm from the center of rotation at the elbow joint.

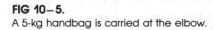

FIG 10–5.
A 5-kg handbag is carried at the elbow.

10.2A

How large a force *(B)* must the biceps muscle generate to counteract the torque produced by the weight of the handbag?

10.2B

How large is the reaction force *(R)* produced at the humeroulnar joint?

DISCUSSION *10.2*

Will moving the handbag closer to or further from the joint appreciably affect forces acting on the joint itself? Would placement of a handbag or other relatively lightweight object closer to the joint serve to protect a fragile or already damaged joint?

GRASP

Manipulation of materials requires the ability to direct variable amounts of force in specific locations. The wrist and hands together with the forearm provide a stable base of support for the thumb and fingers. The tendons of the thumb and fingers can accommodate many materials with a wide variation in force.

The Wrist

The wrist acts primarily to position tools and materials that are manipulated by the fingers and thumb. Most muscles that act to move the wrist originate on or near the distal end of the humerus. The forearm provides a large area for muscle mass so that the tendons of the wrist muscles can provide the strength needed for stabilization.

The wrist joint is formed from eight small bones with a semicircular placement around the central **capitate** bone. The bones are joined together by ligaments forming an arch with its concave surface lying at the base of the palm and its convex surface on the back of the hand. They provide a strong and stable surface for muscle attachment and 360 degrees of movement.

On the palmar surface, the hook of the **hamate** and the **pisiform** bones are connected by the **flexor retinaculum** to form a **carpal tunnel,** which contains and protects the median nerve, artery, and vein. It also contains the ten tendons of the flexor carpi radialis, the finger flexors, and the long flexor of the thumb. If these tendons become irritated, their sheaths and other connective tissue may become swollen and put pressure on the median nerve. This causes tingling and numbness in the thumb and first two fingers. In prolonged cases it can cause the grasp to become weak.

It is important that muscles acting on the wrist work in **synergy** with finger muscles since many of the muscles that move the fingers also act on the wrist. **Extensor carpi radialis longus** and **brevis** and the **extensor carpi ulnaris** enable a powerful grip by maintaining a position of wrist extension even when the fingers are tightly gripping an object. The **flexor carpi radialis** and **flexor carpi ulnaris** hold the wrist in neutral or flexion while the fingers are extended for delicate work. The tendon of flexor carpi ulnaris contains the pisiform bone and holds it stable for independent movement of the little finger.

PROBLEM 10.3: WRIST FORCES NEEDED TO USE A HAMMER

In Figure 10–6 a 0.45-kg claw hammer forms a 28-cm lever from the hammer's center of gravity to the axis of motion in the wrist. When hammering on a level surface the wrist moves from neutral, when the hammer is at 45° to the surface, into 30° of ulnar deviation when the hammer strikes a nail and lies parallel to the surface. When hammering overhead (Fig 10–7), the wrist moves from 30° of ulnar deviation when the hammer is at 45° from the overhead surface into neutral when the hammer strikes the nail. The radial and ulnar wrist muscles are approximately 2 cm from the axis of motion in the center of the wrist.

10.3A

How much force is needed from what muscles to lift the hammer to a 45° angle from a level surface?

10.3B

When hammering overhead how much force is needed from what muscles to lift the hammer into contact with the nail?

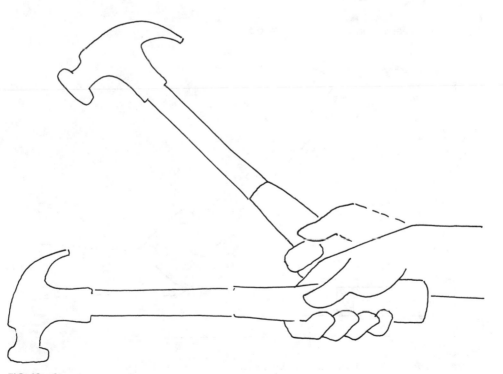

FIG 10–6.
A 0.45-kg hammer is used to hammer on a level surface.

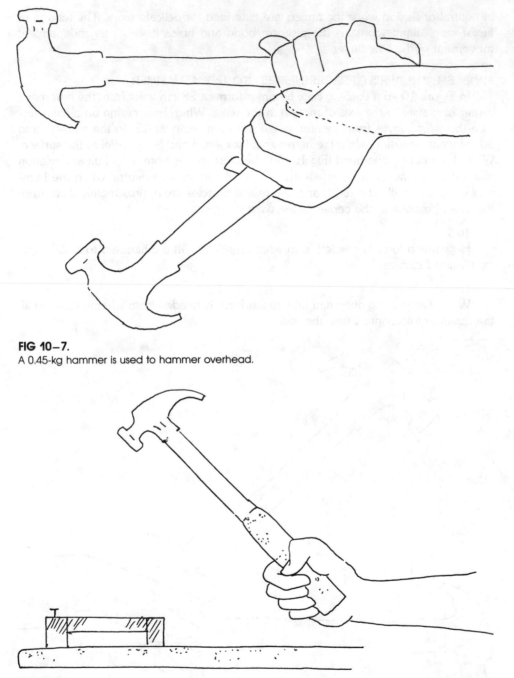

FIG 10–7.
A 0.45-kg hammer is used to hammer overhead.

FIG 10–8.
Hammering work done primarily with wrist muscles.

10.3 Discussion

What changes about this task when hammering is done overhead? Which requires more force from the wrist muscles? Since this problem involves simply lifting the hammer into position, how will adding force to the hammer change the way the various muscle groups respond to the task?

PROBLEM 10.4: DIFFERENCES IN LIFTING WORK WHEN USING TWO STYLES OF HAMMERING

Hammering work is usually done with a combination of wrist and elbow muscles. Figure 10–8 shows wrist muscles as **prime movers** and elbow muscles as **stabilizers;** Figure 10–9 shows elbow flexors as prime movers with wrist muscles as stabilizers. A 80-kg carpenter whose forearm measures 25 cm from elbow to wrist uses a 0.6-kg hammer with a lever handle of 20 cm from the center of gravity to the wrist joint. The carpenter works 6 hours a day and drives in approximately 3,000 nails with 9,000 hammer strokes, lifting the hammer head about 60° from the work surface with each repetition. To lift the hammer, the wrist goes from about 30° of

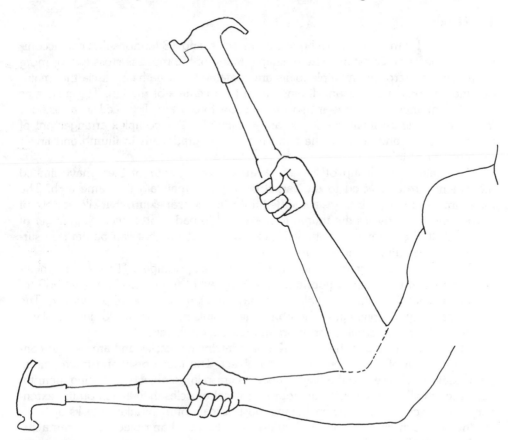

FIG 10–9.
Hammering work done primarily with elbow flexors.

ulnar deviation into neutral, while the elbow moves from about 90° to 130° of flexion. Lifting work is calculated by multiplying weight times height times the number of repetitions. The formula for lifting work is $L = mg \times h \times r$.

10.4A
How much work is done if wrist muscles are the prime movers?

10.4B
How much work is done if elbow muscles are the prime movers?

10.4 DISCUSSION
Which muscles are more efficient as prime movers? Why might one group of muscles be used over another? How would materials affect the way a job is done, and how much work is required? What effect would position have on the type and amount of work done? What type of positions would decrease the amount of work needed?

The Hand

The hand is made up of 19 bones, 25 muscles, and 18 tendons that can accommodate objects of almost any size or shape. Many of the muscles cross two or more joints. Tendons crossing multiple joints are contained in sheaths of fascia that maintain the tendons at a constant distance from joint centers of motion. These sheaths keep the moment arm constant so that muscle forces are displaced at a distance from the muscle belly without losing any magnitude. The complex arrangement of muscles, bones, and fascia in the hand makes fine gradations in thumb and finger movement possible.

The palm is made up of five **metacarpal** bones. Four of these have limited movement, are connected to the carpal bones, and maintain the same arch. The metacarpal of the thumb forms a **saddle joint** with the **trapezium** that allows 360° of movement. This enables the thumb to make pad-to-pad contact with each finger of the hand. It also permits a controlled grasp for any object that can be partially surrounded by the thumb and fingers.

Each of the four fingers is made up of three small **phlanges.** They join the metacarpal bones at the **metacarpophalangeal** joint. All of the fingers can have 360° of movement, but the index and little finger have the largest range of positioning. The thumb has only two phlanges. The **phalangeal** joints move about 90° in one plane, which is sufficient to provide for grasp and release of objects.

Muscles originating in the palm are called **intrinsic** muscles and are used to control the position of the fingers around an object. The four dorsal and three palmar **interossei** muscles spread the fingers apart to grasp large objects and bring them together for smaller objects. Like the four **lumbrical** muscles they attach on the **extensor hood mechanism.** They enable the most delicate of manipulative tasks by holding the fingers in extension while they are flexed around an object at the **metacarpophalangeal** joint.

Because of the **abductor, flexor,** and **opponens digiti minimi** muscles the little finger has an increased ability to wrap around an object. The thumb has more specific positioning movements provided by the **abductor** and **flexor pollicis brevis** as well as the **adductor** and **opponens pollicis.** These muscles together with the **first dorsal interossei** enable the control of the pad-to-pad contact between thumb, index, and little finger that is essential for any delicate manipulation of tools or materials.

The **extrinsic** muscles of the hand provide for strength of grip. These originate on the bones of the forearm and have more muscle mass for added strength. The **flexor digitorum profundus** attaches to the **distal phalanx** of each finger and causes flexion of all finger joints. The **flexor digitorum superficialis** attaches to the **middle phalanx** of each finger to provide additional strength in finger flexion at the **proximal interphalangeal** and metacarpophalangeal joints. The thumb has the **flexor pollicis longus** muscle, which attaches to the distal phalanx of the thumb. All of these extrinsic flexor muscles will flex the wrist as well the fingers unless they are blocked by the synergistic action of the wrist extensors.

Release of objects is provided for by the **extensor digitorum** muscle, which attaches to the extensor hood mechanism of each finger. Independent action of the index and little fingers is provided by separate muscles, the **extensor indicis** and the **extensor digiti minimi.** In the thumb, the **extensor pollicis longus** and **brevis** together with the **abductor pollicis longus** facilitate release of objects. Just as with the extrinsic flexor muscles, the extrinsic extensors will extend the wrist unless blocked by the synergistic action of the wrist flexors.

PROBLEM 10.5: OBJECT SIZE AND GRIP FORCE

An employee with carpal tunnel syndrome work in a warehouse at a job that requires repetitive handling of produce averaging 8 cm in diameter. Maintaining grasp on the produce requires an average of 4.4 kg of pressure. The client demonstrates a full hand grasp in the clinic (Figure 10–10). However, observation at the work site reveals that most of the time the produce is held in a partial hand grasp where contact is made primarily with the distal phlanges of the fingers (Fig 10–11).

Measurements are taken of the two grasps, and both involve 70° of abduction of the thumb. In the whole hand grip, the grip force is applied at approximately a 45° angle to the tendon along the middle phalanx. In the partial hand grasp, the grip force is applied at approximately an 80° angle to the tendon along the middle phalanx. The tendons lie 0.5 cm from the axis of motion at the finger joints.

10.5A

The flexor digitorum profundus provides most of the grip strength in the partial grasp. How much force is required of the flexor digitorum?

10.5B

How hard would the flexor digitorum profundus have to work in the full hand grasp?

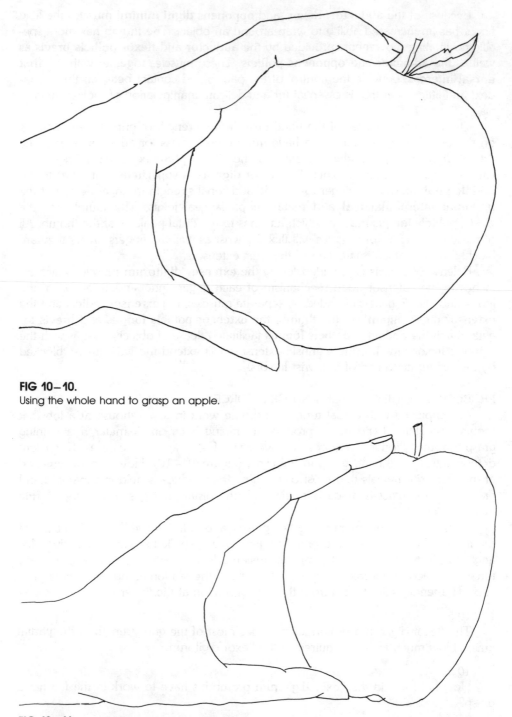

FIG 10–10.
Using the whole hand to grasp an apple.

FIG 10–11.
Using a partial hand grasp to hold an apple.

10.5 DISCUSSION

Is there a significant difference in the amount of force needed for the two different grasps? How would this affect a carpal tunnel syndrome? What could be done to reduce the amount of force needed to perform this job?

SOLUTIONS TO PROBLEMS

SOLUTION TO PROBLEM 10.1: DESIGNING AN OVERARM SWITCH FOR A CLIENT WITH LIMITED SHOULDER STRENGTH

In order to solve this problem the amount of force available in the anterior and middle deltoid fibers must be determined. These two forces are combined by using the parallelogram method explained in Chapter 6. The resultant force is the amount of power available for operation of the switch.

10.1A: "FAIR" MUSCLE GRADES

The force of the anterior and middle fibers of the deltoid muscle is calculated by using the formula for the second equilibrium condition, $\Sigma M = 0$. In Figure 10–12, D

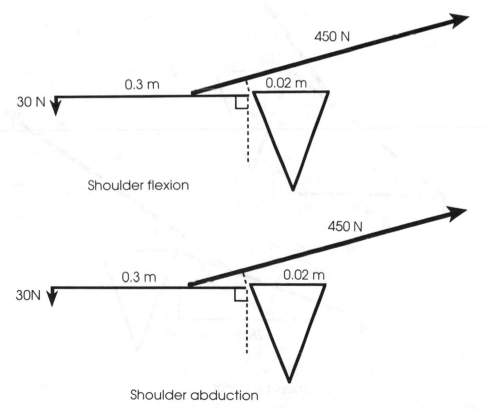

FIG 10–12.

Fair muscle grades in the anterior and middle deltoid muscles indicate 450 N of force available for this client.

is the force of the anterior or middle deltoid fibers, and R is the force of gravity acting on the arm. The formula is *(R × RMA) − (D × DMA) = 0*; 4.8% of 70 kg gives the approximate weight of the arm (2.88 kg). At 90 degrees the arm's center of gravity lies 30 cm from the axis of motion.

$$(30 \text{ N} \times 0.30 \text{ m}) - (D \times 0.02 \text{ m}) = 0$$
$$9.0 \text{ Nm} - 0.02 \, Dm = 0$$
$$9.0 \text{ Nm} = 0.02 \, Dm$$

D = 450 N for the anterior or middle deltoid with fair muscle grade

10.1B: "Poor" Muscle Grades

In Figure 10–13 moment arms for shoulder flexion and abduction are calculated with sines. At 70° of shoulder flexion, the arm's center of gravity lies 28 cm

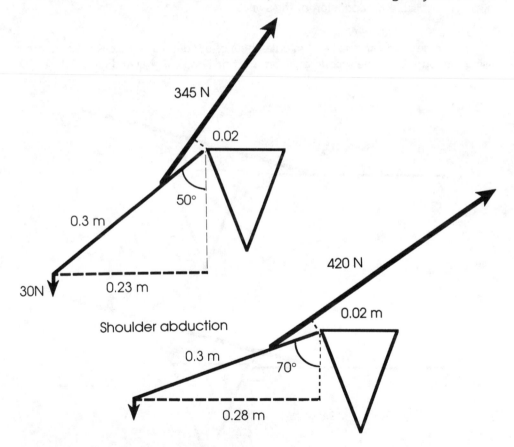

FIG 10–13.
For this client poor muscle grades indicate 420 N of force available in the anterior deltoid and 345 N of force available in the middle deltoid.

from the axis of motion (sin 70° = a/30 cm). At 50° of abduction, the arm's center of gravity lies 23 cm from the axis of motion (sin 50° = a/30 cm).

(30 N × 0.28 m) − (D × 0.02 m) = 0
8.4 Nm − 0.02 Dm = 0
8.4 Nm = 0.02 Dm
D = 420 N for the anterior deltoid with poor muscle grade

(30 N × 0.23 m) − (D × 0.02 m) = 0
6.9 Nm − 0.02 Dm = 0
6.9 Nm = 0.02 Dm
D = 345 N for the middle deltoid with poor muscle grade

10.1c: Combined Anterior and Middle Deltoid Fibers

The "fair"-grade anterior and middle deltoid fibers each pull with a force of about 450 N at an angle of approximately 30° from each other. In Figure 10–14 these forces make up two sides of a parallelogram. The resultant is a diagonal connecting the opposite corners. The resultant force is calculated by drawing a graphic

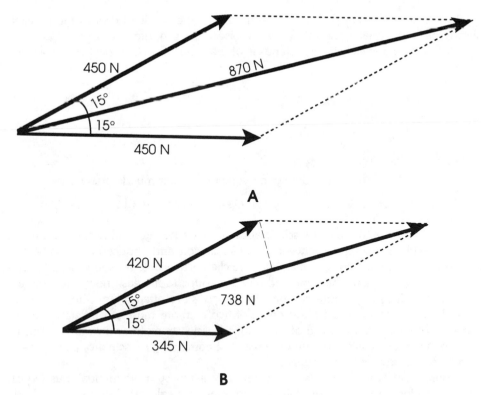

FIG 10–14.
A parallelogram is used to find the amount of force available for midrange shoulder flexion and abduction in clients with "fair" **(A)** and "poor" **(B)** muscle grades.

representation or by using mathematics. A drawing of the parallelogram is essential for a graphic solution and helpful to a mathematic one.

Graphic Solution.—Figure 10–14 shows the vectors representing the force of the anterior and middle deltoid fibers at a 30° angle from each other. The parallelogram is completed by drawing the remaining two sides as dotted lines. The line that runs between the deltoid forces and connects the two opposite corners is the resultant force. If drawn to scale it can be measured to give an approximation of the force available for operating the switch.

Mathematic Solution.—Where both sets of muscle fibers pull with equal force, bisect the parallelogram to get two right triangles with a hypotenuse of 450 N and one angle of 15°. The base of these triangles will be half the resultant force. Use cosines to determine the sides of the adjacent angles (cos $A = b/c$). See Figure 10–14, A.

$$R/2 = 450 \text{ N cos } 15°$$
$$R/2 = 435 \text{ N}$$
$$R = 870 \text{ N for midrange movement with "fair" muscle grade}$$

Where muscle fibers pull with different forces, the resultant divides the parallelogram into two equal triangles. These are bisected again into two unequal right triangles. These triangles have hypotenuses of 345 and 420 N, respectively. See Figure 10–14, B.

$$R_a = 420 \text{ N cos } 15°$$
$$R_a = 405 \text{ N}$$
$$R_m = 345 \text{ N cos } 15°$$
$$R_m = 333 \text{ N}$$
$$R = 405 \text{ N} + 333 \text{ N}$$
$$R = 738 \text{ N for midrange movement with fair muscle grade}$$

DISCUSSION OF PROBLEM 10.1: DESIGNING AN OVERARM SWITCH FOR A CLIENT WITH LIMITED SHOULDER STRENGTH

Both "poor" and "fair" muscle grades produce nearly double the amount of force available in midrange between shoulder flexion and abduction. Placement of the switch in this midrange will maximize the client's available muscle power. Generally people use motions that combine muscle groups to increase power for any activity. In muscle testing, these combination motions are often referred to as "substitutions" because they utilize the strength of two or more muscles or muscle groups and do not give a true picture of individual muscle strength. Awkward or unusual movements in an activity are often the result of combining muscle groups to get additional power from weaker muscles.

Approximate values of muscle force are calculated by using manual muscle testing and goniometry. Force for "fair" muscle grades is calculated by using the body weight as a means for estimating the weight of the body part that is being lifted. Force for "poor" muscle grades is calculated by first measuring the available range of motion and then measuring or calculating the body part's center of gravity from the axis of motion at the end of that range. For "good" and "normal" muscle grades extra weight is added at the center of gravity for the body part being lifted to calculate the maximum amount of force available for a movement. These estimates may be useful when evaluating and designing adaptive equipment.

SOLUTION TO PROBLEM 10.2: FORCES OPERATING ON THE ELBOW JOINT WHEN A LOAD IS APPLIED TO THE FOREARM

To find the weight of the forearm, multiply the person's total body weight by the percentage of the forearm and hand to that weight. A table of percentages of body weight is found in Appendix C.

$$60 \text{ kg} \times 0.02 = 1.2 \text{ kg}$$

Locate the center of gravity in the forearm by using the table found in Appendix C.

$$0.43 \times 30 \text{ cm} = 12.9 \text{ cm from the elbow to the center of gravity in the forearm}$$

10.2A: FORCE OF THE BICEPS MUSCLE

Use the second equilibrium condition to solve for the force of the biceps in Figures 10–15 and 10–16 ($\Sigma M = 0$).

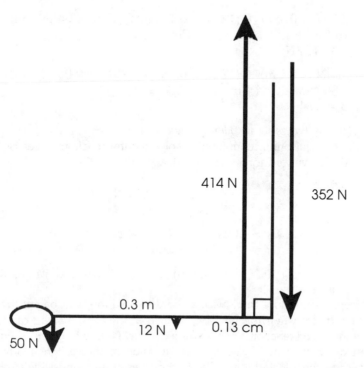

FIG 10–15.
The biceps must produce 414 N of force when a 5-kg handbag is held at the wrist. This produces a 352 N reaction force on the elbow.

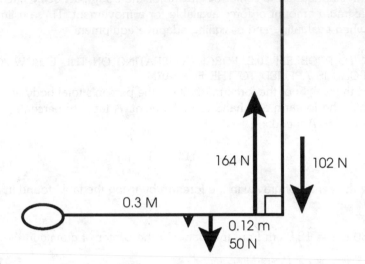

FIG 10–16.
The biceps must produce 164 N of force when a 5-kg handbag is held at the elbow. This produces a 102 N reaction force on the elbow.

$$(50 \text{ N} \times 0.3 \text{ m}) + (12 \text{ N} \times 0.13 \text{ cm}) - (B \times 0.04 \text{ m}) = 0$$
$$15 \text{ Nm} + 1.56 \text{ Nm} = 0.04 \, B\text{m}$$
$$B = 414 \text{ N}$$

$$(50 \text{ N} \times 0.1 \text{ m}) + (12 \text{ N} \times 0.13 \text{ cm}) - (B \times 0.04 \text{ m}) = 0$$
$$6.56 \text{ Nm} = 0.04 \, B\text{m}$$
$$B = 164 \text{ N}$$

10.2B: Reaction Forces on the Humeroulnar Joint

Use the first equilibrium condition to solve for the reaction forces on the elbow joint ($\Sigma F = 0$). Downward forces are negative.

$$R - 50 \text{ N} - 12 \text{ N} + 414 \text{ N} = 0$$
$$R = -352 \text{ N (downward)}$$

$$R - 50 \text{ N} - 12 \text{ N} + 164 \text{ N} = 0$$
$$R = -102 \text{ N (downward)}$$

Discussion of Problem 10.2: Forces Operating on the Elbow Joint When a Load Is Applied to the Forearm

The biceps works more than twice as hard to hold the handbag at the wrist. The reaction force triples when the handbag is held at the wrist instead of closer to the elbow. The increased reaction force is more destructive to a fragile or damaged joint. To prevent destruction of fragile joint tissue, even relatively light loads should be moved closer to the affected joint. Placing loads as close as possible to the affected joints is a principle of joint protection based on joint reaction forces.

The Upper Extremity 137

SOLUTION TO PROBLEM 10.3: WRIST FORCES NEEDED TO USE A HAMMER

Use cosines to find the moment arm for the hammer when it is 45° from the surface (cos 45° = b/0.28 m).

10.3A: HAMMERING ON A LEVEL SURFACE

Force is needed to move from 30 degrees of ulnar deviation to neutral in Figure 10–17.

(4.5 N × 0.28 m) − (r × 0.02 m) = 0
r = 1.26 Nm/0.02 m
r = 63 N to lift the hammer away from the nail with radial wrist muscles

10.3B: HAMMERING OVERHEAD

Force is needed to move from 30° of ulnar deviation to neutral in Figure 10–18.

(4.5 N × 0.20 m) − (u × 0.02 m) = 0
u = 90 Nm/0.02 m
u = 45 N to lift the hammer to the nail with ulnar wrist muscles

10.3: DISCUSSION

Less force is required to lift the hammer to the nail than to lift the hammer above the level surface because the moment arm is less. In order to get efficient hammering, added force must be provided. This added force comes from the ulnar

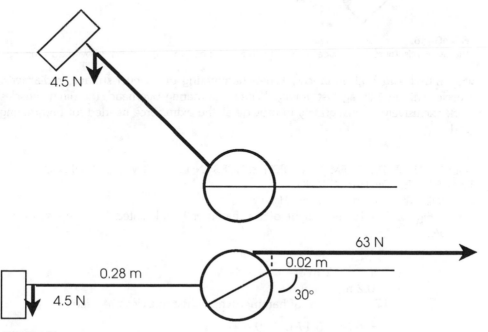

FIG 10–17.
The radial wrist muscles produce 63 N of force to do a hammering task on a level surface.

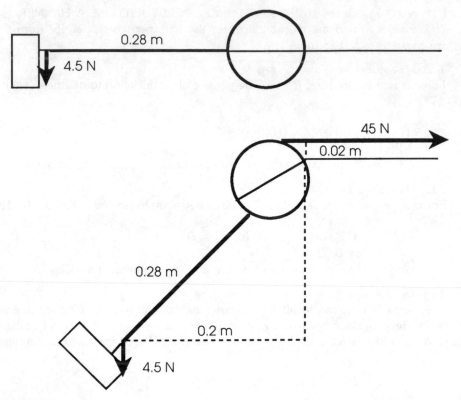

FIG 10–18.
The ulnar wrist muscles produce 45 N of force to do a hammering task on an overhead surface.

wrist muscles in both instances. When hammering on a level surface, radial wrist muscles will only lift against gravity. When hammering overhead, the ulnar muscles work exclusively against gravity to provide all the extra force needed for hammering work.

SOLUTION OF PROBLEM 10.4: DIFFERENCES IN LIFTING WORK WHEN USING TWO STYLES OF HAMMERING

10.4A: WRIST MUSCLES AS PRIME MOVERS

In Figure 10–19 the height of the hammer is calculated by using sines: sin $A = a/c$.

$\sin 60° = 0.2 \text{ m}/c$
$c = 0.2 \text{ m} \times 0.8660$
$0.17 \text{ m} = \text{height of hammer when wrist muscles are used}$

$L_W = 6 \text{ N} \times 0.17 \text{ m} \times 9,000$
$L_W = 9,180 \text{ Nm/day}$

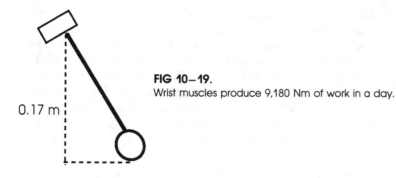

FIG 10–19.
Wrist muscles produce 9,180 Nm of work in a day.

0.17 m

10.4B: ELBOW FLEXORS AS PRIME MOVERS

In Figure 10–20 the height of the hammer is calculated by using sines: $\sin A = a/c$

$$\sin 60° = 0.45 \text{ m} \div c$$
$$c = 0.45 \text{ m} \times 0.8660$$
$$0.39 \text{ m} = \text{height of the hammer when elbow muscles are used}$$

$$L_e = 6 \text{ N} \times 0.39 \text{ m} \times 9,000$$
$$L_e = 21,060 \text{ Nm/day}$$

DISCUSSION OF PROBLEM 10.4: DIFFERENCES IN LIFTING WORK WHEN USING TWO STYLES OF HAMMERING

More than twice as much work is done in a day when the elbow flexors are used as prime movers. The wrist muscles are more efficient for hammering work. Using

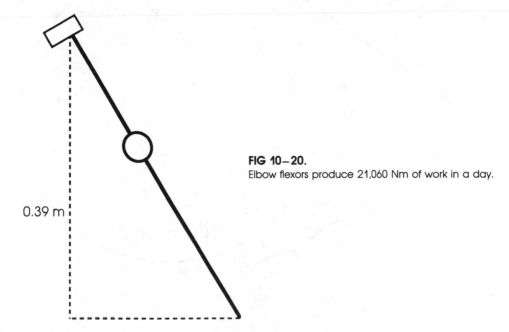

FIG 10–20.
Elbow flexors produce 21,060 Nm of work in a day.

0.39 m

the forearm for hammering imparts greater force on the head of the hammer. In general, hammering work is done by the wrist muscles, but when extra force is needed, the elbow muscles and even shoulder muscles may be used for a hammering job. With larger nails and hardwood or other dense materials, increased effort is required. Placement of the materials determines which muscles are used. In situations where hammering must be done at shoulder level or above, the ulnar deviators of the wrist as well as elbow and shoulder flexors and abductors are needed. They will be working entirely against gravity. This requires even more work. Whenever possible, tools such as a hammer should be used in a gravity-assisted position.

SOLUTION TO PROBLEM 10.5: OBJECT SIZE AND GRIP FORCE
    Use cosines to solve for the force of the flexor digitorum in grasping in Figures 10–21 and 10–22.

10.5A: *Partial Hand Grasp*

$$\cos 80° = F_p /44 \text{ N}$$
$$F_p = 44 \text{ N/cos } 80°$$
$$F_p = 253 \text{ N}$$

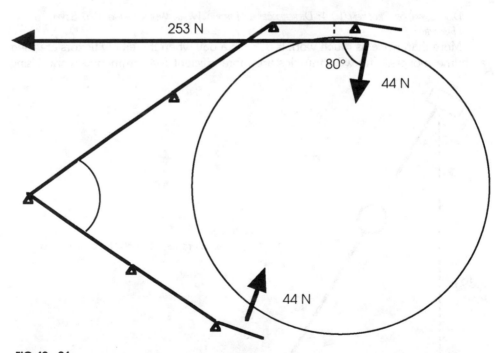

FIG 10–21.
When a partial hand grasp is used to hold an apple, it produces a force of 253 N.

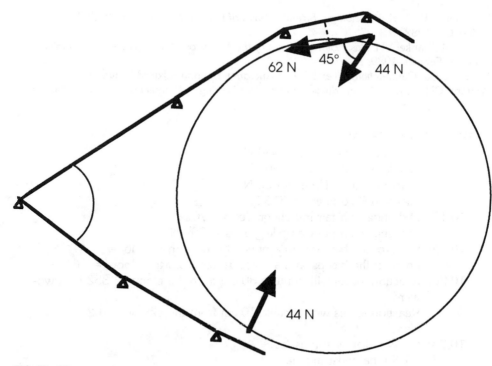

FIG 10–22.
When the whole hand is used to grasp an apple, it produces a force of 62 N.

10.5B: WHOLE HAND GRASP

$$\cos 45° = F_W/44 \text{ N}$$
$$F_W = 44 \text{ N}/\cos 45°$$
$$F_W = 62 \text{ N}$$

10.5 DISCUSSION

The amount of force needed for a partial grasp is four times that needed for a whole grasp. Repeated use of the partial hand grasp during work would aggravate an already-existing carpal tunnel syndrome where swelling in the tight carpal tunnel reduces the amount of room available for tendon movement. Using a whole grasp on the produce would reduce the stress caused by muscle forces on the flexor tendons.

BIBLIOGRAPHY

Boehme R: *Improving Upper Body Control: An Approach to Assessment and Treatment of Tonal Dysfunction.* Tucson, Communication Skill Builders, 1988.
Caillet R: *Low Back Pain Syndrome,* Philadelphia, FA Davis Co, Publishers, 1988.

Luttgens K, Wells K: *Kinesiology: Scientific Basis of Human Motion.* New York, WB Saunders Co, 1982.

Nordin M, Frankel VH: *Basic Biomechanics of the Musculoskeletal System.* Philadelphia, Lea & Febiger, 1989.

Romanes GJ: *Cunningham's Textbook of Anatomy.* London, Oxford University Press, 1972.

Wiktorin CH, Nordin M: *Introduction to Problem Solving in Biomechanics.* Philadelphia, Lea & Febiger, 1986.

ANSWERS TO PROBLEMS

10.1A: Anterior deltoid fibers = 450 N

Middle deltoid fibers = 450 N

10.1B: Anterior deltoid fibers = 420 N

Middle deltoid fibers = 315 N

10.1C: Midrange with fair muscle grades = 870 N

Midrange with poor muscle grades = 709 N

10.2A: Force of the biceps with a purse 30 cm from the elbow = 414 N

Force of the biceps with a purse 10 cm from the elbow = 164 N

10.2B: Reaction forces with a purse 30 cm from the elbow = 352 N downward

Reaction forces with a purse 10 cm from the elbow = 102 N downward

10.3A: 6.3 N radial wrist muscles

10.3B: 45 N ulnar wrist muscles

10.4A: 9,180 Nm/day

10.4B: 21,060 Nm/day

10.5A: 253 N

10.5B: 62 N

Chapter 11

The Lower Extremity

People walk in an upright position with their hands left free to explore and manipulate the environment. This means that the lower extremity must carry the weight of the body and move it from place to place. The lower extremities also help maintain balance and equilibrium.

The legs connect with the rest of the body at the hip joint in the pelvis. This joint provides stability as well as mobility. The knees bring the body closer to or farther from the ground. The ankles and feet support the entire weight of the body and form a base from which movement can take place.

WEIGHT BEARING

The bones of the lower extremity must be able to carry the weight of the rest of the body as well as absorb and adapt to the added forces produced by movement. These bones are very sturdy, and many have curves and arches that increase their ability to handle large amounts of force and stress. Muscles and ligaments must be able to sustain large forces efficiently over extended periods of time.

Weight-Bearing Structures of the Lower Extremity

The pelvis is composed of eight bones that form a somewhat triangular shape around an oval opening. The structure of the pelvis makes it a particularly stable base from which movement of the legs and the trunk can take place. The sacral vertebrae of the spine make up the posterior part of the pelvis. The spinal ligaments together with the curves formed by the structure of the spine allow an upright posture to be maintained with minimal muscular activity.

The hip joint is a classic ball-and-socket–type joint where the ball-like head of the **femur** is firmly seated in the cuplike **acetabulum** of the pelvis. Its position is further maintained by a series of ligaments that form a tough, fibrous joint capsule. The **iliofemoral ligament** makes up the front of this capsule between the **greater** and **lesser trochanters** of the femur. When there is muscle weakness, the body's center of gravity may be positioned behind the hip joint. With this maladaptive alignment the iliofemoral ligament can support the weight of the trunk when standing with minimal muscular activity.

To provide surfaces for movement the knee has large portions of the femur and **tibia** covered with smooth cartilage. Two semicircles of fibrous tissue called **menisci** fill gaps between the femur and tibia and provide extra lubrication throughout the range of motion. The tibia and femur are joined together by the **anterior** and **posterior cruciate ligaments** and the **medial** and **collateral ligaments.** The anterior portion of the joint capsule is further enhanced by the **patella,** which is embedded in the tendon of the muscles that hold the knee in extension.

At first glance the knee appears to move only in one plane, bending and straightening the leg. A more thorough examination reveals that in order to carry and move a person's weight the knee must rotate and glide. This rotation tightens the cruciate ligaments and the joint capsule. A combination of rolling, gliding, and rotation **"locks"** the femur into the seat of the **tibia** so that minimal movement will occur when the knee is extended and bearing weight.

Seven **tarsal** bones form a dome shape where the foot attaches to the leg at the ankle. The **talus** is wedged between the tibia, which bears the weight of the body, and the **fibula,** which serves as a point of attachment for many of the muscles of the lower portion of the leg. It lies on the **calcaneus,** which forms the heel of the foot. The tarsal bones attach to the five **metatarsal** bones that make up the midfoot. The toes are made up of **phalanges,** much like the fingers, with the big toe having only two phalanges and the other toes each having three phalanges.

The foot is able to support the weight of the body because of its arches, which act like springs. The **longitudinal arch,** which runs lengthwise, and the **transverse arch,** which runs widthwise, together make up the hollow that exists between the heel and the ball of the foot. These arches can absorb the forces that are created by standing and moving.

Weight-Bearing Muscles of the Lower Extremity

In order to achieve an upright posture three muscle groups must have sufficient strength to lift the weight of the body against gravity. If these muscles are weak, a person may develop a maladaptive balance on the bones and ligaments. These adaptations may permit standing but not smooth transitions into or out of a standing posture.

Hip Extensors
The **hamstrings,** which act to flex the knee, can also initiate hip extension. The **gluteus maximus** assists in moving to standing from sitting and stooping positions as

well as when jumping and running. It pulls the leg behind the pelvis when in the standing position and has the strength to move the head and trunk forward when the legs and feet are stabilized against a resistive surface. The tensor fasciae latae flexes the hip, but it joins the gluteus maximus to become part of the **iliotibial band,** which runs down the outside of the leg and attaches below the knee for added stability.

Knee Extensors

The **quadriceps** extend the knees and flex the hips. The quadriceps are made up of four muscles; the **vastus lateralis, medialis,** and **intermedius** all originate on the shaft of the femur and are a major force when moving from standing to sitting or when going up and down stairs. The **rectus femoris** originates at the pelvis and works with the iliopsoas to flex the hip. The tendon of the quadriceps muscles surrounds the patella, or kneecap, which provides a fulcrum for added power.

Plantar Flexors

Movement that takes place at the ankle and points the toes downward or pulls the body up on the toes is called **plantar flexion.** Ankle movement that pulls the toes upward toward the leg is called **dorsiflexion.** The plantar flexors use the foot as a lever to lift the entire weight of the body. The prime movers are two muscles, the **gastrocnemius,** which arises on the femur and also acts to bend the knee, and the **soleus,** which arises on the tibia and fibula and acts solely on the ankle joint. The two muscles together make up the **triceps surae,** which attaches to the calcaneus with the **tendo calcaneus,** also known as the "Achilles tendon." This tendon supports the weight of the body when standing. The triceps can lift the body onto the ball of the foot when necessary for reaching and moving. The gastrocnemius and soleus are assisted by several other muscles. Among these are the **flexor hallucis longus,** which attaches to the distal phalanx of the big toe and is important in the final push off when walking or running, and the **flexor digitorum longus,** which attaches to the distal phalanges of the four smaller toes and is important for adapting to the ground for a better weight-bearing surface when walking or running.

The Standing Posture

The muscles described above are needed to assume a standing position. The lower extremity is aligned so that a standing posture can be maintained with an extension synergy. The normal extensor synergy involves anterior pelvic tilt, hip extension, the quadriceps, and the gastrocnemius. Body alignment and synergistic movement make efficient use of minimal muscular effort (Fig 11–1).

PROBLEM 11.1: MUSCLE FORCE NECESSARY FOR LIFTING WEIGHT ONTO THE BALL OF THE FOOT WHEN REACHING

In Figure 11–2 a person weighing 60 kg must shift her weight onto the ball of the right foot to reach into an overhead cabinet. When assuming this position the person's center of gravity is to the left of the spine at about L3, approximately 8 cm

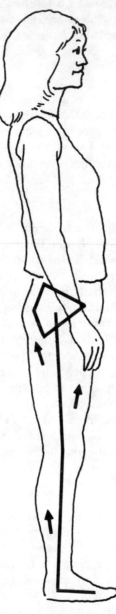

FIG 11–1.
Standing posture can be maintained with minimal muscular activity.

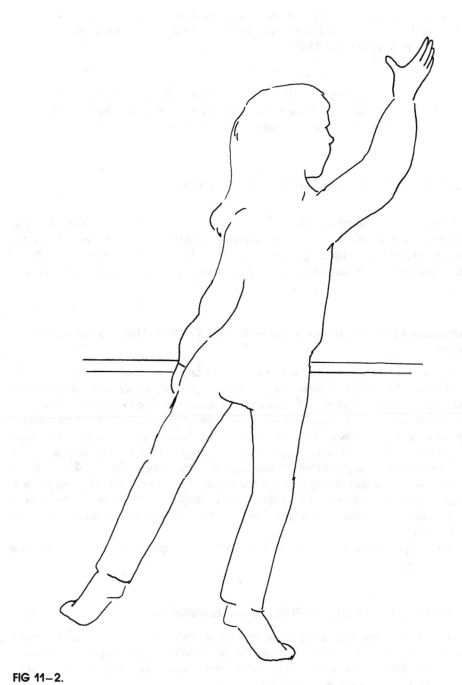

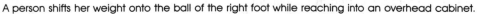

FIG 11–2.
A person shifts her weight onto the ball of the right foot while reaching into an overhead cabinet.

from the axis of motion at the metatarsophalangeal joints. If the gastrocnemius and soleus muscles are lifting the entire weight of the body, how much force will they exert? What type of lever is this?

Discussion

Does the anatomic structure of the lower extremity give it a mechanical advantage in this type of situation? Why would such an advantage be useful? What other activities would be assisted by this anatomic advantage?

BALANCE AND EQUILIBRIUM REACTIONS

Because body weight is shifted by the muscles of the lower extremity, the relationship of these muscles to the axis of motion is constantly changing. Muscles of the lower extremity may perform opposing motions such as flexion and extension or abduction and adduction, depending on their relationship to the axis at the moment of action.

Relationships Between Bones, Ligaments, and Tendons That Contribute to Balance

The head and the neck of the femur form an angle of about 125 degrees to the shaft. Figure 11–3 shows how this angle makes it possible to maintain balance while standing on one foot. It enables the mechanical axis of the leg to run in a straight line from the hip through the knee and ankle while providing hip muscles with a longer lever arm for added power. An angle of less than 125 degrees is called **coxa vara** and produces a "knock-kneed" appearance. An angle of more than 125 degrees is called **coxa valga** and produces a "bow-legged" appearance (Fig 11–4,A–C).

The axis of motion changes in the knee joint throughout the range of motion. Flexion, extension, and rotation at the knee contribute to balance. If the knee is locked, balance and ability to respond quickly to a change in the center of gravity will be impaired.

Multiple joints and arches of the foot allow for adaptability when moving over uneven surfaces.

Muscles Used for Maintaining Balance and Equilibrium

The muscles attaching around the hip, knee, and ankle operate with ligaments to maintain the stability of the joint capsules by actively responding to forces placed on the joint. Muscle fibers can adapt themselves in anticipation of as well as in response to forces incurred in movement.

Anticipatory adaptation is most evident when receiving an unexpected jolt such as that due to a step that is shorter or longer than it appeared to be visually. Ancient

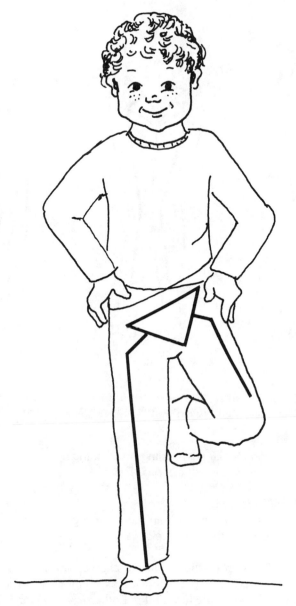

FIG 11–3.
The neck of the femur forms an angle that makes it possible to balance on one leg.

Romans protected their temples and palaces with long flights of stairs where one step would be shorter or longer than all of the others. Invading armies would invariably trip on this step and give the defending armies a chance to act.

When standing, the center of gravity in the body does not remain stationary; there is some constant fluctuation of active muscle groups. Muscle groups in the

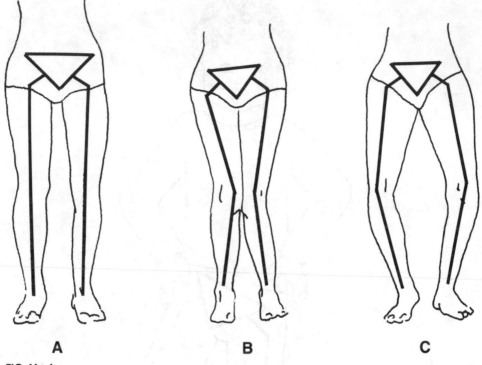

FIG 11–4.
The angle at the neck of the femur affects the appearance of the legs. **A,** the normal angle is 125 degrees. **B,** an angle greater than 125° produces coxa vara. **C,** an angle of less than 125° produces coxa valga.

lower extremity are continually responding to a changing center of gravity as the body moves in and out of various positions.

Pelvic and Hip Movements

Muscles attached to the pelvis and hip move the leg if the trunk is held stable or move the pelvis and trunk if the leg is held stable.

Anterior Pelvic Tilt/Hip Flexion.— In the chapter on the head and trunk, the **iliopsoas** muscle was discussed because it helps maintain a lordotic curve in the back. The iliopsoas also bends the hips and pulls the pelvis forward. When sitting the iliopsoas maintains anterioposterior trunk balance in relation to the legs. The **rectus femoris** of the quadriceps can pull the pelvis forward into an **anterior tilt** to increase the arch of the back. Other muscles that tilt the pelvis forward or flex the hip are the tensor fasciae latae and sartorius.

Posterior Pelvic Tilt/Hip Extension.— The hamstrings and quadriceps move the pelvis when the feet are on the ground. The hamstrings can pull the pelvis backward into a **posterior tilt** and cause the lower part of the back to flatten its lordotic curve. When the hamstrings are tight, they contribute to a rounded back when sitting, especially when sitting on the floor a long time. Poor movement patterns occur when there is an imbalance in the strength of the hamstrings and quadriceps.

Hip Abduction and Adduction.— The **gluteus medius** and **minimus** together with the **adductor group (adductor magnus, longus, and brevis** as well as the **pectineus** and **gracilis)** maintain lateral stability in trunk balance over one leg in walking, running, and other movements. They are also important in maintaining active sitting balance where side-to-side and diagonal weight shifts may be required. The two gluteal muscles pull the trunk away from the midline of the body, and the adductor group pulls it back toward the midline.

Lateral and Medial Rotators of the Hip.— Six small muscles hold the femur firmly in the hip joint. These muscles perform like ligaments but have the ability to sense motion and adapt to forces. The **obturator internus** and **externus, gemellus superior** and **inferior, quadratus femoris,** and **piriformis** all originate on the lower part of the pelvis and insert on the greater trochanter of the femur. The neck of the femur provides these muscles with a longer lever arm for added strength. All these muscles can laterally rotate the femur to assist in turning the thigh outward or balancing the pelvis over the leg.

The hip abductors are active in medial rotation of the femur: they turn the thigh inward and assist in diagonal balance and weight shifts. The adductors attach along the shaft of the femur. This positions them at varying lengths from the mechanical axis of the leg. Depending on the position of the femur in relation to its axis of motion, some of their force will involve rotation as well as adduction. The direction of rotation is determined by the position of the femur in relation to the axis of movement.

PROBLEM 11.2: FORCES OPERATING ON THE HIP WHILE REACHING OVERHEAD

In Figure 11–5 person weighing 60 kg must balance on the ball of the right foot in order to reach into an overhead cabinet. When assuming this position the person's center of gravity is to the left of the spine at about L3, approximately 8 cm from the axis of motion at the hip where balance is being maintained primarily by the hip abductors. The hip abductors are 5 cm from the axis of motion. For the upper extremity the distance from the center of gravity to the hip joint is as follows: 45 cm in the hand, 40 cm in the forearm, and 25 cm in the upper portion of the arm. How much force will the hip flexors need to exert to maintain balance?

Discussion

Does the outstretched right arm increase or decrease the force needed for balance? What would happen if the left hand were stretched out to the side of the body?

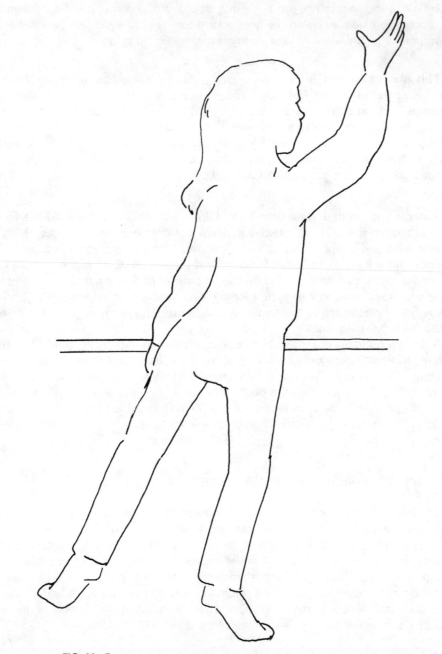

FIG 11–5.
Balance is maintained by the hip flexors when reaching overhead.

Inversion and Eversion of the Foot

Inversion and eversion movements help the foot to gain purchase on uneven ground and allow body weight to shift from side to side when standing or moving.

The **tibialis anterior** and **posterior** pull the sole of the foot inward into **inversion.** They originate on the tibia and insert onto the medial tarsal bones. This helps to maintain the arch of the foot and shift the weight of the body onto the lateral side of the foot. This movement is also called **supination.** The tibialis posterior assists in plantar flexion, and the tibialis anterior raises the toes into dorsiflexion for walking.

The **peroneus longus** and **brevis** pull the sole of the foot outward into **eversion.** These muscles originate on the fibula and insert onto the lateral tarsal bones. They shift the weight of the foot medially. This motion is also called **pronation.** The two muscles also help plantar-flex the foot.

Toe Movements

The foot has a number of intrinsic and extrinsic muscles similar to those of the hand. The **lumbricals** and **interossei** flex the metatarsophalangeal joints and extend the phalangeal joints so that the toes remain in contact with the ground during standing and moving. This action helps to maintain balance. The **flexor hallucis brevis** and the **extensor hallucis longus** perform this same function for the large toe since that toe has no lumbrical or interosseus muscles. Intrinsic and extrinsic toe flexors, extensors, abductors, and adductors also assist in maintaining balance by allowing the toes to grip the ground.

MOVEMENT

Many muscles in the lower extremity cross two joints and therefore have more than one action. Dual action is useful in movements like running and walking that require simultaneous hip extension and knee flexion. It enables the feet, ankles, knees, hips, and pelvis to work together in a variety of movement patterns ranging from crawling and walking to running, jumping, skipping, hopping, and dancing.

Moving From Sitting to Standing

The **hamstrings** originate on the **ischial tuberosity** of the pelvis and continue down the back of the leg to attach on the **tibia.** They are particularly useful in movements such as walking that require simultaneous knee flexion and hip extension. Generally the hamstrings are short enough that the knees will have to be flexed in order to bend over and touch the floor. They assist the quadriceps and gluteus maximus into standing from sitting, stooping, or bending positions. Along with the gluteus maximus they provide most of the power when bending over. They do this by slowly lengthening in an eccentric type of contraction.

The **semitendinosus** and **semimembranosus** attach on the **medial epicondyle,** which allows them to rotate the tibia inward and provide for the locking motion of the knee. When one foot is on the ground, these two muscles rotate the pelvis outward. The **biceps femoris** attaches to the **lateral epicondyle** of the tibia so that it rotates the tibia in the opposite direction and helps to unlock the knee. The **popliteus** muscle, a single-joint knee flexor, provides most of the force for "unlocking" the knee from this position.

When acting together the hamstrings allow for rotation of the knee when it is bent to enable the foot to get adequate traction and torque for movement.

PROBLEM 11.3: COMING FROM SITTING TO STANDING DURING A TOILET TRANSFER

Figure 11–6 shows a 70-kg person seated on a toilet. Because this person is fearful of falling she tries to come to standing from an erect sitting posture or with a posterior pelvic tilt. This places the center of gravity 33 cm from the axis of motion in the knee. In Figure 11–7 she leans forward and tilts the pelvis anteriorly. This brings

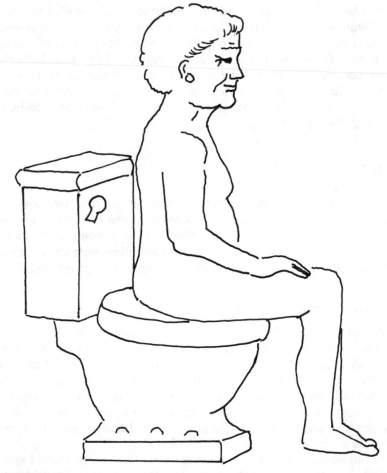

FIG 11–6.
A person tries to stand up from an erect sitting posture.

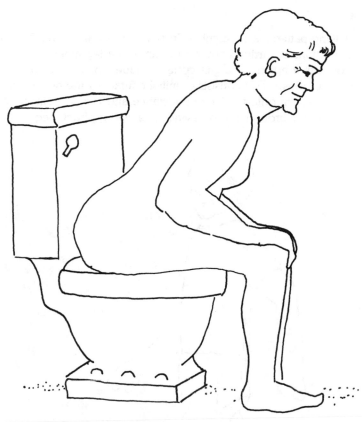

FIG 11–7.
A person tries to stand up by leaning forward from a sitting posture.

the head over the knees so that the body's center or gravity will be 22 cm from the axis of motion at the knee. The moment arm for the quadriceps muscle when the knee is at 90 degrees is 5 cm.

11.3A
How much force must the quadriceps exert to rise from an erect posture?

11.3B
How much force must the quadriceps exert to rise when leaning forward with the head over the knees?

DISCUSSION
Is it possible to rise to standing from an erect sitting posture? Would using the hands to push off from the knees or from armrests make rising to standing any easier? If so, how would it make it easier?

Normal Gait

Normal walking patterns are described in terms of a **gait cycle.** A full gait cycle is the series of motions occurring between the time one leg makes contact with the floor until it contacts it again. The gait cycle is made up of two phases. The first phase is the **stance phase.** This consists of initial contact of the heel on the ground, shifting the body's weight onto the leg in midstance and terminal stance, and finally bringing the heel off the ground into preswing. The **swing phase** begins with the toe

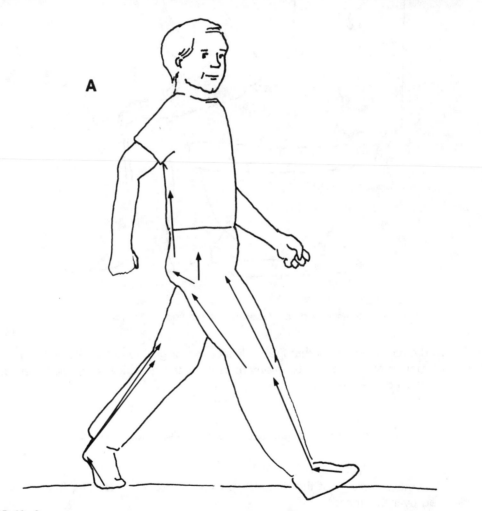

FIG 11–8.
Stages in a normal gait cycle. The right leg is in stance phase, and the left leg is in swing phase. **A,** the right heel makes initial contact, and the left foot is in preswing. **B,** the right foot is in midstance, and the left foot is in midswing. **C,** the right foot moves into terminal stance as the left foot is in terminal swing.

leaving the ground, accelerates into midswing, and decelerates into the terminal swing.

In **initial contact** and **loading** (Fig 11–8A) the knee and hip extensors keep the supporting leg stable in order to carry the weight of the body. Hip stabilizers like the gluteus medius maintain the body's alignment over the supporting leg. Weight shifts medially onto the inside of the supporting foot via the supinators. Dorsiflexors prevent the toes of the supporting leg from slapping the ground, and they raise the toes of the opposite leg off the ground into **initial swing.** On the side of the swinging leg, the erector spinae contracts, and the arm swings forward to counterbalance the trunk as the pelvis progresses forward to initial contact. Hip flexors pull the swinging leg up off the ground to initiate a forward progression.

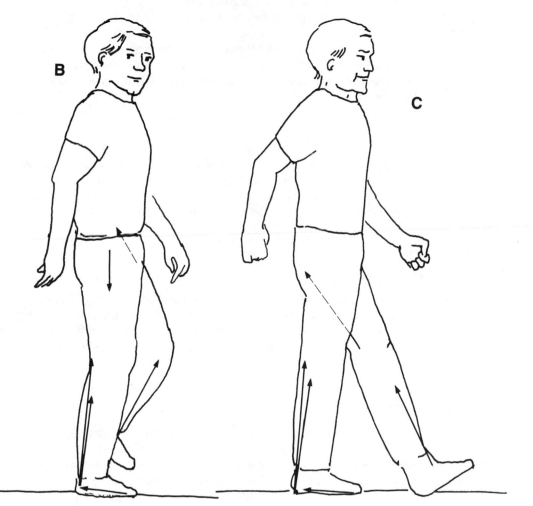

FIG 11–8 (cont.).

In **midstance** (Fig 11–8,B) knee extensors carry the weight of the body while the plantar flexors keep the body from falling forward. Balance over the supporting leg is maintained by the hip stabilizing muscles including the tensor fasciae latae, which also stabilizes the knee. Weight is rolled onto the inside of the foot, over the arch, to absorb the shock of impact. On the swinging leg dorsiflexors pull the toes completely off the ground into **midswing.**

In **terminal stance** (Fig 11–8,C) body weight is supported by the plantar flexors while the swinging leg propels the body forward. Balance is maintained over the supporting leg by the hip stabilizers, and weight is shifted onto the inside of the foot for added stability. Power for pushoff is provided through the flexor of the great toe. The iliopsoas brings the swinging leg forward into **terminal swing,** while the hip extensors control the momentum of the swing. Knee extensors keep the leg straight in preparation for initial contact, and dorsiflexors keep the foot from slapping the ground.

As weight is shifted in **preswing,** the erector spinae, lower abdominals, pelvic hip stabilizers, and hip abductors contract to stabilize the trunk and counterbalance the movement of the pelvis. Plantar flexors and toe flexors provide the final pushoff before leaving the ground.

Running

Running follows a sequence similar to normal gait. However, both feet are off the ground during the midpoint of the running stride. More muscle force is needed to raise the body off the ground and propel it with greater speed. There are consequently greater forces on impact that must be absorbed by the lower extremity and spine.

Jumping and Hopping

Jumping and hopping require greater muscle force from the knee and hip extensors as well as the plantar and toe flexors to propel the body into the air. Strong hip stabilizers are critical to maintain balance over one leg in hopping and are also important on impact when jumping. The adductor longus and brevis also act to flex the hip when jumping.

Crawling and Climbing

The **sartorius** runs diagonally from the ilium to the medial epicondyle of the knee. It bends the hip and knee while rotating the knee away from the body in a manner characteristic of "tailor sitting" or highland dancing. The sartorius is active in normal gait movements. Simultaneous hip and knee flexion are especially useful when crawling, marching, and climbing stairs. When crawling or climbing, the sartorius can position the legs so that the quadriceps and gluteus maximus are in an ideal position for propelling the body forward or upward.

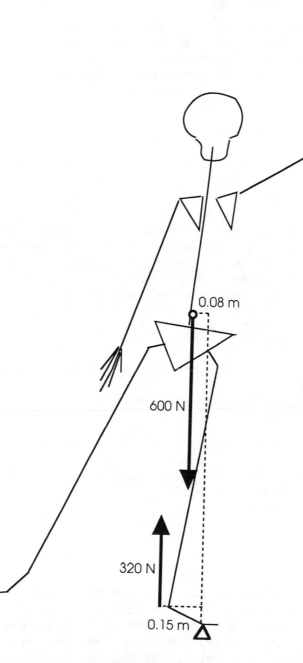

FIG 11–9.
The gastrocnemius and soleus exert 320 N of force to raise the total body weight up onto the ball of the right foot while reaching into an overhead cabinet.

SOLUTIONS TO PROBLEMS

SOLUTION TO PROBLEM 11.1: MUSCLE FORCE NECESSARY FOR LIFTING WEIGHT ONTO THE BALL OF THE FOOT WHEN REACHING

In Figure 11–9 the force of gravity acting on the body falls closer to the axis of motion than the force of the muscles acting against gravity. This makes this action a second class lever. Use $\Sigma M = 0$ to solve the problem.

$(600 \text{ N} \times 0.08 \text{ m}) + (x \times 0.15 \text{ m}) = 0$
$x \times 0.15 \text{ m} = -48 \text{ Nm}$
$x = -320 \text{ N}$ for the gastrocnemius and soleus pulling upward
as a second-class lever

Discussion

A second-class lever gives a mechanical advantage to the muscles. They can exert about half the force of gravity to raise the body's weight to reach an overhead shelf. This type of anatomic structure conserves energy in weight-bearing activities like rising from a sitting position. Energy conservation is important in locomotion types of activities like walking and running, but in these activities the body's center of gravity shifts ahead of the axis of motion, thus making the calf muscles act as a first-class lever rather than a second-class lever (Fig 11–10).

SOLUTION TO PROBLEM 11.2: FORCES OPERATING ON THE HIP WHILE REACHING OVERHEAD

In Figure 11–11 use $\Sigma M = 0$ to solve the problem.

$(600 \text{ N} \times 0.08 \text{ m}) - (4 \text{ N} \times 0.45 \text{ m}) + (9 \text{ N} \times 0.40 \text{ m}) + (16 \text{ N} \times 0.25 \text{ m}) - (x \times 0.05 \text{ m}) = 0$
$48 \text{ Nm} - 1.8 \text{ Nm} + 3.6 \text{ Nm} + 4 \text{ Nm} - (x \times 0.05 \text{ m}) = 0$
$48 \text{ Nm} - 9.4 \text{ Nm} - (x \times 0.05 \text{ m}) = 0$
$x \times 0.05 \text{ m} = 38.6 \text{ Nm}$
$x = 38.6 \text{ Nm}/0.05 \text{ m}$
$x = 772 \text{ N}$

Discussion

The outstretched right arm decreases the amount of force needed by the hip abductors because it provides a clockwise torque. The hip abductors are also working clockwise. If the left hand is stretched out, it would shift the body's center of gravity further away from the spine, thereby creating a longer lever arm and increasing the counterclockwise torque on the hip. The hip abductors have to increase their amount of force to match the counterclockwise torque. The position of the upper extremities can affect balance. The upper extremities are often used to maintain balance or to decrease the amount of work that must be done by the lower extremities in balancing activities.

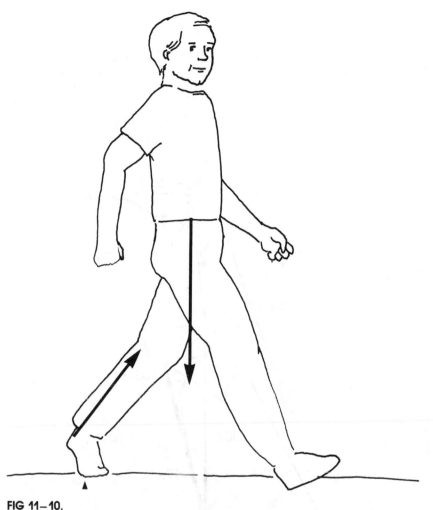

FIG 11–10.
When walking the triceps surae acts as a first-class lever to propel the body.

SOLUTION FOR PROBLEM 11.3: COMING FROM SITTING TO STANDING DURING A TOILET TRANSFER

Subtract the weight of the lower extremities from the total body weight, and use $\Sigma M = 0$ to solve the problem.

$$2 (0.097 + 0.045 + 0.014) (70 \text{ kg}) = 21.84 \text{ kg}$$
$$70 \text{ kg} - 22 \text{ kg} = 48 \text{ kg} = \text{weight of body to be lifted}$$

11.3A: COME TO STANDING FROM AN ERECT SITTING POSTURE (Fig 11–12)

$$(480 \text{ N} \times 0.33 \text{ m}) + (x \times 0.05 \text{ m}) = 0$$
$$x + 0.05 \text{ m} = 158.4 \text{ Nm}$$
$$x = 158.4 \text{ Nm}/0.05 \text{ m}$$
$$x = 3,168 \text{ N}$$

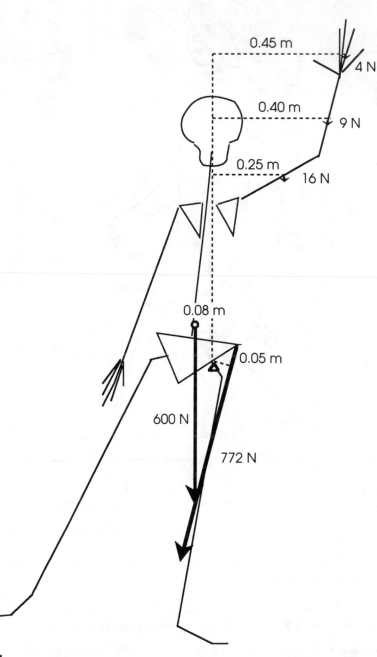

FIG 11–11.
The hip abductors exert 772 N of force to maintain balance when reaching into an overhead cabinet.

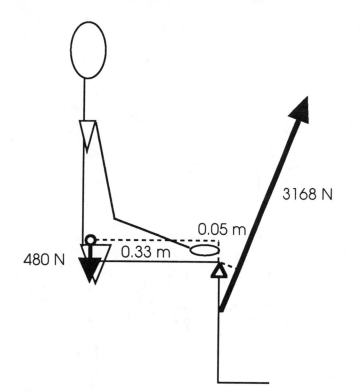

FIG 11–12.
The quadriceps must produce 3,168 N of force to stand from an erect sitting posture.

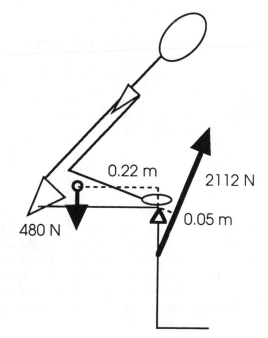

FIG 11–13.
The quadriceps must produce 2,112 N of force to stand when leaning forward.

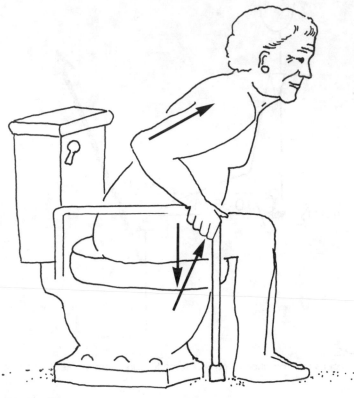

FIG 11–14.
Pushing off on armrests reduces the load on the quadriceps.

11.3b: Come to Standing by Leaning Forward (Fig 11–13)

$$(480 \text{ N} \times 0.22 \text{ m}) + (x \times 0.05 \text{ m}) = 0$$
$$x + 0.05 \text{ m} = 105.6 \text{ Nm}$$
$$x = 158.4 \text{ Nm}/0.05 \text{ m}$$
$$x = 2{,}112 \text{ N}$$

Discussion

It takes 1,000 N more force to come to standing from an erect sitting posture. For most people this is impossible. It still takes considerable strength in the quadriceps to come to standing when leaning forward. Using the upper extremities to push off would make standing easier (Fig 11–14). The force of pushing down with the hands on the knees or on armrests creates a reaction force that acts in the same direction as the quadriceps force. People with weak quadriceps benefit from leaning forward and using armrests when coming to a standing position from sitting.

BIBLIOGRAPHY

Boehme R: *Improving Upper Body Control: An Approach to Assessment and Treatment of Tonal Dysfunction.* Tucson, Communication Skill Builders, 1988.

Caillet R: *Low Back Pain Syndrome.* Philadelphia, FA Davis Co Publishers, 1988.

Luttgens K, Wells K: *Kinesiology: Scientific Basis of Human Motion.* New York, WB Saunders Co, 1982.

Nordin M, Frankel VH: *Basic Biomechanics of the Musculoskeletal System.* Philadelphia, Lea & Febiger, 1989.

Romanes GJ: *Cunningham's Textbook of Anatomy.* London, Oxford University Press, 1972.

Wiktorin CH, Nordin M: *Introduction to Problem Solving in Biomechanics.* Philadelphia, Lea & Febiger, 1986.

ANSWERS TO PROBLEMS

11.1: 320 N for the gastrocnemius and soleus pulling upward as a second-class lever

11.2: 772 N for hip abductors pulling counterclockwise

11.3A: 3168 N when sitting erect

11.3B: 2112 N when leaning over

Appendixes

Appendix A

Review of Mathematics

WORKING WITH VARIABLES IN AN EQUATION

When there is an undetermined value in an equation, the first step is to isolate this variable on one side of the equals sign. Add, subtract, divide, or multiply equally on both sides of the equation so that the numbers on one side cancel out and leave the variable to stand alone.

PROBLEM 1

$$8x = 48$$
$$x = 48/8$$
$$x = 6$$

When numbers and values in an equation involve both addition/subtraction and multiplication/division, isolate these different functions with parentheses, and then move what is surrounded by parentheses as a whole.

PROBLEM 2

$$0.3x + 0.25 \times 4 - 16 = 0$$
$$0.3x + (0.25 \times 4) - 16 = 0$$
$$0.3x = 16 - (0.25 \times 4)$$
$$0.3x = 16 - 1$$
$$x = 16 \div 0.3$$
$$x = 50$$

When numbers and values in an equation are isolated by parentheses, solve them to remove the parentheses.

PROBLEM 3

$$5(x - 4) + 10 = 45$$
$$5x - 20 + 10 = 45$$
$$5x = 45 + 10$$
$$5x = 55$$
$$x = 11$$

PROBLEM 4

$$12x - 6 - 2(4x \times 8) = 0$$
$$12x - 6 - 8x - 16 = 0$$
$$4x = 6 + 16$$
$$4x = 22$$
$$x = 5.5$$

To work with fractions a common denominator must be found.

PROBLEM 5

$$\frac{x}{3} + \frac{1}{2} = \frac{3}{4}$$
$$\frac{x}{3} = \frac{3}{4} - \frac{1}{2}$$
$$\frac{x}{3} = \frac{(2 \times 3) - (4 \times 1)}{8}$$
$$\frac{x}{3} = \frac{6 - 4}{8}$$
$$\frac{x}{3} = \frac{1}{4}$$
$$x = \frac{3}{4}$$

SIMPLE GEOMETRY

The following formulas and concepts are used to solve simple problems in geometry. It is helpful to understand how they work because they are frequently used in biomechanics.

Supplementary Angles.—A line intersected by another line forms two angles that equal 180° when added together (Fig A–1).

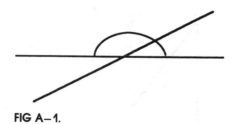

FIG A—1.

Alternate Angle.—When two parallel lines are intersected by a third line, the angles on opposite sides of the intersecting line will be equal (Fig A—2).

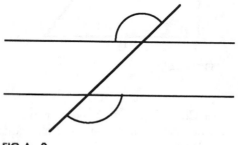

FIG A—2.

Sum of the Angles.—All the angles of a triangle added together equal 180°.

Outer Angle.—An angle outside of a triangle will equal the two opposite inside angles (Fig A—3).

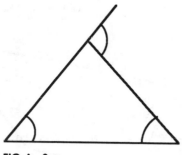

FIG A—3.

Right triangle.—A right triangle has one angle of 90 degrees. This is specified by a boxlike marking in the 90° "right angle" (Fig A—4)

Pythagorean Theorem.—In a right triangle, the horizontal and vertical sides are multiplied by themselves and when added together will equal the diagonal hypotenuse multiplied by itself. The hypotenuse is generally assigned the letter "c": $c^2 = a^2 + b^2$.

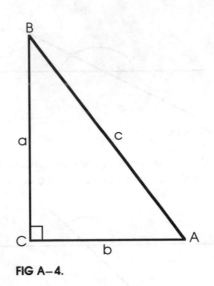

FIG A–4.

PROBLEM 6

In the parallelogram ABCD in Figure A–5, side a is 5 cm, and side b is 8.5 cm. Angle A is 40°. Line *e* divides the parallelogram into two equal triangles. Line f divides ABC into two right triangles. What are the values of the angles in each right triangle?

Angle *A* (intervening angle) = 40°
Angle *A* (bisected) = 20°
Angle *B* (alternate angle) = 140°
Angle *B* (bisected) = 70°
20 + 70 + 90 = 180°

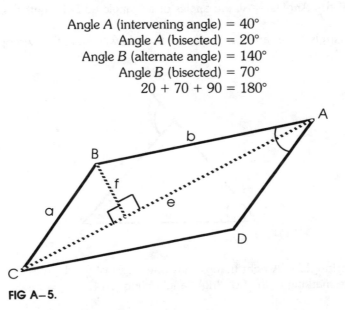

FIG A–5.

PROBLEM 7

In the right triangle *ABC* in Figure A–6, side *a* is 4 cm, and side *b* is 3 cm long. How long is hypotenuse *c*?

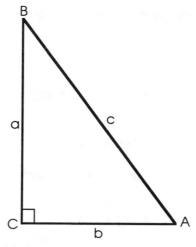

FIG A–6.

$$c^2 = a^2 + b^2$$
$$c^2 = 4^2 \text{ cm} + 3^2 \text{ cm}$$
$$c^2 = 16 \text{ cm} + 9 \text{ cm}$$
$$c^2 = 25 \text{ cm}$$
$$c = 5 \text{ cm}$$

BASIC TRIGONOMETRY

Trigonometry uses the ratio of known angles to known sides in triangles to figure out the values of unknown sides and angles. Through the use of trigonometric functions these values can be determined with very little information. By making imaginary triangles in space, on land, or between body parts numerical values for distances and forces can be determined even if they cannot be actually measured. The usefulness of these concepts is obvious when doing problems in biomechanics.

Trigonometric functions were determined by ancient peoples and were used in the building of the pyramids. They are used today to compute the distances of stars and other astronomic objects. Understanding their derivation is a complex mathematic feat. As with the pyramids themselves, it is easier to accept them as a marvelous fact of nature rather than to understand why they work.

Sines, cosines, and tangents are names given to a fixed set of ratios of angles to sides in right triangles. Use sines and cosines when given the value of the hypotenuse and a side and or an angle of a right triangle. Use tangents and cotangents when given the value of two sides or a side and an angle of a right triangle. Scientific calculators have these ratios built into their memory chips. A table of sines, cosines, tangents, and cotangents is found in Appendix B.

Sine.—In a right triangle the sine of an angle is the ratio of the opposite side to the hypotenuse.

$$\sin A = a/c$$

Cosine.—In a right triangle the cosine of an angle is the ratio of the adjacent side to the hypotenuse.

$$\cos A = b/c$$

Tangent.—In a right triangle the tangent of an angle is the ratio of the opposite side to the adjacent side.

$$\tan A = a/b$$

Cotangent.—In a right triangle the cotangent of an angle is the ratio of the adjacent side to the opposite side.

$$\cot A = b/a$$

PROBLEM 8

In the right triangle *ABC* in Figure A–7, side *a* is 4 cm, and side *c* is 8 cm. How large is angle *A?*

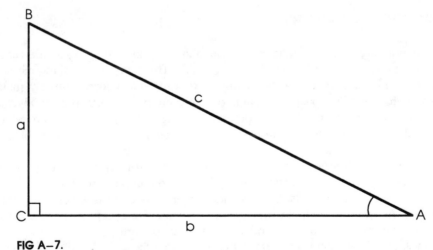

FIG A–7.

Since the value of side *a* and the hypotenuse are given, use sines to solve this problem.

$$\sin A = a/c$$
$$\sin A = 4 \text{ cm}/8 \text{ cm}$$
$$\sin A = 0.5$$
$$A = 30°$$

PROBLEM 9

In the right triangle *ABC* in Figure A–8, the hypotenuse is 12 cm, and angle *A* is 15°. How long are the sides?

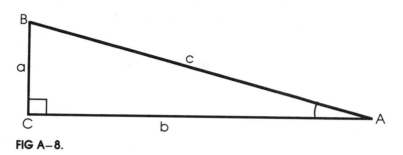

FIG A–8.

Since the hypotenuse is given and the value of both sides is needed, use sines and cosines to solve this problem.

$$\sin A = a/c$$
$$\sin 15° = a/12 \text{ cm}$$
$$a = 12 \text{ cm} \times \sin 15°$$
$$a = 12 \text{ cm} \times 0.259$$
$$a = 3.11 \text{ cm}$$
$$\cos A = b/c$$
$$\cos 15° = b/12 \text{ cm}$$
$$b = 0.966 \times 12 \text{ cm}$$
$$b = 11.59 \text{ cm}$$

Supplementary Angle.—When one line intersects another, they make up two supplementary angles. The sines of both supplementary angles are equal to each other.

$$\textbf{sin } A = \textbf{sin } (180° - A)$$

The cosine of one angle will be equal to the negative cosine of the other angle.

$$\textbf{cos } A = -\textbf{cos } (180° - A)$$

Sines and cosines can be used when working with triangles that are not right triangles.

Sine Theorem.—With two angles and an opposite side or two sides and an opposite angle it is possible to figure out the values for the rest of any triangle because sides are proportional to the sines of their angles.

$$a/\textbf{sin } A = b/\textbf{sin } B = c/\textbf{sin } C$$

Cosine Theorem.—With three sides or two sides and an adjacent angle it is possible to figure out the values of any triangle because of the relationships between them.

$$a^2 = b^2 + c^2 - (2\ bc \times \cos A)$$

PROBLEM 10

In the triangle *ABC* in Figure A–9, side b = 6.0 cm, side c = 9.0 cm, and angle A = 60°. How long is side a?

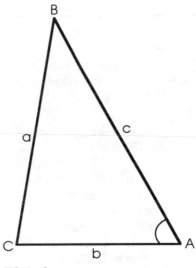

FIG A–9.

Since two sides and an adjacent angle are given, use the cosine theorem to solve this problem.

$$a^2 = b^2 + c^2 - (2\ bc \times \cos A)$$
$$a^2 = 6^2\ \text{cm} + 9^2\ \text{cm} - [2(6\ \text{cm} \times 9\ \text{cm}) \times \cos A]$$
$$a^2 = 36\ \text{cm} + 81\ \text{cm} - (108\ \text{cm} \times 0.5)$$
$$a^2 = 63\ \text{cm}$$
$$a = 7.9\ \text{cm}$$

Appendix B

Table of Trigonometric Functions

Degrees*	Sines	Cosines	Tangents	Cotangents	
0	.0000	1.0000	.0000		90
1	.0175	.9998	.0175	57.290	89
2	.0349	.9994	.0349	28.636	88
3	.0523	.9986	.0524	19.081	87
4	.0698	.9976	.0699	14.301	86
5	.0872	.9962	.0875	11.430	85
6	.1045	.9945	.1051	9.5144	84
7	.1219	.9925	.1228	8.1443	83
8	.1392	.9903	.1405	7.1154	82
9	.1564	.9877	.1584	6.3138	81
10	.1736	.9848	.1763	5.6713	80
11	.1908	.9816	.1944	5.1446	79
12	.2079	.9781	.2126	4.7046	78
13	.2250	.9744	.2309	4.3315	77
14	.2419	.9703	.2493	4.0108	76
15	.2588	.9659	.2679	3.7321	75
16	.2756	.9613	.2867	3.4874	74
17	.2924	.9563	.3057	3.2709	73
18	.3090	.9511	.3249	3.0777	72
19	.3256	.9455	.3443	2.9042	71
20	.3420	.9397	.3640	2.7475	70
21	.3584	.9336	.3839	2.6051	69
22	.3746	.9272	.4040	2.4751	68
23	.3907	.9205	.4245	2.3559	67
24	.4067	.9135	.4452	2.2460	66
25	.4226	.9063	.4663	2.1445	65
26	.4384	.8988	.4877	2.0503	64
27	.4540	.8910	.5095	1.9626	63
28	.4695	.8829	.5317	1.8807	62
29	.4848	.8746	.5543	1.8040	61
30	.5000	.8660	.5774	1.7321	60
31	.5150	.8572	.6009	1.6643	59
32	.5299	.8480	.6249	1.6003	58
33	.5446	.8387	.6494	1.5399	57
34	.5592	.8290	.6745	1.4826	56
35	.5736	.8192	.7002	1.4281	55
36	.5878	.8090	.7265	1.3765	54
37	.6018	.7986	.7536	1.3270	53
38	.6157	.7880	.7813	1.2799	52

(Continued.)

Degrees*	Sines	Cosines	Tangents	Cotangents	
39	.6293	.7771	.8098	1.2349	51
40	.6428	.7660	.8391	1.1918	50
41	.6561	.7547	.8693	1.1504	49
42	.6691	.7431	.9004	1.1106	48
43	.6820	.7314	.9325	1.0724	47
44	.6947	.7193	.9657	1.0355	46
45	.7071	.7071	1.0000	1.0000	45
	Cosines	Sines	Cotangents	Tangents	Degrees

*Note: With angles above 45° be sure to use the headings that appear at the bottom of the columns.

Appendix C

Body Segment Parameters

Measurements of the human body are needed to solve most problems in biomechanics. Whenever possible, actual measurements should be taken. Statistical research data is used for proportional weight and center of gravity in each body segment, since actual measurement cannot be made on living subjects.

The primary data for average body weights and centers of gravity was taken from a study done on eight elderly male cadavers (Dempster WT: *Space Requirements of the Seated Operator,* WADC technical report 55–159. Ohio, Wright-Patterson Air Force Base, 1955.) These data have been revised by other researchers to make allowances for differences in age and gender; however, Dempster's data continue to be widely used. Adaptations of these data, presented in Table C–1 and

TABLE C–1.

Proportional Percentages of Body Segments to Total Body Weight

Body Segment	% of Total Body Weight
Head and neck	7.9
Trunk with head and neck	56.5
Upper arm	2.7
Forearm	1.5
Hand	0.6
Thigh	9.7
Lower leg	4.5
Foot	1.4

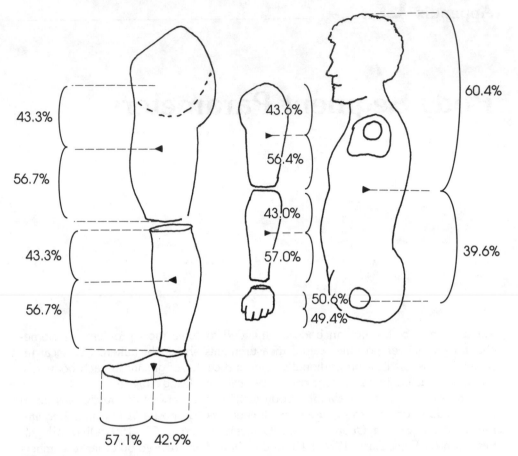

FIG C–1.
Center of gravity for each body segment as a percentage of distance from the end of the body segment.

Figure C–1, give an estimate that is adequate for most problem-solving in the occupational therapy clinic. More exact data may be obtained by consulting with bioengineers or human factors specialists.

Figure C–1 provides the percentage of distance from either end of each body segment to that segment's center of gravity. These measurements are used to determine the moment arm in problems involving torque. Table C–1 gives the proportional weight of each body segment. This information is used to calculate torque.

Appendix D

Converting from English to Metric Equivalents

Most cultures have required a commonly understood system of weights and measurements that allows for sharing of information and trade goods. Like those of the Babylonians, Egyptians, and Romans, the English system of weights and measures developed from body measurements. The more variable digit, palm, span, and cubit became a more uniform inch, foot, and yard through royal decrees. This system was used wherever English was the language of trade from the 17th through 19th centuries.

In the early 18th century the French attempted to establish a uniform system of measurement that would be used throughout Europe and European territories. The British refused to be involved in developing the new system so it was developed entirely by French academicians. The new system was based on the meter, a measurement that was $\frac{1}{10,000,000}$ of the distance from the North Pole to the equator on a line passing through Paris.

TABLE D–1.

Common British to Metric Conversions

British Unit	×	= SI Unit	×	= British Unit
Length				
Inches (in.)	2.54	centimeters	0.3937	inches
Feet (ft)	0.3048	meters	39.37	inches
Yard (yd)	0.9144	meters		
Mile	1.609	kilometers		
Mass				
Pounds (lb)	0.4536	kilograms	2.205	pounds
Slug	14.594	kilograms		
Force				
Pound-feet (lb-ft)	4.4482	Newtons (N)	0.2248	pounds

There was a great deal of resistance to the new system even in France, but by the 19th century the system caught on among scientists because it was possible to reliably reproduce units of measurement. The system was revised and modernized by the General Conference of Weights and Measures in 1960. It is called *Le Systeme International d'Unites* (International System of Units), which is abbreviated as SI.

Since the "metric" system is used by most of the world it is the system of measurement used throughout this book. Table D–1 gives the most common conversions needed for biomechanics.

Appendix E

Commonly Used Formulas in Biomechanics

To Determine the Length of Unmeasurable Body Segments or Moment Arms

When one angle and one side or the hypotenuse of a right triangle are known:

$$\sin A = a/c \text{ for an angle and an opposite side}$$
$$\cos A = b/c \text{ for an angle and an adjacent side}$$

To determine angles when two sides of a right triangle are known:

$$\tan A = a/b$$
$$\cot A = b/a$$

When two angles and an opposite angle or two angles and an opposite side of any triangle are known:

$$a/\sin A = b/\sin B = c/\sin C$$

When three sides or two sides and an adjacent angle of any triangle are known:

$$a^2 = b^2 + c^2 - (2\,bc \times \cos A)$$

TO DETERMINE FORCE (LINEAR MOTION)

$$F = [\text{force} = \text{mass} \times \text{acceleration (gravity)}]$$

TO DETERMINE FORCE EQUILIBRIUM

$$\Sigma F = 0 \text{ (the sum of all forces equals 0)}$$
or
$$\Sigma F_x = 0 \text{ (all horizontal forces equal 0)}$$
and
$$\Sigma F_y = 0 \text{ (all vertical forces equal 0)}$$

To Determine Torque (Rotary Motion)

$$\text{Torque} = \text{force} \times \text{moment arm}$$

To Determine Moment Equilibrium

$$\Sigma M = 0 \text{ (the sum of clockwise and counter-clockwise torque equals 0)}$$
or

EFA × EMA = RFA × RMA (effort force × effort moment arm = resistance force × resistance moment arm)

To Determine Stress

Stress = force × tissue length × tissue width

To Determine Work

Lifting work:

L = mg × h × r (lifting work = mass × gravity × height lifted × number of repetitions)

Carrying work:

C = mg × d × r (carrying work = mass × gravity × distance × number of repetitions)

Occupational Standards and Guidelines

Human activities are limited by the biomechanics of the human body. These limits have been the subject of numerous studies since the 1970s. There are no absolute standards currently available as each study has some variance with others. Certain guidelines for specific actions are accepted by the National Institute of Occupational Safety and Health. Some of these guidelines are presented here. NIOSH expects to issue a revision of these guidelines in December 1991.

GRASP AND PINCH

Power grip   225 N (50 lbf) maximum
Pinch   45 N (10 lbf) maximum 30 N (7 lbf) repetitive work

PULLING

Fingers alone   40 N (9 lbf) maximum
Fingers and wrist   144 N (32 lbf) maximum

HORIZONTAL PUSHING AND PULLING

Standing/entire body   225 N (50 lbf) maximum
   Truck and cart handling
   Moving equipment on wheels
Standing/upper body/arms extended   110 N (24 lbf) maximum
   Leaning over something to move an object
   Pushing at or above shoulder height

Kneeling   188 N (42 lbf) maximum
   Removing or replacing components
   Working in confined areas such as a tunnel
Seated   130 N (29 lbf) maximum
   Operating vertical levers
   Moving objects on conveyors

VERTICAL PUSHING AND PULLING IN STANDING

Pull down from overhead
   Hook grip   540 N (120 lbf) maximum
   Power grip (5 cm/2 in. diameter handle)   200 N (45 lbf) maximum
Pull down from shoulder level   315 N (70 lbf) maximum
Pull up
   25 cm/10 in. above floor   315 N (70 lbf) maximum
   Elbow height   148 N (33 lbf) maximum
   Shoulder height   75 N (17 lbf) maximum
Push down/elbow height   287 N (64 lbf) maximum
Push up/shoulder height   202 N (45 lbf) maximum

Appendix G

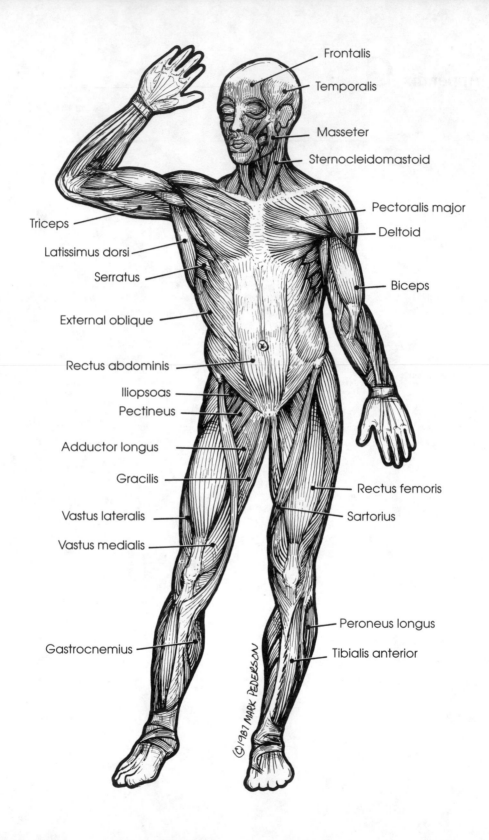

Frontalis

Temporalis

Masseter

Sternocleidomastoid

Pectoralis major

Deltoid

Triceps

Latissimus dorsi

Serratus

Biceps

External oblique

Rectus abdominis

Iliopsoas

Pectineus

Adductor longus

Gracilis

Rectus femoris

Vastus lateralis

Sartorius

Vastus medialis

Peroneus longus

Gastrocnemius

Tibialis anterior

©1987 MARK PEDERSON

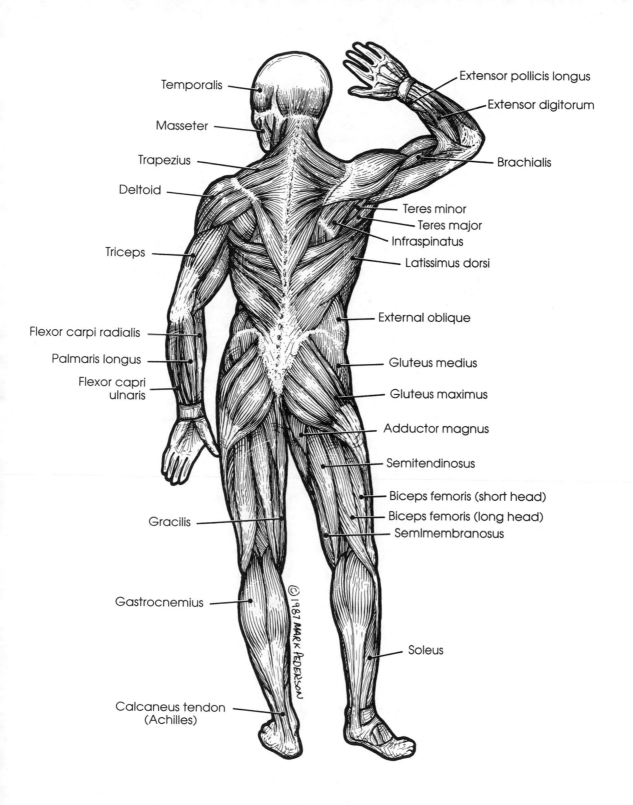

Temporalis

Masseter

Trapezius

Deltoid

Triceps

Flexor carpi radialis

Palmaris longus

Flexor capri ulnaris

Gracilis

Gastrocnemius

Calcaneus tendon (Achilles)

Extensor pollicis longus

Extensor digitorum

Brachialis

Teres minor

Teres major

Infraspinatus

Latissimus dorsi

External oblique

Gluteus medius

Gluteus maximus

Adductor magnus

Semitendinosus

Biceps femoris (short head)

Biceps femoris (long head)

Semlmembranosus

Soleus

© 1987 MARK PEDERSON

INDEX

THE LIBRARY
HAMMERSMITH AND WEST
LONDON COLLEGE
GLIDDON ROAD
LONDON W 14 9BL

081 741 1688

SHAWNA CANON

SEVEN YEARS
AWESOME
LUCK

D0817139

Seven Years Awesome Luck copyright © 2019 by Shawna Canon

All rights reserved.

No part of this book may be reproduced in any form or by any electronic or mechanical means, including information storage and retrieval systems, without written permission from the author, except for the use of brief quotations in a book review or as otherwise allowed by U.S. fair use laws. Names, characters, places, and incidents are either the product of the author's imagination or are used fictitiously. Any resemblance to actual events, locales, or persons, living or dead, is coincidental.

Published by Headcanon Press

headcanonpress.com

Second edition, January 2021

Cover design by Lou Harper

PROLOGUE

Through the darkness and pouring rain, Jacqueline stared up at the mansion and thought, *I was expecting more gingerbread.*

Maybe that wasn't a sensible thought, but if Jacqueline were in a sensible state of mind, she wouldn't be here. She would have thrown out the letter as soon as she'd received it instead of driving four hours with her six-year-old because she couldn't find a sitter, running out of gas half a mile from her destination because she was too distracted to pay attention to the fuel gauge, then walking the remaining distance rather than waiting and calling for help like a normal person. Clearly, her mind wasn't working right.

Desperation did that, though.

There was a wrought-iron gate between her and the mansion, so she pushed the call button, hoping someone was still awake to answer.

"Mom, I'm cold," said her son, his teeth chattering audibly.

"I know, Trick. I'm sorry. We're almost inside." *I hope.* They were both wearing coats, but it hadn't been raining when they'd left home, so she hadn't prepared for the downpour. Now they were drenched through, and her hands were so cold, she could hardly feel her fingers—or his. Despite the near numbness, she kept her hand clenched tightly around his so he wouldn't run off. With Trick, that was always a risk.

A harsh buzz cut through the air, and a tinny voice asked, "Who is it?"

Jacqueline jumped at the sudden sound. "H-hello? My name is Jacqueline St. Andrew. I was… told you could help me." She should have practiced what she would say if she got this far so she wouldn't sound like a lunatic or con artist. The small doubt that had been lingering in her mind since she'd read the letter—the one that told her this was a cruel prank—surged to the forefront, and she couldn't quite get the rest of the words out. There was a small bubble near the speaker, which she took for a camera, so with the hand that wasn't holding onto Trick, she dug the letter out of her pocket and held it up to the lens.

The presentation of her evidence was met with silence. Jacqueline didn't need to read it again to know what it said or how crazy it would look to the person in the mansion. It had come in an envelope with no return address and no mailing address, only her name. The letter read: *This woman is a witch. She can help you in ways modern medicine cannot.* Below that was a street address. The letter had been signed, *A Friend.*

A wild goose chase, Jacqueline thought miserably as the seconds wore on with no answer from the house. When she got home, she was going on a manhunt for whoever had sent her here.

The gate unlatched. "Come in," said the voice from the speaker.

Hope surged through Jacqueline. "Thank you!" She stuffed the letter back into her pocket and pushed the gate open. "Come on, Trick. Let's get inside."

It was another hundred feet to the front door of the mansion, but she hardly noticed the distance even though her feet ached with every waddling step. If this woman really could help her, she was willing to walk naked over hot coals.

When she and Trick reached the front door, it was already open, a woman standing on the threshold. "Hurry inside, you two." The woman was thin, tall, and looked around eighty years old, her white hair cut short in a sophisticated style.

Trick pulled Jacqueline forward, and she let him go so he could run inside the warm house. It wasn't the safest thing in the world to do, but at this point there was little that could make Jacqueline turn back.

"You poor dears," the old woman said, offering a hand to help Jacqueline in.

Jacqueline took it only long enough to get into the foyer, not wanting to be rude, and the woman released her to close the door. "Thank you," Jacqueline said as her own teeth started to chatter.

"There's a fire through here." The old woman guided her through the main hallway and into a huge living room. The furniture was elegant and plush, and the fireplace was big enough for a large dog to stand in.

Trick was already in front of the fire, holding out his hands.

"Let me take your coat," said their host, peeling Jacqueline's drenched coat off of her with minimal cooperation needed from its wearer.

"Thank you," Jacqueline said again. "Trick, take your coat off."

The boy obeyed, yanking it off so that the sleeves turned inside-out, and huddled closer to the fire.

The old woman draped the two coats over wooden chairs near the fire. "I don't have any clothes that would fit you two, but I have extra robes that would work. If you'd like, I could put your clothes in the dryer for you."

Jacqueline weighed the danger of getting undressed in a stranger's home to the danger of hypothermia if they stayed in wet clothes. She looked around, but she didn't see or hear anyone other than the old woman in the house.

As if sensing the direction of her thoughts, the old woman chuckled. "I live here alone. You're perfectly safe."

Jacqueline relented, and soon she and Trick were wrapped in warm robes and sitting in front of the fire. She'd already toweled off Trick's hair so it wasn't more than damp and was working on drying her own. "Thank you again for seeing us," Jacqueline told the old woman. "I'm sorry for coming so late. The letter got me so excited, I sort of took off without thinking it through."

"Perfectly understandable." The old woman was in a chair across from Jacqueline, pouring tea from a set on the coffee table. She slid one cup to Jacqueline's side of the table and sat back, sipping her own.

Jacqueline finished wringing the water out of her hair and set the towel aside. "Are you really a witch?"

"I am," said the old woman.

Jacqueline eyed the tea still on the coffee table. "Witch as in Wiccan, witch as in Hogwarts, or witch as in 'double, double toil and trouble'?"

The witch laughed. "The third one, if that's how you want to differentiate it. My magic is a purely secular practice and doesn't involve wands. Although it is something that's in the blood. Not just anyone can be what I am."

Jacqueline nodded acknowledgment of the information, and she didn't take the tea.

"Tell me why you're here. I assume it has to do with your baby."

One of Jacqueline's hands slid over her large belly. "There's a problem with him. The doctors say he won't survive. They're so sure, they won't even try to save him. I don't know who else to ask."

"You poor thing. You must be so frightened."

Angry and frustrated was more like it, though Jacqueline couldn't deny there was a good amount of fear. It didn't seem wise to let the witch see that part, though. "Can you help me?"

"Of course, child. Witches have been helping women with difficult pregnancies since the dawn of time. Or the dawn of magic, anyway, whenever that was." She got up, setting her empty cup on the table. "Wait right here. I may already have what you need in my storeroom."

The witch left the room, and Trick started playing with the fire poker.

"Trick, put that back. It's dangerous."

"No, it's not," he protested, but he put it back. "I'm bored."

"Are you warmed up yet?"

"Yeah. Can I have some cookies?"

Even if this worked, they had another four-hour drive back home—after they called for roadside service, which could take another hour or more at this time of night. Trick could sleep on the way back, but they did need some food. The witch was friendly enough that she probably would offer food if they asked, but Jacqueline was wary of taking anything from the witch. If witches were real, then all those fairy tales warning about them had to come from somewhere, right? Of course, people used to think redheads, albinos, and other people who fell slightly outside the norm were evil, too, so maybe those stories were meaningless. This witch had been nothing but kind so far. Maybe Jacqueline was just being paranoid.

The witch returned, holding a small, silver goblet. "Drink this, dear."

Jacqueline took the goblet, which was half full of a thick, moss-green liquid that smelled strongly of the forest. "What's this?"

"It's what you came here for."

"Is it… a magic potion?" Jacqueline asked, hardly believing she was really saying those words.

"That's correct."

"What's in it?"

"Oh, you don't want to know," the witch said cheerfully. "But it will work. I promise."

"This will save my baby?"

"Drink that, and I guarantee your baby will be born healthy and hale."

There was a chance this was all some trick, but Jacqueline was too desperate to be cautious about this. Her baby would die without help. The worst this potion could do was kill her, and she was willing to risk her life for her baby. Besides, the witch hadn't given her any reason to mistrust her yet. Before she could second-guess herself, Jacqueline chugged the potion as quickly as she could.

The taste was revolting. As soon as she lowered the goblet, the witch offered her the cup of tea she hadn't touched yet. She'd already crossed the line now, so she drank the tea to get the taste of potion out of her mouth.

She could feel... something in her belly. It wasn't bad or painful, but it was strange. Did that mean the potion was already working?

"Now, then," the witch said, returning to her seat across from Jacqueline, "let's discuss payment."

Jacqueline got an altogether different and more unpleasant feeling in her gut. This was what she got for being reckless. How stupid of her not to think of that before drinking the potion! Of course the witch wouldn't help her out of the kindness of her heart. That wasn't how people—witches or otherwise—operated.

"How much do you want?" Jacqueline asked. She didn't have much money, but she could probably get a loan if necessary.

The witch laughed lightly. "Oh, dear girl, do I look like I need your money?"

Jacqueline glanced around the room. "No, I suppose not. What do you want, then?"

"Your son."

Jacqueline's heart nearly jumped out of her body. A horrible weightless feeling started in her chest and swam through her head. "W-what?"

"Your son," the witch repeated calmly.

"No!" Jacqueline cried, her hands instinctively moving to cover her belly. "I didn't ask you to save him just to lose him!"

The witch laughed as if Jacqueline had made a joke. "Not that one." She pointed at Trick. "That one."

Jacqueline turned her horrified gaze on her oldest son. Trick had been dozing by the fire until her outburst a moment ago, and now he was watching the two of them in confusion. "You... you want Trick?" she asked.

"Is that his name?" The witch sounded pleased. "Yes, he'll do nicely."

I guess the fairy tales were right, Jacqueline thought as she stared at the witch, her heart pounding so hard that her pulse was a drumbeat in her ears.

Trick was less concerned. "Do for what?"

"Nothing untoward," the witch assured him. "Don't worry; I'm not going to eat you."

"Nothing *untoward*?" Jacqueline repeated.

"I'm a very old woman," the witch said. "Much older than I look. I don't expect I'll be around much longer. I simply want some companionship in my final days."

"Then get a pet."

"Witches don't have pets," the witch explained. "We have familiars. And humans make the best familiars."

Now Jacqueline was confused. "Wait, what? I thought 'familiar' was another word for 'pet'."

"Oh, it's much more than that. A magical bond exists between a witch and their familiar. A mere pet could never compare."

"It's not that I'm not sympathetic about your loneliness problem, ma'am, and I'm very grateful for your help, but I'm not going to give you my son. That's just crazy."

The witch's pleasant smile shifted slightly. It was still a smile, but suddenly it was much less pleasant. "I'm afraid you don't have a choice. You've already taken the potion, and you have nothing else to give me that I want."

An air of danger permeated the room. Jacqueline's skin itched. She wanted to jump up, grab Trick, and flee the house. But the two of them were wearing nothing but the witch's bathrobes, her car was out of gas, and it was the middle of the night. Never mind the fact that she was heavily pregnant and moved about as fast as a three-legged elephant.

The witch understood the position Jacqueline was in as well as she did. "Your son won't be hurt, and I won't keep him forever. I'm not a monster."

"How long?" Jacqueline asked. Her throat was so tight that the words came out in barely a whisper.

"How does seven years sound?" the witch proposed. "That

should be plenty for my needs. And then you can retrieve him, and he can go about his life. Seven years isn't so much, is it?"

It was to a six-year-old, but in the grand scheme of things, no. It wasn't much. The witch had Jacqueline over a barrel; she could have demanded a lot more. "W-what will you do with him?"

"Pamper him, feed him, pet him," said the witch.

"*Pet* him?"

"He'll be a cat, of course."

"What?!" Jacqueline shrieked.

Trick's eyes lit up. "What?!"

The witch addressed her more receptive audience. "Yes, sweetie. A witch's familiar is an animal. So I'll turn you into a cat first, then make you my familiar. You won't have to go to school or do chores or any such unpleasant things. How does that sound?"

Trick jumped to his feet. "That sounds awesome!"

"Good!" said the witch. "It's settled, then."

"It is not settled," Jacqueline growled.

The witch directed her gaze at Jacqueline, her eyes suddenly hard as diamonds, even though she continued to smile. "Would you rather take your chances on my bad side?" A beat later, she blinked, her expression softening. "I'm just a lonely old woman asking for a companion to dote on in my last days. Would you deny me that?"

As the witch pointed out, Jacqueline really didn't have a choice. *I shouldn't have brought him with me,* Jacqueline thought, far too late. Though if she hadn't, maybe the witch wouldn't have helped her at all. "How do I know this isn't all some elaborate ruse to kidnap Trick?" she asked. "I haven't actually seen you do any magic yet."

"A good point," the witch acknowledged. "What if I change him into a cat before you go? Will that convince you of the honesty of my intentions?"

"I… guess so," Jacqueline said, not sure what other answer she could give.

Ten minutes later, Jacqueline walked alone out of the mansion, shaking with shock and guilt.

CHAPTER
ONE

Seven years later

Trick St. Andrew had seen dead bodies before. He'd *made* dead bodies before. They were delicious. His favorites were finches, but mice were pretty tasty too. Though as much as he liked eating his prize, the best part was stalking and killing it.

So it wasn't like Trick had never seen a dead body before, but this was the first time he'd ever seen a dead *human* body, and that made it interesting.

Crouched beneath a bush, he crept forward, paws silent on the dirt, and peered at the sky through gaps in the leaves. It was getting dark, but the sun hadn't set yet. The graveyard was quiet and empty except for the big man digging a hole and the dead body sprawled out next to it. Would it get dark before the man finished?

Curiosity killed the cat, Trick reminded himself, except that was totally not true. He'd been curious lots of times, and it hadn't killed him yet. He knew it would be safer to wait until full dark, when his black fur would make him nearly invisible and he could sneak up for a closer look without the big man seeing him. The end of Trick's

11

tail twitched impatiently, rustling some of the bush's lowest leaves. He didn't have time to wait. His mom was expecting him soon.

That thought put him in a bad mood and made him reckless. *I'm doing it*, he decided. Staying low to the ground, he snuck out from beneath the cover of the bush and crept through the grass toward the dead body. A quick look, then he'd go. It was pretty dark, even if the sun wasn't quite down yet. The digging man probably wouldn't see him.

He kept it slow, one paw at a time, the short-cropped grass brushing his belly. The air smelled of freshly-turned dirt, the man's sweat, and rot. Not much, though. The corpse was fresh.

Trick edged up on the man's right side, aiming for the corpse's head. What would it look like? Stiff and inhuman, or like a sleeping person? Did dead people look any different from dead animals?

The man stood in the hole as he dug, only his head and shoulders above ground level. Each time he jammed the shovel into the earth, he let out a stiff grunt, and then dirt flew up out of the hole.

Trick slipped behind a headstone. A moment later, he left its cover to very carefully creep closer to the dead body. In front of the hole was another headstone. It had a name on it. The first name was easy to read, but the last name was so long that Trick's eyes skipped right over most of the letters. There were numbers, too. Dates. Trick didn't pay much attention to the date normally, but today was different. The second date on the headstone was—he counted back —seven days ago?

That was weird. The dead body had to be less than seven days old or it would have stunk a lot more.

He was only a few feet away from the corpse when the digging man hauled himself out of the open grave and brushed a hand off on his pants. Trick flattened himself against the ground and froze.

"That should do it," the big man grunted to himself, wiping his forehead with his arm. He moved to the other side of the corpse—so close to Trick that he thought the man might step on him—and planted a boot on the body's shoulder. "Sorry, buddy." He shoved with his boot, rolling the corpse into the hole.

It landed with a big, hollow thud. Trick's ear twitched. The sound was wrong. Not a dirt sound at all. His curiosity stronger than ever, he crawled toward the edge of the hole and peeked over. There was a wooden coffin at the bottom of the hole. The body had landed on it face up. Trick leaned closer to see. The corpse was a man, maybe around Mom's age, bald with a beard and a big nose. One eye was closed, the other half-open.

Yeah. Dead humans looked a lot like dead animals. Just an empty lump of meat.

The dirt under Trick's right front paw slid into the hole, and he had to scrabble back before he fell in.

"Hey!" cried the big man, right beside him. "Get outta here!" The man swung the shovel at Trick, but he darted away, tearing through the grass back toward the bushes. Only after he'd gotten well away from the grave did Trick glance over his shoulder to see that the man wasn't following. The man wasn't even looking at Trick. He was shoveling the dirt back into the grave, eyes darting around like he was afraid someone might be watching.

Trick ran out of the graveyard without seeing any other people and started down the hill back toward the main part of town. The sun was getting low, but he could probably make it back before dark.

Agreste was a small town. He didn't know how many people were in it or anything, but he knew it was big enough to be interesting and small enough that he could get around without constantly being bombarded by big, loud things. And most of the people, when they saw him, either ignored him or talked nicely to him. Some even gave him food. That big man was a lot meaner than most of the people Trick ran into around here.

Downtown, he loped down the sidewalk beside an old movie theater, then ducked into an alley. It was a shortcut that saved him a couple blocks on his way home, which was good because he was likely already gonna get yelled at as it was.

Halfway down the alley, the rustle of feathers drew his attention to the edge of one of the roofs, where a red-tailed hawk sat watching him. Trick eyed the hawk, wondering if he should turn back the way he'd come or run on and hope the hawk didn't make a move.

Dang bird, he thought to himself. This wasn't the first time he'd caught the hawk watching him. Or *a* hawk, anyway. He couldn't really be sure it was the same hawk, and it didn't make any sense that it would be. Trick and his family had only moved into Agreste a week ago, but he'd been spotting hawks watching him for years, even back in Three Sisters. None of them had ever actually tried to snatch him, but those talons were sharp, and he knew that he was still small, even for a cat.

He crept forward carefully, keeping his eyes on the hawk, which peered down at him with a cool gaze as if it didn't care at all what he did.

Something shifted behind him, then the direction of the wind changed, and he caught a scent that froze his feet and raised his hackles. *Fox.*

His heartbeat sped up as he considered what to do. *Caught between a hawk and a fox. Not good. Not good.* Trying to act casual, he started down the alley again, ears pricked for the fox that he knew was trailing him, eyes darting to the hawk every second or two as he scanned the alley for an escape.

A wire fence butted up against one wall of the alley, blocking off a driveway or something on the other side. It hadn't been put up very well, and the edge at the corner was loose. It was a small gap, but he was a small cat. The hawk could still fly over, but if he could… *Yes. That's it.*

Cats were predators, but they were also prey, and even though Trick hated to think of himself as prey, he knew that was what he had to be for this to work.

Activate prey drive, he thought, breaking into a sprint toward the gap in the fence. As he'd expected, he heard the scuffle of claws on pavement as the fox behind him bolted out from where it had been hiding, determined to catch him before he got through to safety. Energy surged through Trick's body as he ran, paws light as air on

14

the ground, practically flying. A second later, the hawk screeched and dove toward him. He heard them both, the fox and the hawk, and knew that if he took even a moment to glance toward them, he'd be dead. He could practically feel the hawk's talons in his back and the fox's teeth on his tail. From somewhere inside him, he dug out another burst of speed.

He reached the fence and threw himself at the gap, wriggling with all his might through the hole between the wire and the brick of the building, and tumbled out on the other side. A screeching cry and sharp yip came from behind him, and he spun to see the fox and the hawk locked in vicious combat, tumbling together against the wire fence, which rattled loudly as the two bodies beat against it.

Take that! Try to eat me, huh? He spared a moment to meow tauntingly at them, enjoying his victory. Even with the fox snapping at its neck, the hawk took the time to turn its head and pierce him with a glare. Its talons were buried in the fox's side. The fox was a lot bigger than the hawk, but those talons …

Trick didn't really want to wait around to find out which of them would win. Or whether the winner would be satisfied with its kill or if it would want some kitten for dessert. He slipped through a cracked-open back door into the building, hurried through what turned out to be an antique store, and got shooed out the front door by the shopkeeper.

———

The fox was tough; Julia had to give it that. But then, for an animal like a fox to hunt this far into town, it had to be either young and stupid or desperate and hungry. For several minutes, as she beat her wings against the fox's face and raked its side with her talons, Julia thought this might be the end of her. Cut down in her prime in some alleyway by a dumb animal.

How embarrassing that would be.

And then, finally, the sun set. It had been gradually getting darker as she trailed the kitten boy on his way home, and it would take another half hour for full dark to set in, but Julia knew it—*felt* it —the moment the sun dipped below the horizon.

The fox jerked back with a start. Well, tried to jerk back. Really more lurched backward against the brick wall, limping on legs whose tendons had been cut and bleeding profusely from the gouges in its side. It tried to run from the human who had suddenly appeared where the hawk had been a moment ago, but it couldn't get to its feet.

Julia got up off her side and shifted into a crouch, her own flesh scratched and torn, though not nearly as badly as the fox's. The injuries stung, and she hissed out a curse, both from the pain and from the distraction which had made her fail in her directive. Even still, annoyed as she was at the fox—and at that blasted, stupid boy —the wild panic in the fox's eyes, the pained sounds it made, and the way it scrambled hopelessly to flee on dysfunctional limbs stirred a swell of pity inside her.

The fox wouldn't live long, either dying from shock, killed by a stray dog, or slowly succumbing to its injuries. Julia would mercy kill it now if she had some weapon that would let her do it cleanly. She glanced around the alley, looking for both a weapon and anyone who might see her, and found neither. But she could see a canvas flour sack sticking out of a nearby dumpster.

With a growl of annoyance, she stood, body stinging with all the cuts and shallow punctures the fox had managed to give her, and got the bag. Careful not to get herself bitten again, she scooped the panicked fox into the bag and tied the bag closed. The fox cried and fought like crazy, but she figured it would either settle down soon or pass out from the pain. Maybe it would live long enough for her to get where she was going, or maybe not. It wasn't like Kester needed another familiar, especially not some dumb fox. Best case, it'd get released into the wild to maybe try to kill her or the kitten boy again. It didn't matter. Julia had bigger problems to worry about.

Like how she was going to get across town as an injured, naked woman with no possessions except a bag full of screaming fox.

———

Julia's master lived on the farthest edge of Agreste in a four-bedroom house on two acres of lush, green land with a small river a stone's throw from the back porch. The house was a sprawling single-storey, with brick pillars and façade at the front setting off the green-painted wood of the rest of the house and a brown-shingled roof.

Hidden by the moonless night, Julia walked carefully down the driveway, a cut on the sole of her right foot making her limp. The front porch light was on, and when she knocked, the door opened instantly. He'd been waiting for her, as she knew he would be.

"Julia! Are you all right?" Kester's eyes searched her face, then flitted over her body and noted how cold she was. Reaching an arm around her shoulders, he pulled her inside and shut the door. "Come in and warm up, dearest one." He led her to the fireplace and pushed her down onto a footstool in front of a crackling fire. With a cock of his head, sapphire blue eyes moved to the sack in her hand. "Why have you brought me this?"

Julia shrugged and held it up for him. The fox wasn't moving anymore. "Thought you could save it. Might be too late."

He took it, opening the top to peer inside. "Hmm. You may be right. I'll have a closer look." His concerned gaze swept over her again, taking in the cuts and scratches. His frown dug little furrows into his brow: creases he didn't normally have. At thirty-six, he showed no signs of aging, aside from having filled out so as to become even more handsome. Kester had been beautiful at eighteen, when she'd first met him, and he'd only grown more so with time.

Unlike Julia, who was dirt-plain as a human and would probably start getting gray hairs and wrinkles as soon as she hit thirty next year. That was the way things always seemed to go.

"After what it did to you, why save it?" he asked, genuinely curious.

She shrugged again.

"Such a sweet girl. What a soft heart you have. All right, go get a hot shower, and I'll see if this beast can be saved."

After she got out of the shower and put on some flannel pajamas, Julia went back into the large, open living room. She didn't recognize any of the furniture, but she liked it. When he'd bought the house a few days ago, Kester had paid a designer to furnish it for them. While the design was stylish and elegant, it was also minimalist and comfortable, with soft cushions on the couch and more seating than the two of them were ever likely to need.

Kester was sitting in one of the armchairs with his feet propped on a footstool and a laptop resting on his thighs, his head tilted down so the edges of his wavy blond hair hid his eyes. The fox lay curled in a tight ball on the floor near his feet, gauze wrapped around its ribs. It looked up when Julia entered the room, nothing but calm disinterest in its expression.

"What did you do to it?" she asked, a trickle of annoyance winding through her. Did he mean to keep it as a house pet?

"Only a calming spell. I'll lift it when the poultice has finished healing its wounds."

So, he didn't mean to keep it. Good. She sat in a chair across the seating area from him. Now that the fox was saved, she wondered if it was smart of her to have bothered. "It tried to kill the boy. It might again."

Kester looked up from his computer and stared at the fire, tapping his fingers on the arm of his chair. "That's a good point. I should probably kill it to be safe."

Julia sighed. "I did carry it all the way here."

His fingers moved to the keyboard, and Julia listened to more tapping for a few minutes. "There's a wildlife sanctuary about two hours away," he said at last. "I'll drop it off tomorrow. If I don't lift the calming spell, they should see that it can't go back into the wild and may give it a home. Does that please you?"

She gave him a small, tired smile and nodded.

"Good." He set the laptop aside. "You did well protecting the kitten boy from the fox, though I'm disappointed you weren't able to see him safely all the way home."

Julia bowed her head. "I'm sorry, Master."

He held up a hand. "I'm not blaming you, only expressing my current feelings. I would have had a hard enough time sleeping tonight without knowing whether or not he changes, but to not even be sure he's home when the time comes—not to mention alive..." He tapped his finger against his chin. "We'll have to watch the house. Jacqueline will no doubt have all the curtains drawn, but if the boy is missing, she'll go out to search for him. Hmm." He checked his watch. "We don't have much time." He stood and held out his hand for Julia. "Come. I'll mend you, then we need to go."

"It's not that bad," Julia protested, but she was already getting to her feet and reaching for his hand.

He made a dismissive sound and took her to his laboratory.

———

Trick's mom was buzzing around the house like a bee, and Trick sat on the top perch of his cat tree, staying out of the way. When Trick had made it home, Mom had been standing in the open doorway, watching for him. A look of worry had turned into annoyance and relief when Trick had scooted past her feet into the house, and he'd gotten a really long lecture about being on time and how important tonight was. He had mostly tuned her out, and she'd gone back to cooking dinner.

The dinner was laid out on the dining room table now, dishes covered with lids and foil to keep them warm. The garlicky scent made Trick's nose twitch. Mom had made spaghetti with salad and garlic bread, which she swore Trick used to love even though he hadn't had it in seven years. As Trick had found out soon after he'd been turned into a cat, cats were carnivores, which meant they had to eat meat in order to live. Mom, though, was a vegetarian. She always made faces when preparing the meat for Trick's dinners, especially when handling the livers and kidneys and stuff. Which was so silly. Meat was just dead stuff, and dead stuff was just... stuff that wasn't alive anymore. Nothing lived forever, which meant everything died at some point, so dead stuff was as normal and natural as plants and sunshine. Trick didn't understand what Mom's problem was. But she had been very excited to make a meat-free meal tonight.

She fiddled with the three place settings, fidgeting and pacing and adjusting forks every few seconds. Trick watched his mother from his perch in the living room, annoyed at how excited she was. She was so sure she was right, and Trick was afraid maybe she was.

"It's almost time," Mom said, coming in from the dining room. "Trick, get off of that. You can't be sitting there when you change back."

I'm not going to change back, Trick thought, willing it to be true. *The time's going to pass and nothing will happen and I'll be a cat forever. So there.*

His little brother was sitting on the couch, kicking his feet in boredom. "Mom, can I go read yet?" he asked.

Trick didn't understand him. What six-year-old boy wanted to *read*? Why did *anyone* want to read? Who wanted to stare at scribbles on a page when there was a whole world of adventure out there? Maybe it was because Brother wasn't a cat. Poor kid. Life probably *was* a lot more dull when you had to obey all the rules that humans did.

"Landon!" Mom said, turning on the boy like he'd said something outrageous. "Aren't you excited to see your brother for the first time?"

Brother frowned in confusion and pointed at the top of the cat tree. "Trick's right there."

"As he really looks," she insisted. "Not as what that witch made him."

"But he's always been like that," Brother said.

She sat on the couch beside him. "Do you remember what I told you before? About how you were in trouble before you were born, and Trick let himself be turned into a cat by a witch in order to save you?"

"Witches... are made-up," said Brother, not sounding super convinced about that.

"Most people think so, but there really are some of them around. The sneaky witch gave me a potion to save you, then wanted Trick to be her familiar for seven years as payment. She died a year later, so I was able to bring Trick home early, but he was still stuck as a cat."

Trick yawned and stretched, then got up and lay down with his back to them.

"And tonight is seven years?" Brother asked.

"Yes." Mom checked the clock. "Very soon, Trick will be human again, and we can all go on with our lives."

Trick turned his head and meowed at his mom.

"Why are you in such a bad mood?" she asked him. "Aren't you excited to get your life back?"

The end of Trick's tail twitched in exasperation. He couldn't explain to her that he didn't want to be human again, that he hoped the witch had intended to remove the spell herself instead of it undoing itself automatically after the seven years were up as Mom believed. Hopefully, he'd never be able to tell Mom that because if he could tell her that, it meant he could talk, and talking meant being human, and who needed that?

She stood and picked Trick up. He had an impulse to hiss and lash out with a paw, but he could never hurt his mom, so he let himself be picked up and set on the floor between the couch and the curtain-covered windows. For a second, he thought to run into his room and hide. But if the change was coming—and it definitely *wasn't*—then it wasn't something he could hide from. Better to stay here and let Mom see that she was wrong, that Trick was meant to be a cat and no amount of optimism and regret and spaghetti could make him a boy again.

So Trick sat on the rug in front of his mom and brother and waited.

Mom didn't do a countdown. Things had been so weird when the witch had turned Trick into a cat, they hadn't gotten an exact time on when it had happened. But Mom watched Trick with wide, unblinking eyes, her body perched literally on the edge of her seat.

Minutes passed. Then a few more. As his nervousness was beginning to turn into happy relief, a feeling flowed through Trick like being stretched in a taffy pull. Everything felt weird and wrong, and the world lurched around him. He heard Mom cry out and Brother squeal, and Trick himself let out a yowl that morphed into a boyish scream. And then he was suddenly very cold. He looked down at his pale, hairless body in horror. His fierce claws had turned into fragile, dull little caps for his fingertips; he was defenseless. His whiskers had fallen out, and the world around him felt far away and blurry. His senses were muffled. And his tail—an entire limb—was just *gone*.

He screamed at the top of his lungs.

"My baby!" Mom cried, pulling a throw blanket off the back of the couch and kneeling to wrap Trick in it, hugging him so tightly he could hardly breathe. He trembled with rage and loss as his mom held him. She pushed him out to arm's length and looked into his eyes. "You're so big!"

He was. Big and awkward. He was probably slow, too. He couldn't believe this. It had actually happened.

"Look, Landon!" she said, pulling the blanket tight around Trick's body. "It's your big brother!"

The little boy's eyes were wide, and he pushed back into the couch cushion instead of coming over to them.

Trick sucked in breaths faster and faster as Mom wrapped him in another tight hug.

Outside, in a car across the street, Julia sat with Kester, watching and listening. They couldn't see anything past the closed curtains, but they had the car windows open, so they'd heard the first scream. When the second one came, sounding like neither a woman nor a young boy but like something between a teenager and a tortured cat, Kester turned to Julia, a broad grin on his beautiful face. "Well," he said, "this should be fun."

CHAPTER
TWO

It was dark under the blankets, where the world shrank to nothing but a pocket of warmth and safety around Trick. This was better. Better than out there in the house with his mother's demands. Better than the outside world with all its rules and expectations.

But it wasn't perfect. Nothing could ever be perfect again. The soft expanse of his bed was now barely big enough for him to fit. He'd had to shift around for several minutes before finding the exact center, where his long, awkward limbs wouldn't slip off the edge. He couldn't even tuck his limbs in properly or form a decent ball. All he could do was lie there in a position that wasn't very comfortable, limbs curled under him with his belly not even touching the mattress. The feel of skin on skin irritated him, and he kept squirming to alleviate the feeling, unsuccessfully. It was quiet except for the too-loud sound of his own breathing, and eventually he fell asleep.

He awoke to a world of orange glow, the sun shining through the blankets surrounding him. His body was stiff, his neck ached, and he couldn't feel his lower limbs. That last fact made him panic and jerk. He tumbled off of the bed, landing with a thud and a surprised yelp on the floor. The numbness in his hind limbs turned to pain like a thousand needles, and he yowled and swatted at them, wondering if invisible insects were attacking him. Maybe the swatting worked because the pain receded soon, and he could feel his whole body again.

His whole stupid, awkward, human body.

He fought with the blankets to disentangle himself, then stood on all fours. Immediately, everything felt wrong. His legs were too long or his arms were too short, and his balance was all off. Experimentally, he took a step, but no, this wasn't going to work. When he'd run into his room after becoming human, he thought he'd done it on all fours, but he'd been in such a panic, he couldn't really remember.

Human, he thought. *Walk like a human.* But how? He'd learned it once already, when he was very young. It couldn't be that hard to learn it again.

As Trick stood in his room on all fours, trying to figure out how to get upright, his brother appeared in the open doorway to Trick's bedroom.

"What are you doing?" Brother asked.

Trick let out a soft, annoyed growl. If Brother wasn't going to help, why didn't he go away?

He didn't go away, so Trick tried to ignore him. Carefully shifting his weight to his hind legs—his *legs*—he bent into a squat and grabbed the dresser next to him with his forepa—*hands*. Using the dresser for balance, he stood.

Wow. He was so high off the ground. The floor hadn't been this far away the last time he'd been human, he was sure of it. He could see the whole room, his whole domain spread before him. Sure, it was a small domain, but it would do for now. Even his brother, who'd always seemed like a giant—albeit a smaller giant than other humans—stood well below him.

A deep sense of satisfaction settled into Trick's chest. This standing upright thing was all right.

Trick took a step forward but overbalanced and almost fell. His hand shot out to catch himself on the door frame, and Brother skittered back like he was afraid Trick would fall on top of him. With the help of the wall, Trick took a few steps forward, then back, then to the side, finding his balance. It went quicker than he'd expected. He'd had excellent balance as a cat, and his body still knew what balance was. Getting used to the new shape and center of gravity was the hard part. By the time he was halfway down the hall, he could walk without even needing to brace himself against anything.

He went into the bathroom and climbed up onto the toilet.

As a cat, when he'd been outside, he'd gone to the bathroom wherever he wanted to like a normal cat. But when Mom had brought him home after the witch had died, she'd told him that she was not going to be cleaning up a litter box when she knew he had the mental capacity of a human. "Real cats can use the toilet," she'd told him, "so I'm certain you can figure it out." And then she'd shown him some YouTube videos of how to potty train a cat. Since he'd had the intelligence of a seven-year-old human at the time, even though he was in a cat's body, it'd been a simple thing to learn to hop onto the toilet seat and balance himself to go.

Unfortunately, after seven years as a cat, he'd kind of forgotten how to use the toilet like a human would. So when he tried to balance himself with feet and hands on the toilet seat, his hand slipped, and he crashed to the floor and smacked his head against the bathtub. Letting out a yowl of pain and anger, he got to his feet and glared at the toilet. In a fit of pique and rebellion, rather than spending five seconds trying to work out how to use a toilet, he squatted in the bathtub to do his business.

He was already safely hidden under his blankets again when he heard his mom's startled cry of disgust. She didn't come into his room and yell at him, though. Maybe she was giving him time to adjust. Maybe her feelings were hurt because he'd run away last night and not eaten the spaghetti she'd made. He didn't really care what the reason was. He was just happy to be left alone.

Several hours later, he ventured out again to drink some water and discovered that Mom had removed his water bowl. He walked out to the kitchen, hoping she'd left one out in there, but he couldn't find one, and she wasn't around to get him one. Brother was in the living room reading, but when Trick started searching the kitchen for water, he came in and watched silently.

Since Mom hadn't left any water out for him, Trick would have to get some for himself. He bumped the lever on the water faucet with his hand and put his face under the spout, lapping at the flow of water that came out. It was a lot messier than it should have been, and by the time he'd slaked his thirst, most of his face was wet and it had gotten into his hair, which stuck to his skin irritatingly. He stood upright and pushed the lever down to turn it off. Water dripped down his face and all the way down the front of his furless torso in a cold, wet line. When he turned away from the counter, he saw Brother sitting at the kitchen island, watching him.

They stared at each other for a long while, and then Brother got up from the bar stool and pulled a plastic cup out of a cabinet. He filled it with water at the sink, then took it back to the island and resumed sitting. "Like this," he said, slowly lifting the cup to his mouth and taking a sip, then lowering it.

Trick eyed him skeptically. He'd been watching his mom and brother eat and drink for years. He understood the concept. That wasn't the problem.

Brother patted the bar stool next to him. Trick didn't move at first, then the boy's eyes narrowed and Trick felt a tiny electric shock in the soles of his feet which made him jump. Once he was no longer rooted to the spot, there wasn't much point in not going to sit beside his little brother.

Trick didn't analyze that strange little shock. He knew it came from his brother. He wasn't sure if their mom paid enough attention to spot things like that, but Trick was observant, and he'd noticed over the last few years that things always seemed to end up going the way his brother wanted them to, sooner or later.

As soon as Trick started lifting his foot to climb onto the seat of the stool, Brother said, "No."

Frustrated, Trick tried to lash his tail. Remembering he no longer had a tail made him even more annoyed, and he ended up frozen for a second with one hand on the top of the stool and his foot in midair. *Sit like a human,* he told himself. Looking at his brother in order to copy him, Trick slid his butt onto the bar stool.

There. Sitting like a human.

It felt weird.

The boy slid the cup of water in front of him. Trick reached toward it and used the pads of his—*palm* of his hand to nudge the cup over. It slid about an inch. He nudged it again. Another inch. He kept nudging it, watching it slide toward the edge of the island. Not too much farther…

Brother reached across Trick and picked up the cup, setting it back where he'd put it before. When Trick touched the cup to nudge it again, Brother held on to the top of the cup with one hand and used the other to separate Trick's thumb from his other fingers and wrap Trick's hand around the cup.

Oh, right, his thumb.

Thumbs were weird.

Trick flexed his fingers, making them curl around the cup. He tried to get his thumb to press in where Brother had put it so he could grip the cup, but it didn't work. His thumb kept twitching back to the side, sliding out of place, and when he tried to tell it to go back around the other side of the cup, he couldn't get it in the right place on his own.

Behind them, the front door opened. Trick gave up on trying to pick up the cup and turned to watch his mom come in. After she closed the door and dropped her purse, she looked through the open archway into the kitchen at them.

"Trick!" she snapped. "Why are you still naked?"

Trick tried to twitch his tail in response, but when he sent the signal from his brain to his muscles, the muscles weren't there to receive it. He considered what the human equivalent would be. A shrug. That was what he wanted. But when he tried to send the right signal from his brain to his body, he ended up pushing his shoulders backward like he was puffing out his chest. No, that wasn't right at all. How could there be so many of his own muscles that his brain didn't know how to use?

"For heaven's sake, Trick," Mom said, coming toward them. "You're not a cat anymore. And you're not a little boy anymore, either. You're thirteen—a teenager." She shook her head, her eyes drifting around his face and chest. "My goodness, you've grown so much."

"Are you sure he's my brother?" the smaller boy asked her. "He doesn't look much like either of us."

Mom raised an eyebrow at him. "I was there, so yes, I'm sure." She shrugged. How easy she made it look. "I wish you boys had taken after me, but you both look like your fathers, so..." She shrugged again.

Trick watched her carefully and tried to shrug back. He couldn't quite get there, but at least his shoulders twitched a little more in the right direction.

The motion caught his mother's attention. "You know, most thirteen-year-old boys would be embarrassed to sit there in front of their mothers with no clothes on."

Trick tried another shrug. He almost got it that time.

His mom sighed. "I left some clothes in your room earlier. Go get dressed."

Sliding off the bar stool, Trick stood in front of his mom long enough to see that even though he was a lot taller now, her head was still higher than his, which kind of annoyed him. He drifted off down the hall. When he turned into the bathroom, he heard his mom say, "Oh, no. Landon," and a moment later, his little brother was in the bathroom with him.

"It's gross to pee and poop in the bathtub," Brother said. Trick really didn't have any rebuttal to that. "Mom wants me to make sure you don't do it again."

Trick wasn't sure what kind of response Brother was expecting, so he just stared down at him.

"Do you want me to show you how to do it?" Brother asked.

Trick stared at him.

"Why don't you talk?" Brother asked.

It hadn't occurred to Trick that he should have tried. He hadn't had anything to say yet. He opened his mouth and tried to form some words—any words, really—but all that came out were strange tones from the back of his throat.

Brother pointed to the toilet. "Sit on it like you did the bar stool if you need to poop. To pee, lift the seat and aim."

Trick narrowed his eyes at him. *Aim?*

The look in his little brother's eyes grew cautious. "Maybe you should sit for now. I'm pretty sure peeing on the wall would make Mom even madder than peeing in the bathtub."

There was definitely something unnatural about humans peeing from the same position they ate from, but when Trick was done, there wasn't a mess and his brother seemed satisfied.

Trick went back to his room, crawled under his blanket, and fell asleep. When his empty stomach woke him a few hours later, he felt colder than he had been before. Sticking his face out from under the blanket, he noticed two things right away: the scent of cooking meat, and the crisp bite of cold air. The coldness sent him back under the covers, curling the blanket around himself. But the scent of meat made his stomach growl. Carefully, as if by moving slowly he might get the cold to not notice him, he slipped out from under the blanket. Cold air washed across his exposed skin, raising bumps, making what little hair he had left on his body stand on end.

Why is it so cold?

He spotted the clothes Mom had left in a folded pile on his dresser and let out a soft hiss. She had turned up the air conditioner to force him to get dressed. *Well played, Mom.* There was nothing for it. She'd won this round.

Trick got to his feet and prodded the pile of clothes until they fell on the floor. A sweatshirt, sweatpants, and briefs. He ignored the briefs and struggled to put the shirt and pants on. Which was hard because he still couldn't get his thumbs to work like he knew they should. After a lot of scrambling around on the floor and some frustrated hissing and groaning, he finally got the darn things on. He was still mad, but he was also warm now, so when he went into the dining room (really an extension of the kitchen), he sat down at the chair Mom had already pulled out for him without giving her the satisfaction of a comment.

She didn't return the favor. "There," she said, looking across the table at him. "Don't you feel better?"

He grumbled unintelligibly and leaned down to eat the chicken on his plate.

"Trick!" she said sharply. "Utensils."

Trick looked at the knife and fork lying beside his plate, then poked at them.

"I don't think he can use his thumbs yet," Brother said from Trick's right.

"Really?" Mom asked, sounding concerned for once. "Is that true, Trick?"

Instead of answering, Trick tried to pick up the fork. His thumb kept twisting the wrong way or not responding at all, so he couldn't get a grip. Eventually he got the fork curled against his palm with his fingers, holding it in a fist.

"Oh, sweetheart, here." Mom reached over and cut his food into pieces. "I'm sorry. I didn't think it would be so hard for you to adapt to your human body again. There, you should be able to pick those up with your fork and eat. Okay?"

His failure to grasp his fork and her insistence on him not eating straight off the plate had put Trick in a bad mood, so he spared her a dirty look and stabbed at one of the pieces of meat. He only knocked it off the fork twice before he got it in his mouth.

"I'm sorry, Trick," Mom said, "but we don't have the time to let you ease into this. I've already registered you for school. It starts on Monday."

Trick blinked, not sure he'd heard her right. School? She was sending him to school? It wasn't enough that he'd been forced into this cold, awkward body, but now he had to spend all day reading and obeying rules?

He didn't realize he was breathing fast until Brother put a hand on Trick's forearm. "I'm going, too. It'll be okay."

"It'll be fine, Trick, you'll see," said Mom. "Landon won't be at the same school as you, but yes, he'll be going to school as well. Now that you're human again, you'll really need to buckle down and catch up. You know you never paid enough attention to the lessons I tried to give you." The reprimand in her tone didn't make Trick any happier about the situation. He *had* paid attention... most of the time.

Trick moved his tongue around, grunting out sounds, trying to force the word out. "Uh... oh... ayoh... un... *No*." He panted with the effort, but he was pleased with himself. He'd said a word. That deserved a reward. Ignoring the fork in his hand, he grabbed a big bite of meat off the plate with his teeth.

His mom shook her head. "It's been seven years since I've heard my baby speak, and what's the first thing he says? Is it, 'I love you, Mom'? Is it, 'Thanks for taking care of me while I was tiny and vulnerable'? Of course not. The first thing my son says to me after seven long years is, 'No'." Trick kept chewing, not answering. "That was your first word as a baby, too. But I'm sorry, Trick; this isn't up for discussion. You're going to school. That's the whole reason we moved to a new town, remember? You've got your life back, and now it's time to start living it. We'll get you ready in time."

"No," Trick repeated, clearer than before.

"It's happening," she said as she got up to adjust the thermostat. "Tonight, Landon and I will start helping you remember how to use your human body. You'll be ready by school on Monday. And in case you're thinking of sabotaging your own progress, you should know that you're going to school on Monday whether you're ready or not."

Trick shoved more food into his mouth and refused to look at her.

"Okay, Trick?" she asked pointedly.

He didn't answer. What good were words anyway, if they couldn't get him out of school?

"Trick?" his mom prompted.

He let out a low sound of acknowledgment and wondered

where he could find the nearest witch. He wanted his body and freedom back.

————

As the sun dropped lower toward the horizon, Julia flew back to Kester's house and through the window he kept open for her. There was still some time before sunset, when she'd regain her human body, so she perched on the back of the couch in the living room.

Across the seating area, Kester looked up from his laptop with mischief dancing in his eyes.

She cocked her head inquisitively.

"I've got a plan," he said with a boyish grin.

She knew he would have, sooner or later. He couldn't hear her thoughts—and she couldn't direct them to him in the same way that he could direct his thoughts to her—but their bond allowed him to sense her intent. So although she couldn't speak, he heard her curiosity.

"Patience, beloved one," he murmured.

Julia rolled her eyes. Kester savored every new development and discovery with a childlike glee that was really a bit tiresome at times. When it wasn't endearing beyond words.

He turned the computer in his lap to face her, and she flapped over to get a closer look, alighting on the footstool. The screen showed the website for the school Jacqueline had registered Trick at. Julia had broken off her observation of the house earlier that day to follow the woman and watch where she'd gone. The magical bond Julia shared with Kester allowed him to see through her eyes at will, so he had seen what she had, and had apparently thought more of it than she did. The page currently on the screen showed a photo of a woman—forty-something, slim, and fairly pretty. With a pang of disappointment that she couldn't hide from Kester but which neither of them acknowledged, Julia understood at least some part of his plan.

"This is the principal," he said. "Tomorrow afternoon, you're to follow her home from school so I can learn where she lives."

Julia nodded acknowledgment of the command and waited to see if he'd tell her any more of his plan.

He didn't. He only stroked the feathers of her head in a fond caress and said, "I've got dinner in the oven. The sun's nearly down. After you change, have a bath, and then we'll eat."

———

The next night, Kester sat silently in his car, patient as a spider. The day had been fairly uneventful, but now it was Friday night, and he had high hopes for the evening. He'd spent much of the day watching Jacqueline and her kitten—and the other boy, of course—through Julia's hawk eyes. To be perfectly accurate, most of the day had been spent periodically checking in on Julia's observation of the house, since Jacqueline persisted in keeping the curtains firmly closed. But around noon, he'd heard the prodding of Julia's interest in his mind and had watched with her from her perch high in a tree as the family of three ventured out into their back yard. The delightful former kitten was awkward and argumentative, but he appeared almost like a real boy. Still lively as ever, too, not that Kester had expected anything less.

After Julia had found the principal's house, Kester had left his familiar at home to pass the time as she would while he went about his own business.

A quarter past ten p.m., Lisa VanBuren, principal of Agreste Junior High, pulled out of her driveway in a cherry red Volkswagen convertible. Excitement hummed through Kester's body, and he wondered if his quest would extend into Saturday. It could be a fun challenge all on its own, seeking out a way to intercept her in some sober, daylight activity. But he was too eager to get on with things to want a challenge. For now, easier would be better.

He drove twenty yards behind her all the way through town, and she never appeared to notice. When she parked on the street, he found a spot three spaces away and watched as she entered a bar with a glowing neon sign reading 'Bruno's'.

Kester waited three minutes before following her in.

Bruno's was not a dive, but neither was it the sort of upscale nightclub only larger cities could boast. The establishment was clean, the music was loud and adequate, and the lighting was stark enough to cast explicit shadows and clearly illuminate faces not hidden in those shadows. Bodies gyrated on the dance floor, mostly thin and young and scantily clad. Even the men weren't afraid to show some skin.

Smiling, Kester unbuttoned his shirt down to the bottom of his sternum. *When in Rome.*

He spotted Lisa as she slid onto a stool and spoke to the bartender. Her dress was short, and her heels were sharp. Kester eyed her from across the room, examining the lines of her body. She was perhaps slightly too thin, too angular, but her waist was small. Ordinarily, she'd be far from his first choice—not with so many much younger women in the room—but she would do well enough. There was, after all, something to be said for experience.

Responding with only a polite smile to the interested gaze of a young blonde, Kester made his way across the room and took a seat on the stool beside Lisa. Her face was as angular as her body, but comely in its way. Her light brown eyes were surrounded by smokey makeup, and her dark hair was twisted up with tendrils teasing her neck. She wasn't endowed with much when it came to her bosom, but rather than try to hide or disguise that fact, she wore a black dress with a neckline plunging nearly to her navel. On her, the look was daring and elegant, where a woman with cleavage would appear cheap and desperate.

Not that Kester had anything against cheap and desperate.

Lisa looked at him askance, needing only a moment to take in his appearance. Kester knew what she saw: incredibly handsome and at least five years younger than her. In other words, out of her league. Probably—she would assume—he was here only for a drink or, more likely, was waiting for someone.

When he turned and locked her in with his gaze, she started slightly. She was interested but wary.

At that moment, the bartender set a drink in front of Lisa, and Kester laid a twenty down. When Lisa didn't immediately protest, the bartender scooped up the cash.

"I'll have one of those as well," Kester said without taking his eyes off of Lisa's.

"An appletini?" asked the bartender.

"That'll be fine," Kester answered.

With a shrug, the bartender got to making the drink.

Lisa smiled, her wariness bleeding away. "I like a man who's secure in his masculinity."

"Likewise," he replied, dipping his gaze lower to appreciate her dress before returning his attention to her eyes.

They fell into light conversation. She had clearly come to this bar with a purpose, so it would have been easy to skip the conversation if that was what he'd wanted, but it wasn't. Not tonight.

When she asked why she'd never seen him here before, he said, "I'm only visiting. My cousin recently moved into town, and I came for a few days to help him get things settled."

She didn't ask any probing questions about where he was from. "You're a good cousin, to take time off work to help him out."

He only said, "I try," not responding to the hinted question about what he did for a living.

She didn't push, which he appreciated. Instead, she let out a breath. "Must be nice."

"What must?"

"Having the time to do that."

"Your job doesn't allow it?"

She grimaced at the mention of her job. "I'm desperate for a vacation, but all I can afford is a night out once a week if I'm lucky."

He grinned playfully. "Then I'll try to make sure this night doesn't go to waste."

Her eyebrow cocked. "How thoughtful of you."

"A gentleman must always keep a lady's needs in the forefront."

Before they could get sidetracked too much with flirting, he took the opportunity to nudge the conversation where he wanted it. "If you'd like to talk about your problems at work, consider me a captive audience."

She laughed. "Yeah, I'm sure that's what you came here for."

"I really don't mind." He kept his full attention on her, not taking his eyes off of hers for a moment. "I'm a good listener."

Lisa considered him skeptically, then shook her head with a smile. "It's a good thing you're not in town long. I get the feeling you could be very distracting."

He grinned and winked. "Very."

As she let out another big breath, some amount of tension left her body. "Normally, I wouldn't. But things have been such a mess lately, it's been hard to get my mind off of it."

"Maybe if you get it off your chest, you'll be able to move on to more enjoyable topics."

She considered the suggestion. "I guess there's no harm. You don't know anyone in town, and it's not like the press haven't already gotten ahold of all the juicy parts. I'm the principal of the junior high. My job's hardly relaxing on the best of days, but things are especially bad right now. One of my teachers has gone missing."

"Missing?" Kester asked, putting a concerned expression on. He'd already read all about this on the internet, but he needed to let her tell it.

"Yes. He doesn't have any family, but a neighbor heard noises in his apartment. When the neighbor went by to make sure Brad was all right, the door was ajar and Brad was missing. He still is. The police haven't been able to find out much yet."

"How disturbing. Do they think he was kidnapped?"

Hopelessly, she shrugged. "They don't know. It's possible, but there's been no ransom demand or anything, though there were some signs of a struggle. Meanwhile, the new school year starts on Monday, and I'm out one eighth grade teacher. I've been scrambling, but there aren't a huge number of good substitutes in a town this small, and we're too far from any other cities for anyone to want to commute. And I don't dare advertise the position permanently before we know what happened to Brad or the press will crucify me."

Kester nodded thoughtfully. "Posting a permanent position at this time could come across as heartless if he's still alive—and ghoulish if he's not."

"Yes, exactly. Never mind that it's *necessary*." She shook her head, irritated. "Great. I came here to forget about work. I don't think talking about it is helping much, after all."

"Perhaps you're wrong about that," Kester said. At her curious look, he added, "My cousin. The one who just moved here. He's a teacher."

Lisa sat straighter. "Really? What a funny coincidence. Where's he work?"

"He doesn't have a job yet. He came here because he wanted a change of scenery. He has some money—inheritance—so he doesn't really need to work. But if you're in a bind, I'm sure he'd be willing to take the position for however long you need him."

"You're kidding."

Kester shook his head.

She bit her lip. "I'd have to see his resumé, of course, and interview him. If everything checks out… Would he really be able to start on Monday?"

"Let's ask him." Kester dismounted from the bar stool and offered Lisa his hand. "I'm staying at his house. Why don't we go over there and you can see if the arrangement will work for both of you?"

She took his hand and stood. "I hate that work is invading my night, but yes, let's do it." When they exited the bar into the cool night, Lisa said, "I'll follow you."

"I'm right there." Kester pointed to his car. He waited until she got safely into hers first, smiling to himself. If Lisa hadn't already decided to go home with him—or take him home—she probably wouldn't have agreed so readily.

Once they'd reached his house and parked, Kester walked Lisa to the door. She didn't try to hide the frown that creased her carefully-shaped brows.

"Something worries you?" he asked.

"Only wondering if someone who can afford this house really wants to put up with a bunch of teens and tweens every day."

Kester chuckled. "My cousin is not intimidated by children." He unlocked the front door and swept out a *ladies first* hand. She hesitated for half a second, then went in. "John!" he called out as they walked through the foyer and into the living room. "We have a guest."

"Oh!" Lisa said with a start when she spotted Julia.

Adorable in flannel pajamas, Julia looked over from the couch, where she sat curled up with a book in her lap. "Hi," she said in a bored way.

"Hello, Julia," Kester said, standing beside Lisa. "Is John in bed yet?"

"He had something to do," Julia answered as Kester had instructed her to before he'd left that night. "Said he'd be back tomorrow."

"Oh," Lisa said. It was a sound of disappointment and awkwardness.

Before she had time to wonder what she ought to do next, Kester went ahead with his script. "Well, I can at least get you his resumé. Julia, do you know where he keeps copies of his resumé?" He gestured between the two women. "Julia is John's girlfriend. Julia, this is Lisa, a school principal. She has a position in which I thought John might be interested."

Lisa relaxed, more comfortable now that she thought she understood the scene better.

Julia got up and headed into another room. "I'll get it." She returned a few seconds later with a piece of paper and handed it to Kester.

He passed it to Lisa. "Here you are."

Lisa looked over it, nodding in approval. Kester wondered if she'd even bother to call the references he'd listed. There would be people on the other end to vouch for 'John' if she did. Falsifying documents, records, and life histories was a hobby of his.

While Lisa was reading, Julia met Kester's eyes with an understanding gaze. Through their bond, he felt the dull ache in her heart. He knew she knew he felt it, but she didn't allow any emotion into her expression, and he indicated no acknowledgment. He could never acknowledge that he knew she ached—or worse, that he knew why. Doing so would quite possibly destroy everything he cherished in this life. So he smiled and nodded and barely stopped himself from stroking her cheek with his hand.

"I'm gonna head to bed," Julia said, leaving without waiting for a response from either of them.

Lisa put the resumé in her purse. "He certainly looks good on paper. I'll call him tomorrow or Sunday. Thanks for the tip."

Kester smirked and stepped closer, his body inches from hers. "My pleasure. I'm sorry for forcing you to do work on your night off. You must allow me to make it up to you."

Lisa eyed him, her gaze turning from professional to hungry.

Hours later, he left Lisa sleeping peacefully in his bed, pulled on a pair of boxers, and went to Julia's room. Her bedside light was on, and she was still reading even though it was long past midnight.

Pushing the discomfort of her dull ache as far out of his awareness as he could, he sat on the foot of her bed, very pleased with himself. "I think we can consider my plan a lock."

"Go well, did it?"

"You have to ask? Julia, you wound me."

She laid the book on her lap. "For a fun challenge, have you ever considered coming up with a plan that didn't involve seducing someone?"

He shrugged one shoulder. "Two birds. Besides, it isn't as if she didn't want to be seduced."

"Would it have stopped you if it were?"

She had him there. "It's only a bit of fun."

"And they're the toys?"

Kester sighed. This wasn't about Lisa. Or not *only* her. "Not toys, dearest one. If you must use childish language, call them... playmates. And I believe I can say with certainty that none of them have ever been left unsatisfied."

"Trust me, I've heard—and seen—that much."

"You're angry with me."

Julia put a bookmark in her book and set it on her nightstand. "Of course not," she lied. "It would be stupid to be angry at you for that. First, because it's like being angry at a cat for clawing the furniture, and second, because it's not my place to disapprove of you, Master."

That was all quite true, though her disapproval still pained him. He got up and, taking the back of her head in his hand, pressed a kiss to her forehead. "Get rest. Tomorrow, I have magic to do."

He went back to his room and lay down, giving plenty of space to the woman lying bonelessly on the other side of his bed, and quickly fell into a contented sleep. When he awoke the next morning, she was gone without so much as a note left on the pillow.

He appreciated that in a woman.

Kester stretched in satisfaction. He decided he was going to enjoy working for Lisa VanBuren.

CHAPTER
THREE

The janitor's closet was dark, and it smelled bad, and the floor was hard, but it was reasonably quiet and totally secluded, so Denneka was happy. Sitting on the cold concrete floor with her back against the wall, squished between a mop bucket and a rack of cleaning supplies, she cradled her phone in her hands, finger reflexively swiping, eyes never leaving the screen. She wasn't in a janitor's closet—not really. She was in Middle-earth, searching for kidnapped hobbits.

With a sudden burst of light, the door to the janitor's closet opened and her brother's voice jolted her unpleasantly back to reality. "I found her, Mom! She's playing on her phone!"

"I am not *playing on my phone*," Denneka protested. "I'm *reading*." She only read on her phone because it was convenient and—usually—easier to hide than a paperback.

"Whatever you're doing, it doesn't look like work, and that's really more the point," said Jonah.

The sharp clicking of footsteps approached, and their mother appeared next to Jonah, who left once the task of dealing with his sister had been handed off. Mom didn't look happy. "Again? Denneka, we need you out there. It's the day before school starts, and all the procrastinators are doing their new school clothes shopping." Mom reached down a hand to help her to her feet, and Denneka couldn't figure out a way to refuse.

Reluctantly, Denneka put her phone in her pocket.

"Nuh-uh." Mom held out her hand. "You can get it back after we close. I need you focused."

Denneka handed the phone to her mom, groaning her annoyance.

"You're worse than Barb," Mom commented after putting the phone in her own pocket. "At least she reads *around* her work."

"But Barb just sits at the register all day," Denneka pointed out. "You don't make her do anything when no one's checking out."

Mom shooed Denneka through the hall. "It's important that customers know there's always someone available to help them check out. Make them wait even a few seconds and they might decide not to buy something." She pushed her daughter through the open doorway into the storefront. "Go help customers."

Things had gotten busy while Denneka had been hiding. The fifteen-hundred-square-foot shopfront, already packed pretty tightly with racks of clothes for all ages, was further crowded with much more than the usual number of customers. As she stood taking stock of the situation, Denneka noticed a woman trying to herd two boys toward the young boys' area. Mom had already gone off to help a mother with a little girl, and Jonah and Alex were both with customers already, so Denneka sighed and headed for the trio.

The mother was auburn-haired and pretty. Almost gorgeous, really, even without wearing makeup and with... well... being mom-aged. Younger than her mom, though, Denneka guessed: maybe mid-thirties. The younger boy had light blond hair and blue eyes so bright that the word 'cherub' came to mind. The other boy had his back to Denneka, but he was close to her height, so she guessed he might be her age. Aside from his height and lean build, all she could see of him was somewhat shaggy raven-black hair.

Glancing down to make sure she was still wearing her name tag, Denneka approached them. "Can I help you with anything?"

"Oh, yes, thank—" The woman stopped short when she looked

at Denneka. "You work here?" Clearly she wasn't used to seeing thirteen-year-old shop assistants.

"Yep." Denneka waved a hand to indicate the store. "Family businesses get to play fast and loose with child labor laws, I guess."

"In that case, yes, we could use some help." The woman looked from her youngest boy to the crowded shop, to Denneka, to the older boy who was ignoring all of them and flipping through a rack of ties.

No, not flipping through them, exactly. He was... batting at them.

Weird.

Sounding a bit overwhelmed, the woman said, "We're new in town, and what with the move and all, I haven't had any chance to get either of the boys new clothes for the school year." Her eyes flitted back and forth between her sons, probably deciding which of them she wanted Denneka to help. Could the older one not shop on his own? Which child to leave to his own devices shouldn't have been a difficult decision here. But the woman hesitated for several more seconds before saying, "Trick."

The older boy turned to face them, and Denneka's breath caught. He was her age all right—and really cute, with the most striking grass green eyes she'd ever seen.

He wasn't looking at her, though. He'd faced his mother without even glancing at Denneka.

"Landon and I are going to be right over there," the woman told him, pointing at the area with the clothes in the younger boy's size. "This girl's going to help you find some clothes in your size. Denneka, is it?" she asked, reading the name tag.

Denneka nodded.

"This is Trick," the woman said as if the boy couldn't introduce himself. Or maybe he wasn't inclined to, given the blank and disinterested way he finally looked at Denneka. "His, um, clothes were all lost in the move, so he'll need pretty much everything."

Denneka's attention had been so much on the woman—and then she'd been so distracted by Trick's eyes—that she only now noticed the gray sweatsuit he was wearing. Yeah, definitely not something he'd want to be seen in public in. "Sure thing."

Looking Trick directly in the eyes, the woman told him, "I'll expect you to have enough clothes picked out by the time we're done. And"—she leaned in to whisper, but Denneka still heard it— "try to act normal."

After she and the younger boy walked away, Trick just stood there, gazing around the room as if he couldn't possibly be less interested in anything, Denneka included.

Several silent seconds later, she asked, "So, do you wanna look at some jeans?"

He met her eyes, but there was no expression on his face, and he said nothing.

His aggressive apathy toward her made her skin itch. *Am I doing something wrong?* she wondered. People often told her to smile more. Not that she didn't like people, but she was usually caught up in her own thoughts. Maybe she wasn't smiling enough. She gave the boy a big smile and hoped it didn't look fake. With as cute as he was, she was sure that if he'd smiled first, a natural smile would have sprung right out of her. But he wasn't smiling at all, so she had to force it a little.

He didn't smile back. Those brilliant green eyes were still locked with hers, but he somehow managed to appear not to even notice her. She could probably dance a jig and he wouldn't seem to notice. She was tempted to do it just to see if she could get a reaction out of him.

"Okay, then," she said, smile still plastered on, and turned to lead him toward the men's jeans. To her mild surprise, he followed her. She stopped in front of the wall with the rack of men's jeans, all folded into cubbies on the wall and organized by style. "So, what kind—" She stopped when she noticed his feet. He was wearing flip-flops. A sweatsuit and flip-flops. Even if his clothes had all been lost in the move, hadn't he at least had on the set he was wearing at the time? She shook the thought away. Not her business. "What style do you prefer?"

He stared at her.

Was he brain-damaged?

No. She could see the intelligence in his eyes. She also saw the boredom. And mild irritation. He was annoyed that she was talking to him.

The smile fell from Denneka's face. *Too good to talk to the nerdy girl, are you?* She was so, *so* tempted to walk away and leave him to his shopping, but if her mom saw her, she'd get in trouble, especially if the boy's mom made a big deal about him not having all the clothes picked out by the time she was ready to leave. Considering his bored attitude, it didn't look like he'd do it on his own. If Denneka got in trouble, her mom might keep her phone even longer, and she was in the middle of a chapter!

So she pressed on.

Denneka pulled two pairs of jeans from the cubbies and held them up. "Boot cut? Relaxed fit?"

His gaze fell to each one, showing no interest.

She pulled down another pair. "Skinny?"

He looked between the three pairs of pants, then to her. "I need… ones that fit."

Denneka blinked at him. Why was he being deliberately difficult? She sighed, trying to keep from sounding annoyed. "Okay. What size do you wear?"

He stared at her like she'd asked him what his favorite flavor of rainbow was.

She stepped back to get a better look at him and took a guess, then tossed him a pair. "Why don't you try these on, and we'll go from there?"

He stepped out of his flip-flops and—before Denneka could fully register that odd thing—pulled down his sweatpants.

She froze in surprise, then reflexively looked around to see who else was watching. No one, thankfully, since they were hidden against a wall by a bunch of racks. When she looked back at Trick, he was pulling the sweatpants all the way off.

"What are you doing?" she whispered urgently.

He stopped with the pants in his hand, giving her a slightly confused look, and slowly reached for where he'd laid the jeans over a rack. Then, still moving slowly and never looking away from her, he began stepping into them.

"Not here!" she whispered and pointed to the clearly marked dressing room not five feet away. "In there!"

Trick looked from her to the door and back to her, then kept trying to put on the jeans. Apparently, he had no intention of going into the dressing room.

Did one of the girls at school send him here to make fun of her? Was someone secretly recording this? She took a hard look around, but she couldn't see anyone.

With a soft thud, Trick fell onto his butt on the floor, his leg flailing with half the pant leg flapping off the end of his foot. He let out a soft hiss of annoyance.

Denneka knelt next to him. "What are you doing?" she repeated. "Stop!"

He obeyed her, but after a second, gave his leg another irritated shake like he was trying to get the pants off.

"You're putting them on backward," she pointed out. This guy was definitely messing with her, and she wasn't happy about it. But she couldn't freak out. If someone was recording her—or if the idea was for him to report back to whoever and tell them what happened —it would only be worse for her if she reacted. She had to remain totally professional.

She pulled the jeans off of his foot, turned them right-way around, and started tugging them onto his legs as if dressing a small child. She tried not to imagine how he was laughing at her behind that mask of boredom and annoyance. He must be a friend or relative of one of the cool kids in her class, and they put him up to this as a bit of vacation fun while he visited.

Except his mom had said they'd just moved here. If that really was his mom. But even if she wasn't, an adult wouldn't be in on something like this, would she?

But if he had really just moved here, and if Denneka was right that they were the same age, then...

No, she couldn't worry about that now.

But her brain didn't stop. In her mind's eye, she saw herself walking into school, saw this Trick guy standing with the cool kids, laughing and talking, normal as could be, and as she passed, they would all turn to her. Someone would make a joke. Those lovely green eyes of his would turn cold and venomous as they all laughed at her.

She almost walked away from him right then. *Professional*, she reminded herself. *It'll only be worse otherwise.* After all, so far, he was the only one who'd done anything to be embarrassed about. Not that he *was* embarrassed. If the goal was to make *her* embarrassed... well, it was working, but she wouldn't show it. If she did, they—or he, though she had a hard time believing he was a lone actor in this —would win.

When she'd gotten the jeans tugged on enough so the bottoms were at his ankles and the tops were scrunched up at his knees, she stood and stepped back. "Now pull them up the rest of the way."

If he asked for help standing, she would lend a hand, but she wasn't going to offer and give him the chance to leave her hanging. He didn't ask for help. Instead, in the most contorted way she could imagine putting on pants, he lay back on the ground and arched his body, shoulders and feet on the ground, to lift his hips high enough to pull the jeans up.

And thrusting his crotch up in the process. She looked away, cheeks burning. His sweatshirt wasn't long enough to cover the white briefs that were, frankly, a little too snug for her liking. She let him struggle on the ground while she kept an eye out for any other customers coming too close. None of them did, though the boy's mom caught her eye, and Denneka gave her a reassuring smile, as if everything was going perfectly well.

When she heard Trick stop moving, she turned back around to see him standing there with jeans in place.

"Are you gonna fasten those?" she asked.

He looked down at the fly, where the zipper was open and the single button still undone. At his side, his fingers flexed, and she noticed that their movement was a little stiff and awkward. He looked up at her.

She crossed her arms.

After a moment, he started working to get the zipper up. He couldn't seem to get the hang of it.

He is really milking this, she thought. After a full minute, Denneka gave up and went to him. "Oh my goodness; here." *If he wants to act like a child, I guess I can treat him like a child.* Her face felt like it was on fire, but she kept her expression stern and was careful to touch nothing but metal and loose fabric as she zipped and buttoned the jeans, pretending he was one of the little boys she occasionally had to help dress. A very big little boy. When she finished, she faced him again with folded arms.

He stared at her. "Why is your face red?"

"This isn't funny, you know," she said before she could stop herself.

The angle of his head twitched. "Why would it be funny?" The guy sure had a talent for deadpan delivery. He didn't sound at all sarcastic, even as he mocked her to her face.

She huffed. "Do they fit?"

He looked down at the jeans, then back to her, giving no response.

"Walk over there, then back to here."

He gave her a skeptical look but did as she instructed.

"Now squat down and stand back up."

He did so.

"Does the fit feel fine? Not too loose or too tight?"

He twitched his shoulders in a jerky shrug.

"Great. Here's two more pairs." She pulled two more of the same size off the wall and shoved them into his arms. Then she led him to a table full of t-shirts and handed him a medium.

He must have been anticipating her action, because he was awkwardly pawing off his sweatshirt before she could tell him to go

49

to the dressing room. But she didn't make a fuss because this was less bad than before, and making a fuss would be more likely to draw attention than acting like this was no big deal.

Trick struggled with getting the t-shirt holes in the right places and pulling it on, and Denneka tried not to notice the shallow grooves outlining his abs.

Because that was probably exactly what he wanted.

Still, when she finally pulled her eyes away from his abs only when they'd been covered by fabric, she found him staring at her again. "Well, that fits," she said, not bothering to get his input on it this time. "Here." She handed him a stack of the same shirt in several different colors and patterns. "Anything else?"

"I need underwear," he said. And then, for some reason that could only be to torment her, he added in a faux-irritated mutter, "My stupid *human* boy parts are all dangly and floppy. They didn't use to be like that. It's annoying. I need underwear to keep them out of the way."

Denneka caught herself gaping at him in surprise and felt the traitorous heat in her face. She snapped her mouth shut, angry at herself for giving him the reaction he was obviously going for. Glowering, she marched to the rack of men's underwear and— guessing the size again—grabbed a package of briefs. Patterned, so at least if he went around pantsless again they'd disguise things a bit. After she shoved that package at him, she added some boxer-briefs for good measure.

He examined the two packages and the photos on the fronts of men modeling the contents. He didn't argue about them, which she decided to take as approval.

Hoping she was finally done, Denneka walked over to where Trick's mom stood with the younger brother in the boys' section. Trick had followed her, so Denneka put on a big smile and gestured toward Trick and his armful of clothes.

The woman beamed at him. "Now you look like a normal boy. Isn't that better?"

It was a weird almost-insult, and Denneka wasn't sure what

could explain it or what sort of response she expected, but it was the sharp, sullen, "No," that Trick gave.

The woman didn't look bothered by the response. "You still need a jacket and shoes. Did you get socks?"

"Socks?" Trick asked, not sounding as if he liked the idea.

"I'll get some," Denneka offered, running off before the woman made Trick go with her. She took a guess and came back with a package of socks that were probably the right size and handed it to Trick. "We don't sell shoes here, but all the jackets are over on that wall."

The woman gestured at a nearby chair. "Trick, set those here and then go over and look for a jacket." Trick did so, wandering away without a backward glance. His mom moved closer to Denneka and said in a quiet voice, "Thank you for helping him. Did he act, um, odd at all?"

Was she in on it? Why else would she expect Trick to have acted weird? What was she getting at? Denneka decided to be honest. "Yeah, kinda. He didn't know to use the dressing room and needed help getting the jeans on."

With a weary sigh, the woman closed her eyes for a couple seconds. "Sorry about that, and thank you again for helping him. He's… gone through some strange things lately. He's having to adjust to… normal life again."

Well, that opened up a whole slew of possibilities and questions. Denneka was ninety-nine percent sure the boy had been messing with her—mocking her—but a small inkling of doubt crept in with his mother's words.

"I'm Jacqueline, by the way," the woman said, "and this is Landon."

The younger boy was standing quietly nearby. With attention now brought to him, he held up a white button-up shirt on a hanger and asked Denneka, "Does this come in red?"

Denneka mentally ran through their current inventory and answered, "No, I'm sorry. Only white and black for that style."

"But I want it in red."

I'm... sorry?" she said uncertainly. "It doesn't come in red."

The boy hummed unhappily and went to the other side of the nearby rack.

Jacqueline was squinting at Denneka. "Are you thirteen?"

Denneka nodded.

"Oh, that means you'll be in Trick's grade, doesn't it? You're going into eighth?"

"Yeah..."

"Oh. Ah, I'd appreciate if you don't mention how odd he was today. Or what I said about him going through some things. I know how rumors can get around, and I really want him to have a fresh start at a normal school life."

What was a normal school life, anyway? People always said 'normal' like it was a good thing. Normal had never been on the table for Denneka, at least not if all the other normal kids had anything to say about it.

But from how Trick had behaved, either the strange things he'd been through were strange on an epic scale, or Jacqueline really was in on the joke and was setting Denneka up for an even bigger fall tomorrow morning. Given the inherent odds of epic strangeness, it was certainly the latter. But Denneka nodded and smiled and said, "Sure, Mrs. uh..."

"Just Jacqueline," she said.

"Okay. Sure, uh, Jacqueline." It felt weird calling an adult by her first name, especially one of her probably-classmates' moms, whether the woman was mocking her or not. "I won't say anything." As if she even had anyone to tell—if Trick's strangeness was genuine, which obviously it wasn't.

"Could you take our stuff up to the counter? We're almost done, but I want to have the boys pick out jackets first."

"Sure." Denneka gathered Trick's clothes up and then added the clothes for the younger boy into the pile.

"This too," Landon said, appearing suddenly from behind a rack and handing her a red shirt.

Denneka carried the whole lot back to the counter, where Barb was chatting with Alex. They were two of the regular, non-family employees. Barb was a motherly lady in her fifties who spent all day planted behind the counter, reading romance novels when she wasn't working the register. Alex was a nineteen-year-old freshly-graduated non-college-student who was charming and good-looking enough that Denneka always got nervous around him for no reason that made any sense.

"That's a cute one," Barb teased, glancing unsubtly toward Trick as Denneka dropped the pile of clothes on the counter.

"That's a jerk," Denneka countered.

Alex chuckled. "Yeah, he may have been teasing you a little."

"You saw?"

Alex's grin was so brilliant, Denneka couldn't look directly at it. Between that and his chatty nature, she understood why her parents had hired him as a salesman. "The crowd thinned out while you were helping him."

"And you didn't help me?"

"Oh, no. It was way funnier to watch you flounder."

"You're a jerk, too."

"You don't mean that."

She didn't.

Since there weren't many customers in the store at the moment, Barb started ringing up the big batch for Jacqueline. A flash of red caught Denneka's eye, and she snatched the shirt right after Barb scanned it.

"What's wrong?" Alex asked.

The red shirt. It was the same as the white shirt the boy had asked her about. She turned it around to show the other two. "I thought this only came in white and black."

Barb shrugged as if to say, *Not my department.* Alex frowned and eventually shrugged. "I thought so, too. Huh. I guess we must have gotten one in red."

The two of them went back to chatting, but Denneka couldn't stop thinking about the shirt. She was sure there was no red version of that particular style.

And yet, there was, right in her hand.

She looked over to where Jacqueline and the two boys were trying on jackets.

Strange things…

"Denneka," Mom called from the doorway into the back of the store. "Can you come help me with something?"

Reluctantly, Denneka set the shirt with the rest of the batch and went to help her mom.

She was absolutely certain that Trick—and even his mom—had been messing with her. Teasing her. Making fun of her the way everyone else other than her family and friends at the shop did.

She was absolutely, positively… ninety-eight percent certain.

CHAPTER FOUR

Trick didn't like car rides. They were way too fast, and he never knew where they were going. Well, that wasn't so bad now that he could see through the windows—Mom had never let him ride outside of a cat carrier, claiming it was for his safety—but he refused to count that as a point in favor of being human. There were *no* points in favor of being human. Riding in cars was simply terrible, and less terrible didn't mean better. As buildings and signs and other cars careened toward them, making Trick grip the edge of his seat for dear life, he wasn't actually all that sure that seeing what was happening outside *was* less terrible than not seeing it.

"Mom. Mom. Mom. Slow down. Slow down, Mom," he said loudly, the same as he'd been saying practically since they'd left the house. Mom had tried telling him to stop at first, saying that it was fine and he was perfectly safe, but he didn't believe that for a second. He saw how fast those other cars were coming at them and how close each one passed by on the left.

When the car finally stopped, Trick scrambled to figure out how to open the door, but the handle wouldn't work. He got the window to roll down and was halfway through it when his mom's hand grabbed the back of his jacket and yanked him down into the passenger seat. "This isn't your stop, Trick."

In the back, Brother gathered his backpack and said goodbye before slipping out. Once his door was shut, Trick's window rolled up and the car pulled back onto the road. "Mom! Slow down! Mom. Mom? Mom!"

She sighed.

Finally, they stopped again, in front of another big building with a bunch of kids milling around, but these kids were bigger than the last ones. Trick tried the door again, but it still wouldn't work. When he pushed the button to roll the window down, Mom said, "For goodness sake, Trick, stop. I'll let you out. Just calm down first."

Trick looked at her and tried to calm down. He did. But how could he be sure this wasn't some kind of ruse and she'd blast off onto the road again at any moment? Plus, sitting still gave him time to notice how uncomfortable his feet were. The velcro on his new tennis shoes was fastened loosely, but he still hated how the shoes pressed against his skin and wouldn't let him feel the ground under him.

She noticed him fidgeting and looked at his feet with a frown. "You're not wearing socks."

Well, no, obviously not.

"I told you to wear socks."

"They feel weird." And anyway, wasn't he making a fine concession by wearing shoes? He thought he was.

"Your feet are going to stink by the end of the day."

That had to be a lie. His feet had never stunk in his life, unless he'd stepped in something. Why would they spontaneously start doing it now?

"I guess it doesn't matter," Mom said. "I didn't bring any with me, and it's too late to go back." Her finger hovered over a button on her door, and her eyes met his. "Please try your best. This whole cat/witch thing is behind us, and I want us all to move on with our lives. To be normal for once. Will you help me have that?"

She kept looking at him, so he looked away but nodded. He wasn't really sure what she wanted or how he could do it, but he guessed he could try.

"Thank you," Mom said and stroked the back of his head onc He wished she'd keep doing it, but she dropped her hand and he heard a click. This time, when he wrapped his fingers around the door handle—his weird, human digits were starting to obey him more reliably—it opened for him. He leapt out of the car, dragging his school bag behind him.

As he approached the front steps, Trick pulled a folded-up piece of paper from the back pocket of his jeans. Mom had told him that most of his classes would be in the same room, but some were in other rooms, so he needed to pay attention to where he needed to be at what times. Which meant he also needed to figure out where to go in the first place. There was a map on one side of the paper, which was easy enough to figure out. He'd long ago gotten used to keeping maps of places in his head, so it was convenient to have one ready-made for this new place. But the class schedule on the other side gave him more trouble.

Apparently Room Thirteen was something called 'homeroom', and it was also named beside most of the subjects on the list. There were different subjects in other rooms listed, but he wasn't sure what the third column meant. He understood the idea of telling time by numbers, but he'd never really gotten the hang of actually doing it. Maybe if he just stayed in Room Thirteen until everyone else got up and left, he'd get to the next class when he was supposed to.

He made an annoyed sound in the back of his throat. How could Mom just throw him into school like this? Couldn't she at least have sent Brother with him to help him find his bearings? The younger boy was so much better at this human thing than Trick was.

As Trick studied the paper, he slowly made his way toward the school entrance, weaving around people without even looking up. He was trying to work out the name of his third class in his head— *Preelgebra? No, wait, there's a dash, so those letters are separate.*—when some girl stepped in front of him. He stepped to the side to get around her, but she moved again, surprising him, and he ran smack into her.

Clumsy humans. Can't they see I'm walking?

She hurtled toward the concrete in front of the school's main ~~ntrance but was caught by a blond guy wearing a puffy vest over a ~~hort-sleeved shirt. "Whoa, Amy, you okay?" He helped put her back on her feet, and Trick tried to slip around them and continue on his way. But even while still helping the girl, the blond guy reached out with one hand and grabbed Trick's shoulder. "Dude. Apologize."

A spike of fear at being trapped shot through Trick, and he tried to growl a warning at the boy, but his stupid throat wouldn't work right and it came out like an impatient hum. His gaze ran from the grip on his shoulder, down the boy's startlingly muscular arm, toward eyes that were almost hidden by the boy's lowered brows.

After trying and failing to pull his shoulder from the boy's grip, Trick said the only thing he could think of. "Why? It's her fault. I was trying to get around her."

"Apologize, noob." The grip on his shoulder tightened painfully.

Trick hissed a fierce warning at the boy, satisfied that he could at least still do that. The boy's eyes widened, and he stepped back, releasing Trick—which was good, because the warning was mostly bluff. Without his claws or sharp teeth, Trick wasn't at all sure what he could do to get away from a predator now if running didn't work. Mom had assured him it shouldn't be necessary here at school, but obviously she didn't know anything about school, since he'd been attacked even before getting inside the building.

The girl he'd bumped into had stepped back from him too, as had another girl standing with them. Trick took the opening, darting into the building before the bigger boy could get his hands on him.

Denneka lingered in the back of the bus after all the other kids got off, hunched down behind the back of the seat like she had been ever since she'd slunk down the aisle half an hour ago. Another summer gone. Another year of school to get through. At breakfast, she'd tried one last time to get her parents on board with the idea of homeschooling her, but they kept saying they didn't have time for that, with them both working full-time at the store. She'd insisted that she didn't actually need them to do it, that she could totally homeschool herself, but they wouldn't go for it. "Plus, it's important for your social development," her dad had added.

Spoken like someone who hadn't been a total reject when he'd been her age. She'd tried explaining that too, but they only ever said she wasn't trying hard enough or that it would get better if she kept practicing. Kinda hard to do in a small town, where she'd been stuck with the same group of kids since second grade after they'd moved to Agreste from a much bigger city. Once kids pegged you as a weirdo, you couldn't really 'socially develop' your way into the cool crowd. Heck, she'd settle for any crowd that wasn't the delinquents at this point.

The bus driver appeared in her line of sight, standing over her while doing his last pass to make sure everyone was off. He didn't look surprised to see her hiding there. "I gotta go park the bus in the lot, Denneka," he said calmly. "And you've got about five minutes before the bell."

She sighed and got up, hefting her backpack onto her shoulders. Stepping off the bus, she saw a lot of kids still milling around. No one ever liked to get to the classroom any earlier than necessary. Which was exactly why she'd tried doing it for a while, but that had left her sitting for ten minutes in a room alone with the teacher, which led to the teacher making awkward attempts at conversation, which was worse than dealing with the other kids.

As she made her way up the broad concrete stairs toward the school entrance, she noticed a lot of people standing still and looking at something. When she saw what everyone was staring at, her stomach clenched. It was that boy from the other day. Trick. And he was standing on the top landing in front of the doors with Amy, Trevor, and Flora.

Together. With Trevor's hand on his shoulder like they were old friends.

So it was just as she'd thought. She didn't realize how much she'd been hoping it wasn't true until she felt the bitter disappointment in her gut.

They hadn't seen her yet, so she ducked her head and tried to continue up the stairs and get past them while they were talking.

When she was about ten feet away from them, Trick suddenly made a weird hissing sound, and the others jerked back from him in surprise. Denneka stopped short, her head reflexively snapping toward Trick at the sound. Disbelieving murmurs floated around her, but Denneka was stunned silent. Was this some weird joke between them, or—that horrible hope reared its head again—had Denneka not read the situation right?

While the others were still staring at him in surprise, Trick pulled away and slipped into the school. Once he was gone, people started moving and talking more normally, but Denneka's brain was still working through what had happened, trying to figure it out, so her feet hadn't started moving again.

So she ended up staring like an idiot at the cool kids Trick had been talking to. Trevor glared toward where Trick had gone like he was thinking of going after him. Amy, for some reason, was glaring even harder than him.

"Dang, that blows," Flora said, sounding weirdly disappointed. She gave the blonde girl a commiserating look. "Sorry, Amy. It's not fair when the cute ones turn out to be weirdos."

"Can it, Flora," Amy ground out between her teeth.

But the comment made Trevor turn and look at Amy with a raised eyebrow. "Hey… why did you step into that guy's way?"

Amy's face turned pink. "What? I didn't!"

"I was standing right here," Trevor countered. "You walked into his path like you were *trying* to make him run into you."

"I was not!"

Flora rolled her eyes and took Trevor's hand. "Honestly, Trev, you can be so stupid sometimes." She leaned closer and whispered something to him. Denneka couldn't make out anything other than what sounded like 'cute' and 'single', but it made both of Trevor's eyebrows shoot up.

"*That* weirdo?"

"I didn't *know* he was a weirdo!" Amy protested in an urgent whisper, eyes darting to see how many people were still looking at them. "He just got here. How was I supposed to know that? He *looks* like a halfway normal person."

"And we haven't gotten a new boy at school for, like, three years," Flora added.

"Can we drop it?" Amy asked, still keeping her voice low. "It's embarrassing. And everyone was watching, so now I'll have to make sure no one thinks I was trying to flirt with--" Then she spotted Denneka staring at them, and her voice and face turned hard. "Can we help you with something, dorkface?"

Denneka frantically shook her head and hurried past them. She really didn't want to be late to her first class, after all.

Trick stood in front of the door to Room Thirteen, double-checking the number against the paper that Mom had given him. While he did sometimes have trouble with knowing what to do with numbers, he'd learned to *identify* numbers when he was young, before he'd become a cat, so he felt like he had a pretty solid handle on that part. But after not paying enough attention had already caused him to narrowly avoid a fight this morning, he wanted to be absolutely sure that he was going into the right room now. Wandering into territory he didn't belong in would surely only get him into another fight.

He flexed the fingers of the hand that wasn't holding the paper. If only he still had his claws, maybe he wouldn't be so nervous.

"Um, excuse me," said a small voice.

He looked to the side—and then down—to see a girl a full head shorter than him hunching like she was trying to make herself even smaller. Seeing someone so obviously weaker than him made Trick feel a bit less scared.

"Are you going in?" the girl asked.

Trick noticed a few other people crowding behind him and the girl, and he slipped into the room before any of them decided to attack him. Pressing himself against the wall just inside the room, he watched the small girl and the others stroll past him like they didn't care that he was there.

He already knew that staying out of the way of others (human or animal) was a good way to avoid getting attacked. The problem was that it was a whole lot harder to do when his body was so much bigger now. Even when he wasn't trying to be seen, even when he wasn't making trouble, people still noticed him. He didn't like that.

Most of the kids were sitting at the weird desk/chair things, so he slid into the nearest empty one. Staying perfectly silent so as to avoid drawing attention, he scanned the room—only to find out that somehow, despite being as still and quiet as he could, he was still drawing attention. There were about a dozen kids in the room and a man at a desk up at the front. At least half of the humans were watching him. There was a group of four girls who kept whispering to each other as they all watched him, definitely conspiring how to coordinate their efforts for an attack, if the sharp interest in their eyes was any hint. A couple guys tossed him a look now and then, sizing him up.

Trying not to display any of the fear he felt, Trick met their eyes, careful not to show weakness but trying not to seem like a challenger. When he'd been a cat, he'd always had to pay attention about what other cat's territory he was in. Even though he'd been a cat for seven years and cats were full-grown at one year old, he'd continued to age at a normal human rate. Which meant that for seven years, he'd actually been a kitten. A bigger kitten, but still a kitten. Which meant that even when he'd tried to claim territory back in Three Sisters, it hadn't taken long for some other cat to come around and claim it over him. Usually some huge tomcat three times his size. Sometimes an adult female only twice his size.

He'd learned very quickly not to try challenging any adult cats for territory, even if it was his territory to begin with, and he'd gotten good at finding out which territory was claimed by the less mean and more tolerant cats. The good thing about being a kitten was that, unless he challenged them, other cats usually didn't see him as any kind of threat and left him alone.

Either humans were different from cats in this way or Trick seemed like much more of a threat as a human than he did as a cat.

When Trick's eyes met those of the human man sitting at the front of the room, a shiver ran down his spine that would have raised his hackles if he'd still had any. His back curved defensively, though it probably only looked like he was slouching in his seat.

The man's mouth split open, showing a hint of teeth. A moment later, the smile was gone. The man had a very bland look. Brown hair, brown eyes, and a face so average it would have been hard for Trick to find a way to describe the man. But that smile and the interested way he watched Trick made Trick want to skitter out of the room.

He looked away, choosing to risk showing weakness in order to break the uncomfortable eye contact, and noticed that he hadn't been the only one taking stock of the man. Of the kids who weren't still watching Trick, most were looking at the man.

Motion from the doorway caught Trick's attention, and he saw another girl come in. The recognition she triggered felt like a calming caress to his insides. Finally, something familiar. He couldn't remember the girl's name—he'd never been good with names—but he remembered her face. She also had brown hair and brown eyes and was a bit boring-looking, but there was something about how she looked that made the tightness in his muscles relax and his racing heart slow down a little.

Her body was tense, her movements quick. Was she as scared as he was? That couldn't be right. She was used to being human. She belonged here. Her eyes met his for a second, then she huddled into an empty seat three spots in front of him.

Trick swallowed nervously. If someone who belonged here was afraid, what were *his* chances of ever getting through this?

Then the aggressive boy who'd attacked him on the way into school and the two girls with him came into the room. Trick's hands curled, but he had no claws and he was sure the man would take their side if the aggressive boy attacked. But he didn't. The three of them gave Trick dirty looks, but they went to the other side of the room and found seats.

Dirty looks, he could handle. Maybe his warning had worked.

A loud bell rang out in the hall, and the man got up from behind his desk and closed the door, trapping them all inside.

———

Denneka watched with everyone else as the unknown teacher moved to stand in front of the whiteboard, hands clasped casually behind his back. They all quieted as he did so, waiting. It was not, as a general rule, so easy to get the attention of a class full of thirteen-year-olds, but any time they got a new teacher was an unusual occasion, worth their full attention.

Besides that, they were probably all wondering what this meant about Mr. Haug.

"Good morning," the teacher said, giving them a pleasant but impersonal smile. "I am Mr. McKenzie. I'll be your homeroom teacher until such time as… I am not."

"Where's Mr. Haug?" asked a boy from the back. Sounded like Ian.

"I'm certain I don't know," Mr. McKenzie said blithely.

"Wasn't he supposed to be our homeroom teacher?" Ian persisted.

Mr. McKenzie's smile fell; he was losing patience. "Quite possibly. I am not privy to the details. Your principal needed a teacher on short notice, and I was available. Now—"

"Where'd you come from, anyway?" Ian asked.

Denneka winced. Ian meant well, but he'd never known when to shut up.

Mr. McKenzie's mouth curled into a smile as he looked at Ian, but unlike the pleasant one from before, this time it was sharp and mocking. "Haven't your parents explained that to you by now?"

This was met with a stunned, confused silence, until he added, "If you have questions regarding human reproduction, please save them for health class."

Half the class erupted into laughter. Not because he'd said anything particularly witty, of course, but because of the smackdown he'd given Ian. Denneka knew better than anyone, if there was one thing some of her classmates loved, it was seeing people they already looked down on being put in their place.

Denneka didn't laugh. She turned to see Ian blushing and sinking low in his seat. She tried to give him a supportive smile, but he didn't meet her eyes. As she started to turn back toward the front of the room, she noticed Trick. He wasn't laughing either. He was sitting stiff and hunched, looking wildly at the sudden outburst from his classmates as if he couldn't understand what it meant.

Mr. McKenzie turned to the whiteboard and, consulting a sheet of paper, sloppily wrote out a seating chart. "When you're in this classroom, you will sit in your assigned seat," he announced, silencing the lingering snickers. "Starting now." He stared at them all expectantly.

After a few seconds, most people got the hint and started getting up and exchanging seats. The chart was alphabetical by last name, putting Denneka near the back of the class, which she was more than fine with. Fortunately, her new seat was vacant when she arrived at it, so she was able to take her place without any awkward interactions with others. Then she waited and watched while the rest of the class took their new seats.

Most of them, anyway.

After everyone else had sat down, Bobby Juarez was left standing by the desk he was supposed to be in, arguing with Trick, who hadn't yet left it.

Well, arguing *at* Trick, really, since Trick wasn't bothering to answer him back. He just stared at the seating chart with his head slightly cocked.

"Is there a problem?" Mr. McKenzie asked.

"The new kid won't get up," Bobby said.

Mr. McKenzie's eyes ran over the room, spotted the empty desk at the front, and consulted his paper copy of the seating chart. "Patrick Andrew," he drawled, leveling an impatient glare at Trick. "Is there some reason you haven't taken your assigned seat?"

Sitting in the back, Denneka couldn't really see Trick's face, but it was a long beat before he responded. "That's not my name."

"Excuse me?" Mr. McKenzie asked in a flat, warning tone.

"My last name isn't Andrew. It's St. Andrew. Which, I'm pretty sure, starts with an S."

That startled a few laughs out of people, but Mr. McKenzie's piercing eyes silenced them instantly. Denneka couldn't really blame him for getting angry. From anyone else, Trick's words would almost definitely have been meant sarcastically. Denneka knew all too well how Trick's mild, blunt words could come across as a particularly flat delivery of sarcastic insults. But now, seeing that he spoke that way to everyone and not just her, she was beginning to think it was merely the way he was.

Mr. McKenzie's face hardened, but before he responded to Trick, he looked down at the seating chart again, then went to his desk and consulted another paper. In the tense silence of the classroom, everyone could hear the teacher's muttered curse. Then he straightened and told Trick, "So it is." He went to the seating chart he'd written on the whiteboard, erased 'Patrick Andrew' and everything after it, and wrote the whole thing out with 'Patrick St. Andrew' in the correct place. Then he turned and glowered at Trick as if it had all been his fault. "You heard him, everyone. Mustn't keep the young master waiting."

Amidst snickers and groans of annoyance, books were shuffled, bags hefted, and everyone behind Wanda Aaron shifted one seat over. Denneka was already picking up her books to move when she noticed that the handful of kids down the list from her weren't moving their things. She looked back at the chart.

And noticed that 'Patrick St. Andrew' was now assigned a seat directly to the right of 'Denneka Sparrow'. The seat she was currently in.

She quickly moved a seat to her left, her heart leaping like a rabbit at a dog race.

While everyone else was still moving, Trick picked up his bag and slipped around the side and back of the room, sliding into the seat beside her so smoothly that if she hadn't been so attuned to him, she might not have even noticed. Inexplicably afraid to look over but unable to help herself, she turned her head.

Those grass green eyes were already watching her, wide and a bit wild. He was slouching as if trying not to get noticed again. "You're that girl. The one who helped me get dressed," he said in a quiet voice.

Not quiet enough to stop the boy in front of him from turning his head to raise an eyebrow at Denneka, though.

"Shh!" Denneka hissed at Trick. "Don't mention it. I mean *that*. Don't mention *that* ever again, okay?"

"Why?"

She let out a frustrated breath. What was this guy's deal? "Just don't."

He didn't respond, but he did keep staring at her. They were mesmerizing, those eyes. So green. Denneka couldn't manage to look away. But while he didn't say anything, the wildness in his eyes gradually eased as the stiffness in his body softened and he sank a little further into the chair.

When his eyelids had begun to very slowly drift closed and he still hadn't looked away from her, Denneka blurted out, "What?"

"The chair's warm," he said contentedly, which made Denneka blush.

———

The bit of peace that Trick had managed to find in all this scary chaos thanks to the familiar girl and a warm seat vanished as soon as the teacher man up front spoke again.

"If everyone is settled," the man said sharply, "why don't we go around the room and introduce ourselves. I collect I am not the only new face to this class. For my benefit, as well as Patrick's, tell us your name and something about yourself."

"Trick," Trick said in a small voice. He really didn't want to challenge the man, but 'Patrick' was what his mom called him when she was especially angry at him.

To his surprise, the man heard him. "Excuse me?"

Trick spoke a little louder. "I go by Trick."

The teacher man snorted. "That's ridiculous. You'll go by Patrick in my class."

And just like that, the man slapped Trick's challenge down and put him in his place. At least he'd done it without inflicting any actual injury.

The aggressive boy and the two girls with him laughed louder than anyone else at the man's words.

The teacher man pointed at the girl in the front left desk, and she gave her name and some other stuff Trick didn't bother paying attention to. He tried to avoid the man's eyes as one kid after another talked about themselves. It was mostly the same. They'd been in this town their whole lives or close to it. They had families who had jobs. He gathered the aggressive boy and two girls had parents who were important somehow, but he didn't quite pay enough attention to work out how. There were words he'd heard before but didn't really understand—mayor, administrator, CEO. He had a vague idea that the words meant the kids' parents held a lot of territory, or something like that.

When the familiar girl stood up to speak, Trick watched her closely.

"Hi, um, I'm Denneka," she said, her eyes on her desk. That wasn't very smart. Trick could tell she was scared, but she wasn't trying to hide it at all. She showed weakness too easily; she might as well have lain on the floor and rolled over. Couldn't she tell how dangerous some of these humans were? "Most of you know me. Obviously. Um, I've been here since second grade. My parents own Sparrows', a clothing shop on Main Street. That's, um, about it." She sat down, and her eyes flicked over to him.

He stared into them until the teacher man said making Trick look at him instead. "Please stand and te. yourself."

Everyone was looking at him. The whole class. Every hu the room had turned in his direction and was watching him. had a strong urge to bolt for the door or maybe even the nea. window.

But Mom had asked him to try, and she'd warned him that something like this might happen and told him what to say. So he swallowed his fear as much as he could, looked into the kids' eyes long enough to not show weakness, and then said, "I'm Trick."

"Don't you mean Patrick?" the aggressive boy said in a loud voice.

Trick met his eyes and repeated, "I'm Trick."

The boy's laughter died.

When Trick didn't continue, the teacher man said, "And... something about yourself, Patrick?"

Trick was starting to really not like that man. He'd already shown his dominance. Did he really have to keep calling him the wrong name? But it wouldn't do Trick any good to challenge him again on that. "I just moved to town with my mom and little brother," he said, trying very hard to remember what Mom had told him to say if he was asked something like this.

"Oh?" said the man. He sounded polite, but there was something... off about his tone. "Where's your father?"

That wasn't one of the questions Mom had prepared him for, so Trick simply told the truth. "I don't know. After my mom got pregnant with me, he left, so I've never met him."

That fact had never struck Trick as something worth getting bothered about, so he was confused by the odd silence that followed his statement. The corners of the man's mouth twitched, and the aggressive boy let out a loud laugh.

"He's such a freak, even his dad didn't want him," said the girl who'd run into Trick, while her friend snickered. Several kids were

some were looking back at him with strange expres-
others had looked away from him entirely.

unfortunate," the teacher man said, but his mouth had
curl up at the edges. "And yet, it begs the question: If your
left, how did you acquire a younger brother?"

another question Mom hadn't prepared Trick for. Just as he
opened his mouth, the familiar girl beside him whispered, "You
don't have to answer that." He looked down to see her brown eyes
wide and filled with... was it fear? No. He couldn't tell. It was so
much harder to read human faces than an animal's body language.
If only they had tails and proper ears to help express themselves.

Since he couldn't figure out what she meant and it seemed like
refusing to talk might be taken as another challenge by the man, he
answered the man's question. "She said she didn't need a father.
Only a..." He searched around, trying to remember the term she'd
used that time—way back when she'd still been trying to give him a
sibling—when he'd caught her in a bad enough mood to answer his
question. "...sperm donor." He hadn't understood what she'd
meant at the time, and even later, after she'd explained to him how
humans mate, he still wasn't sure he did.

The teacher man burst into laughter so sudden and so genuinely
pleased that Trick only blinked and stared at him. A moment later,
some of the kids started laughing, too, but the familiar girl had
turned red and put her hand over her face.

After several seconds, the teacher man's laughter diminished to
a wide smirk, his voice a warm murmur when he said, "Oh,
indeed?" But then he forced the smile from his face, and the
unpleasant scowl returned. "That was a highly inappropriate thing
to say in class, Patrick. I think I shall have to give you a detention.
And on your first day," he said with a *tsk*.

Trick could only stare at him in confusion. What had he said?
He'd only answered the man's questions honestly. And what was a
detention?

Despite the snickering, muttering, and odd looks from around

the room, it seemed like Trick was now allowed to sit back d
he did.

The boy beside him hesitantly stood and introduced him.
When all the kids had talked about themselves, the teacher m
said, "Thank you. Now, it's about time we got started. English
first—"

"Excuse me."

Trick looked beside him to the familiar girl. Her face was still
red, and her hand was in the air, but she was looking directly at the
teacher man.

The man glanced at the seating chart, and then raised an
eyebrow at her. "Denneka, isn't it?"

"Yes."

"You have a question?"

The girl's face got even redder, but she boldly said, "You didn't
tell us anything about yourself, Mr. McKenzie. Shouldn't you intro-
duce yourself, too?"

He considered this, then said, "My name is John McKenzie. I,
also, am new to town. I am your teacher. And… that is all you need
to know." His eyes narrowed and shifted from the girl to Trick and
back. "Except for one more thing. I do not permit interruptions
when I am speaking. Raising your hand is fine, but do not speak
unless I call on you. You also get a detention, Denneka."

"But I didn't know—"

The man's eyebrow went up.

The girl stopped talking and lowered her eyes.

You shouldn't have challenged him, Trick thought at her. Already so
weak, already having shown that weakness so easily, why had she
challenged the man? Unless she hadn't meant it as a challenge. It
had only been a question. But this man seemed to take anything as a
challenge, so staying quiet and not saying anything was obviously
the safest way to go.

That was exactly what Trick planned to do from now on when he
was around this man and especially in his classroom. He would

ught the man would be satisfied with that, but it turned out
n't.

rtway into their first period, the teacher man looked directly at
k and said, "Patrick, would you please read the next section?"

Trick kept his mouth shut.

"Patrick?" the man said after a moment.

Trick met his eyes.

"The next section, please?"

"The last time you wanted me to talk, you didn't like what I
said," Trick pointed out.

"That doesn't mean you get to not participate in class. Just read
what's written and you should be fine."

*'Talk.' 'Don't talk.' 'Talk, but not about that.' 'Talk, but not at that
time.' Why are human rules so complicated?*

Trick looked at the next section in the book. He hadn't read
aloud since he was a little kid, and it felt weird. "The good man
drank his cho... co... late"—wait, he knew that one—"chocolate,
and then went to look for his horse; but passing through an ar...
bower... of roses, he re... mem... bred..."

"Patrick?" said the man.

Trick looked up from the book.

"Are you having some trouble?"

The aggressive boy snickered. "He can't even read."

That wasn't true. Trick could read. Mom had taught him. He
only had trouble with the long words. And the ones he'd never
spoken aloud before.

When he looked down at the familiar girl, her eyes were tight
like she was in pain.

"Hmm," the teacher man hummed impatiently. "All right,
Patrick, that's enough. Amy, please continue."

———

When the bell signaling the end of second period rang, Denneka let
out a sigh of relief. Finally, she'd be able to get away from Mr.

McKenzie for one class before she had to come back. What an irritating man. Asking poor Trick the most inappropriate, prying questions, then giving her detention for something she couldn't have known was against his rules.

It had been worth it, though. After the way he'd harassed Trick, she'd wanted to do something to get back at him, and pointing out that he hadn't reciprocated when it came to sharing was the least she could do.

How weird that he'd so pointedly avoided sharing anything, though. She'd say it was suspicious... if she had anything to suspect him of. Other than being a jerk.

Of course the cool kids had loved him. That was obvious immediately. Why wouldn't they, when he took such enjoyment from bullying the same kids they bullied? Though he hadn't mocked Trick for not being able to read well, for whatever that was worth.

Covered by the general noise and bustle of kids getting their stuff together for their next class, Denneka leaned over to Trick. "He shouldn't have asked you those questions about your family. I think I'll complain to the principal about him. That was way too personal."

"Too personal?" he repeated like he didn't understand what the words meant.

Well, he was a boy. Maybe it didn't bother him like it would bother a girl.

"Never mind." She ducked her head, pretending to sort through her backpack.

He got his things and stood but didn't walk away. When she looked up from her bag, she saw he was staring at a piece of paper. Since she could see the school map on the back, she figured it was his schedule.

"What, um... what class do you have next?" she asked.

"Drama."

A pang of disappointment hit her stomach, and she pushed it aside. How silly could she be? "What room?"

"Twenty?"

"Oh. I have art in Twenty-One. Do you… um… want me to show you the way?" It was a ridiculous offer. Their school was small enough that there was only one hallway, and the room numbers ran in the usual order.

But he sounded slightly relieved when he said, "Yes."

He seemed to be waiting, so she got up and pushed past him. As they left the classroom, they happened to walk by Amy and the others.

"Hey, look," Trevor said. "Weird and weirder."

Amy and Flora laughed cruelly.

Denneka kept her head down and kept walking. When they were well past those three, she glanced behind her to see Trick following on her heels. His expression was passive, as if he hadn't even heard them, though she knew he had to have. Did their taunts really not bother him? She remembered how he'd responded to Trevor in class, insisting he was 'Trick' and not 'Patrick' despite the teacher and Trevor both. He'd done that so coolly, not getting angry or defensive or anything.

Coolly. Yeah. Maybe that was what actual coolness was, not the mean arrogance that Trevor, Amy, and Flora displayed. Maybe Trick was what people really meant when they said 'cool' like it was a good thing.

As she was looking back at him, his green eyes met hers, and her heart fluttered around in her chest like a butterfly. She had to look away so she didn't lose her footing and run into someone.

What was wrong with her? Sure, he was cute, but she'd seen cute boys before. None of them had ever made her feel like she was about to have a medical emergency.

Denneka focused on weaving through the crowd of students, but when she got to the midpoint of the hallway, where the office was, they hit a traffic jam. She looked around, trying to see why people were stopped, and noticed something new pinned to the main bulletin board. Curious, she pressed closer.

It turned out to only be old news, but maybe a lot of kids didn't read the paper. Pinned to the bulletin board was a notice that

Bradley Haug was missing and that any information about his whereabouts should be directed to the police. It had been big news over the weekend after the paper had first reported it, but from the looks of things, there weren't any new developments.

There were so many people crowded around her and talking that she hadn't noticed Trick step up beside her, so close their shoulders were touching, until she turned to go and saw him staring at the photo on the notice.

"Who's that?" Trick asked.

"Mr. Haug," Denneka explained. "He was supposed to have been our homeroom teacher, but he went missing last week. Apparently that's why we got stuck with Mr. McKenzie."

"He's not missing. I know where he is."

"What?" That didn't make any sense. Trick was new to town. He hadn't even known who Mr. Haug was until she'd told him a second ago. How could he know anything about him? Still, she asked, "Where is he?"

"In a grave."

CHAPTER
FIVE

It was definitely the same guy. Even though in the photo he looked a lot more alive than the corpse Trick had seen, he had the same bald head, big nose, and beard. Trick wasn't so good at remembering words or numbers, but faces and places were something he was really good with. So even though the man in the photo was smiling and wasn't as strangely colored as the corpse, Trick was positive they were the same.

Speaking of color, the familiar girl's face suddenly got several shades paler. "What?" she whispered at him.

It was pretty loud and busy here. Maybe she hadn't heard him. He opened his mouth to speak louder, but she slapped her hand over it. Trick jerked back at the sudden attack. Shock and betrayal clouded his mind as he tried to get away from her, but the crowd pressed close, keeping him trapped.

"Sorry!" the girl yelped. "Sorry! I just mean, not here!" She held her hands up, palms toward him. He'd seen humans show him their palms before. It meant something like, *I don't intend to hurt you.* Even though she'd grabbed him, she hadn't actually hurt him like the aggressive boy had when he'd grabbed Trick. Warily, Trick stopped trying to get away (the person behind him was complaining anyway, and he didn't want to get into another fight) and stood watching her. "Follow me," she said. "Please."

He almost didn't, less pleased with her company than he'd been a minute ago. But if he didn't, he'd be left stuck in the middle of this crowd, so he did.

The familiar girl led him out a side door and onto a concrete path beside a nice, big stretch of grass. The warm sun and fresh air instantly made him feel better.

"Sorry about, um, touching you," said the girl. Her face had gone pink again. It seemed to do so now and then for no reason Trick could figure out. He hadn't ever seen other humans change colors like she did. Maybe it was a defense mechanism? Or maybe she was sick? "But what on earth did you mean by Mr. Haug is in a grave? That's—that's—super creepy and morbid!"

"Morbid?" He didn't know that word.

"Yeah! Why would you say that?"

The same reason he ever bothered to say anything, except when Mom told him he should say something else. "Because it's true."

"How do you know? You've never even met Mr. Haug."

"I saw him," Trick explained. "In a grave."

The girl's mouth opened and closed, and she blinked several times. "What?" she finally spat out. "How? When?"

Trick considered his answer. Just before he started to explain, he remembered that this was part of what Mom had forbidden him to say anything about. So he didn't answer. When the girl kept watching him, though, he figured it was probably expected that he say something. "I'm... not supposed to talk about it."

"Talk about *what?*" the girl demanded.

"About when I was a cat."

Whoops.

The girl's mouth fell open again. "When... when you were what?"

"I mean, not that. I mean something else." Those stupid human talking/no-talking rules again.

"What do you mean, when you were a cat? Is that, like, slang for something?"

Nope, no more talking. He might have to talk sometimes to avoid a fight with the teacher man, but he'd seen how weak this girl was, and he was pretty sure he could take her in a fight if he had to.

"Trick? Hello?"

The sun sure was nice. And the grass looked soft. Maybe he could take his shoes off and feel it under his pa—feet. There were some nice trees over there to climb, and—*Ooh! A finch!*

Trick dropped his bag and sprinted toward the finch standing right there on the ground in front of that tree like an idiot. Birds were so stupid sometimes. But delicious. Running was awkward on two legs, but he'd had enough practice at walking by now that he didn't fall on his face. When he judged he was close enough, he pounced, diving at the finch with both fore—hands stretched out and grasping.

But he wasn't as quick as he should have been, and the finch saw him coming a mile away and casually flitted up into the tree. Meanwhile, Trick couldn't stop his momentum and landed face-first on the ground. He pushed himself to his hands and knees, glaring at the bird now perched on a branch.

Stupid big, human body. He was going to have to re-figure his whole hunting technique.

The finch chirped at him. Cocky finch. He'd show it. He crept around the back side of the tree and…

Shoot. He'd have to learn how to climb without claws now, too. Being human was the worst.

Then again, the branch the finch was perched on was a lot closer to him than it would have been when he was a cat, even with him still standing on the ground. Maybe he could jump up and grab it.

He crouched, gaze pinned on the finch, preparing to spring.

"Um, Trick?" said the girl, who was suddenly right in front of him.

Startled, Trick tried to scramble back, but his clumsy body made him fall on his nonexistent tail.

The finch flew higher up the tree.

Trick glared at the girl.

"The, uh… the bell rang. We should get to class before we're late. You still want me to show you where yours is?"

Class. School. Human stuff. How annoying.

Trick got to his feet, walked back to where he'd dropped his bag, and picked it up. He waited for the girl to lead him inside, following her through the hall until she pointed to a room and told him to go there. He verified the number against his schedule to be sure. The classroom was pretty full already, but he was able to find a seat in the back. The human at the front of this one was a woman. He hoped that meant she wouldn't be as territorial toward him as the man had been.

———

Kester John McKenzie was sitting behind his desk in his otherwise unoccupied classroom when the principal came in, closing the door behind her.

"Good morning, John," she said. "Got a moment?" In a pencil-skirted suit, tight bun, and black-framed glasses, she was the perfect picture of an educational professional. Not a hint of flirtation imbued her polite smile.

Not that Kester would expect to see any from her—or any woman for that matter. Not with him looking like he did now. He'd needed to hide himself in plain sight, to make sure that no one who knew him or had ever met him would be able to recognize him. He could have become ugly, but actively repulsing people wouldn't have suited his purposes. So he'd softened and dulled everything about himself, from his coloring to the lines of his face to muscula-ture which he usually kept lean and well-defined with the help of his magic. The change had been so complete that when Lisa had met him for the second (but as far as she knew, first) time, she'd declared that she could barely see any family resemblance to his cousin Kester at all.

"Certainly, Lisa. How can I help you?"

There was nowhere for her to sit other than at one of the students' desks or on top of his. He fought back a smile at the mental image that observation conjured. He didn't know her particularly well, but he could tell she wasn't the type of person to be caught dead taking either option. So, as he suspected she would, she strode closer—close enough to converse, far enough to maintain an appropriate distance from his personal space—and contrived not to appear the least bit awkward by using her hands to gesture slightly as she spoke. "I've had a conversation with one of your students."

That didn't sound good. "Oh?"

"There were some… complaints regarding your behavior. More specifically, your way of speaking to certain students during class."

He waved a hand dismissively, the heavy gold watch on his left wrist an unfamiliar weight. He'd needed a vessel to hold the magic of his current transformation, and the watch was just gaudy enough to not fit in with his boring teacher persona. The incongruity amused him. "Whoever it was, I'm sure they were exaggerating. I'm not a coddler, and some people take that as being mean. Did this student say specifically which comments they didn't like?"

"No, but she implied they were the sorts of comments she didn't feel comfortable repeating."

"*She*, is it? Don't tell me it's that girl who got a detention for speaking out of turn. Clearly, she's overreacting."

"Not her," said Lisa. "Although now that you bring it up, I'd like to talk about that as well. Two detentions in your very first class, John? Don't you think that's a little excessive?"

"I find it's helpful to make a firm first impression. Let the kids know I won't tolerate nonsense or insubordination in class."

She nodded slightly. "I can appreciate that. But now that you've made your statement, you might want to lighten up a little. The boy is brand new to this school, and I'd prefer he not think we're all out to get him. And Denneka is far from a troublemaker. She only had two detentions last year, both of them for persistently reading on her phone when she was supposed to be participating in group activities."

"A nerd, is she?" When Lisa's eyes narrowed behind her glasses, he held up his hands. "Sorry. I didn't realize that word was still considered an insult. I meant to ask if she's bookish."

Lisa considered the question for a moment. "I suppose you could call her bookish, yes. Not particularly studious, but her grades are good enough. From what I've gathered, she prefers fiction. Does quite well in English. She doesn't seem to interact much with others, though, and isn't eager to participate in class. Giving her a detention when she does bother to speak up probably isn't going to help that."

"Are you asking me to retract the detentions?"

"No," she answered. "It wouldn't look good for me to undermine your authority immediately like that. Just... try to ease up from now on. And watch how you speak to them. There are the parents to consider. I can't imagine Trick or Denneka's parents will be thrilled to hear about them getting detention on the first day of class, though some of the other parents could have caused us real grief if you'd targeted their kids to make an example of."

"Oh, I know the kids you mean. Don't worry, they were easy to spot right off. If it makes you feel any better, I think I won them firmly to my side by choosing the... weaker members of the herd to pick off."

Lisa pressed her fingers to her forehead as if rubbing out a headache. "No, that doesn't make me feel better. Those brats already feel too untouchable—and largely are." She shook her head. "Never mind that. What's done is done. But you might want to know how we handle detentions. All detentions for the week are done on Friday after school, and the teacher who hands out the first detention of the week gets to preside over it."

Kester would have laughed at that, maybe even congratulated her for scoring a touch, but he didn't think it would have been in character for 'John', so he forced his face into a scowl and muttered, "I see. Guess it's a good thing I hadn't yet made plans for Friday evening." But he couldn't quite manage to keep himself from being a little cheeky. "Does the principal ever give out detentions?"

"When necessary," she answered. And then her strict professionalism cracked the smallest degree, a tiny hint of the playfulness he knew she had in her showing in the momentary softening of her eyes and quirk of her mouth. "But the policy says the first *teacher* to give one."

She still wasn't flirting with him, only softening a bit to create some goodwill with a new employee. Even knowing that, it was hard for Kester to keep the scowl on his face. "Thus preserving *your* Friday evenings from disruption."

The playfulness vanished as soon as it had come. "You'd better believe it."

He needed to change the subject before he made an allusion to how she spent her Friday evenings. Maintaining his false persona was important to his longer-term goal, no matter how satisfying momentary amusement would be. "Would you like me to call the parents to explain about the detentions?" he offered. "I could probably smooth things over a little."

"That's a good idea. I'll leave you to it." With that, Lisa nodded her goodbye and left.

Kester looked up the contact info for Denneka's parents first. When he placed the call, a woman answered. "Sparrows'. How can I help you?"

"Hello. Is this Mrs. Sparrow?"

"No. Hang on."

He heard muffled voices, then another woman came on the line. "This is Keri Sparrow. What can I do for you?"

"Hello. I'm John McKenzie, your daughter Denneka's homeroom teacher."

"Oh. Hello. Is Denneka okay?"

"She's fine. It's nothing to be concerned about. I only wanted to warn you that she'll have detention this Friday after school, so you may need to make arrangements for her to get home."

Keri let out a breath. "What was it? Reading again?"

"Speaking out of turn."

There was a pause, then, "Denneka? Are you sure?"

"It was a very minor thing, I assure you. Principal VanBuren has already rebuked me for being overly harsh. Though Denneka *did* interrupt me in class, so we thought it was better not to retract the detention."

"Oh. Okay. I guess I can understand that. This won't go on her record, will it?"

He honestly didn't know, but he didn't think he was lying when he said, "No."

"Good. You didn't have to call me, Mr. McKenzie. I'm sure Denneka would have 'fessed up to it herself."

A responsible, well-behaved girl, was she? "Given the circumstances, I wanted to make sure you didn't react too harshly when she did."

"Well, thanks. I don't think I've heard your name before. Are you a new teacher?"

"I recently moved to town. I'm filling in for as long as needed while Mr. Haug is missing."

"Welcome to town. Stop by the shop some time and say hi. Mark and I would like to meet you."

"I'm sure I'll be by sooner or later. Thank you for your time." He hung up and sat back, interlacing his fingers.

Denneka Sparrow had been of absolutely no interest to Kester until he'd seen how Trick looked at her in class. It wasn't wariness and fear, the way he'd been looking at everyone else. It was... *Hmm.* On a human, he'd have said it was indifference. But Trick had only been human again for a few days and hadn't learned to emote like a human. And for a cat, the eye contact and body language would have expressed something at least slightly positive.

There was a connection between the nerdy girl and the kitten boy. So of course Kester simply had to find out what it was and where it would lead.

It was too bad the girl had to be so mundane, though. Normal, boring girl. Normal, boring family. 'Good enough' grades. She was even boring to look at. Kester wasn't sure he'd even bothered looking directly at her until he'd noticed Trick watching her.

That would change, of course. Now. No matter how dull and average Denneka was, Kester's intervention assured that her life was about to take a turn for the interesting. Really, she should thank him.

He dialed Jacqueline's number. It was quite a while before she answered, and when she did, her tone was terse.

"What is it? I'm working."

Kester smiled, picturing her hunched over a keyboard. Had she had time to set up a home office yet, or was she working at the kitchen table? "Hello, Ms. St. Andrew. I'm John McKenzie, Trick's teacher."

A most-likely-involuntary groan came over the line. "What's he done?"

Kester didn't rush to answer, letting her imagination run wild with that for a few seconds. What was the worst case scenario she was imagining? "Nothing to be concerned about. Used some... indelicate words in class. I just wanted to warn you that he received a detention for it, to be served Friday after school, in case you'll need to make arrangements to get him."

"They give detentions for that?"

"I do. Although I've already been warned by the principal that it was too harsh."

"So why did you?"

Because the more I make Trick hate school, the more he'll resist adapting to human life, and the more entertaining it will be to watch him. "I'm new to this school as well. I suppose I'm used to a stricter environment."

"So, can't you cancel the detention?"

"The principal thinks it's best not to. For appearances, mostly."

"What did he say that got him in trouble?"

"I think he was repeating something you'd said, actually. Something about"—Kester could hardly speak through his delighted grin —"a sperm donor."

"What? When did he—" She groaned again, more loudly. "All

right. Crap. That's embarrassing. He's... got some problems under-standing social interaction. So, sometimes, he... overshares."

"I'll keep that in mind."

"If he does, um, anything else that's odd, please don't mind it. He doesn't mean any harm."

"Is he..." What was the term people used? "...on the spectrum?"

"What? You mean autistic? No." She sounded slightly insulted, but when she continued, Kester detected a hint of relief. Still, she didn't quite take the excuse he'd offered her. "I mean, I don't think so. I haven't had him tested. He's just... unusual. He's a good kid, though. He's been homeschooled until now, so he's got to learn everything about school life from scratch. If possible, I'd appreciate it if you took that into consideration when dealing with him. I can hardly get him to go to school as it is."

That sounded promising. Perhaps he ought to lighten up a bit, though. If Trick ended up protesting so much that Jacqueline actu-ally pulled him out of school, Kester would lose his opportunity for personal observation. He didn't really think Jacqueline would ever give in, no matter how much Trick complained, but it was a risk, however small. "For your sake, Ms. St. Andrew, I'll see what I can do." He hesitated then, wondering if he should push his luck. Oh, what was the harm? "Is your younger son as unusual as Trick?"

"How did you know—"

"Since it's the first day of class, I asked all the students to intro-duce themselves and tell me something about them. That was what precipitated Trick's... oversharing."

"Oh. No, Landon's very well-adjusted. I spend so much of my energy dealing with Trick, it's a relief to have one son who's self-sufficient, especially for a six-year-old. I don't have any worries about him at all."

Perhaps you should, Kester thought. But that was enough on that topic for now. "I'll let you get back to your work. Thank you for taking my call, Ms. St. Andrew."

"No problem... sorry, what was your name again?"

"John McKenzie."

"Thank you, John. And please call me Jacqueline."

"I'll do that. Until next time, Jacqueline."

———

"I can help with that if you want, Miss Cutler," Landon offered. The rest of the kids had left as soon as school was over, even though the stuff from the project they'd been doing was only half picked-up.

The teacher, a nice lady with curly blonde hair, smiled at him. "Oh, you're so sweet for offering, Landon. Thank you. I can finish this up, although it would be helpful if you wanted to pop those books back on the shelf before you go."

Landon would have done so even if she hadn't asked. He hated seeing books thrown around and left on the floor. After he finished, he saw that Miss Cutler was nearly done cleaning up. She came over to him, looking in surprise at the shelf. "You alphabetized them?"

"It's what I do with my books at home."

She gave him another smile. Not one like she gave most of the kids, which looked like how an adult smiles at a little kid. For a second, she smiled at him like an adult smiles at another adult.

Maybe it was the tie.

He'd had to dress his best today. The first day of school, especially a brand new school, was an event. First impressions were important. So he'd worn his new red shirt and tan slacks and a blue tie. It was a clip-on, because he hadn't gotten the hang of tying his real ties right, but he thought it still looked pretty good.

Some of the other boys had made fun of him, but they'd been wearing t-shirts with stupid cartoon characters on them, and at recess he'd seen them playing with a dead rat beside the schoolyard fence, so he didn't really care much what they thought.

None of the girls had teased him. Most of them had been really nice to him. Girls usually were.

Miss Cutler gave him a pat on the shoulder, thanked him again, and told him not to keep his mom waiting. Landon picked up his messenger bag and headed out to the front of the school, where Mom had said she would pick him up.

As he came around a corner in the hall, he stopped. Some other boys were blocking his path.

"Excuse me," Landon said, trying to find a gap between them to get through.

One of the boys turned to face him with a sneer. "It's the preppy kid. What do you want, preppy?"

"I just need to get through."

Another boy, much bigger than him, pushed forward to block Landon's path even more. "Why do you dress like that? It's weird."

"I like to look nice," he said simply.

"What are you, a girl?"

"No. Are you?" Honestly, sometimes it *was* hard to tell.

Anger flashed in the big boy's face, and he grabbed Landon's tie and yanked. He'd probably meant to pull Landon off his feet with it, but since it was a clip-on, it only came off in his hand. The boy looked at it stupidly.

"Give that back," Landon said in a darker tone. They were starting to make him mad.

The big boy tossed the tie on the floor and grabbed a handful of Landon's shirt, raising his fist like he meant to hit him.

Landon reached his own hand up to cover the bigger one fisted at his chest, letting his anger out. The boy's whole body jerked, his back curving backward, and he fell to his knees. While he gasped, trying to get his breath, and the other boys pestered him about what was wrong, Landon slipped around them and continued on his way.

His hands were shaking when he got into his mom's car, but she didn't notice.

"How was school?" Mom asked.

"Okay," he said. He hadn't ever hurt anyone that much before.

"Was your teacher nice?"

"Yes." He didn't know exactly what he'd done to the big boy, but he thought it might have had to do with the boy's heart.

"Do you get along with the other kids?"

"Mostly." The boy had been about to hit him. He was only defending himself. Why did he feel bad about that at all?

"Mostly? Any problems I should know about?"

He didn't have any reason to feel bad. The boy had had it coming, and now he probably wouldn't mess with Landon again. Probably the others wouldn't either. And it wasn't like they could tell on him.

Landon relaxed. "No."

CHAPTER
SIX

On Tuesday morning, Denneka waited for the bus at the end of her driveway, as usual, and when it came, she shuffled down the aisle, all the way to the back, also as usual. Somewhere around third grade, it had come to be understood that the back left seat was hers. Even though she didn't get on until at least half the other kids had already been picked up, that seat was always open. And even though she shoved herself into the corner by the window, no one ever sat beside her.

Until today.

The bus had already started moving again and Denneka had pulled out her phone and started reading when she saw movement out of the corner of her eye. She jerked her head up, startled, to see Trick slide into the seat beside her.

He didn't look at her. He didn't sit close enough to be touching her. Nor did he say anything. He was just… there.

"H-hey," Denneka tried.

Trick hadn't said a word to her for the whole rest of the day yesterday, after she'd caught him chasing a bird. At least, it had sure looked like he was chasing a bird. She wasn't sure what else it rightfully could have been, and he hadn't bothered explaining anything to her.

Other than that comment he'd made about 'when he was a cat', whatever that meant. Denneka was afraid it meant that he really was a weirdo. Which upset her so much—not that Trick might be weird, but that she could still consider anyone a weirdo after people had called her that most of her life—that she hadn't tried to talk to him when they'd come back to homeroom. But then he hadn't said anything to her either, and she was afraid he'd been angry at her or maybe decided he didn't want to bother with her.

So she took it as a good sign that he'd come to sit next to her. She hadn't been paying enough attention when she'd gotten on to notice he was riding the bus today, so she hadn't had a chance to worry about whether he'd talk to her or not.

Except he didn't even respond to her greeting. He did turn his head to look at her, and suddenly it seemed that he was *very* close. Even though they weren't touching, she could feel his body heat beside her. His tousled black hair was shiny in the morning sun, and his eyes were green as new grass.

"Good… morning?" she tried again.

His mouth tightened a little, but otherwise he only kept staring at her.

So… he wasn't angry at her, but still didn't want to talk to her? Not sure what else to do, she went back to reading.

He kept staring at her for a while before eventually facing forward.

And that was pretty much how the entire rest of the week went. Trick never said another word—not only to her but to anyone, aside from when a teacher basically forced him to speak by asking him a direct question or something. On Thursday, Denneka even asked him why he wasn't talking, but he didn't answer. However, every morning on the bus he moved from wherever he'd been sitting and followed her to the back seat—until Friday morning, when he was there waiting for her when she got on. Every day at lunch, he waited until she sat down, then ate his sack lunch close by. Not always right next to her. Maybe a few seats down or one table over.

And every afternoon on the bus ride home, he was right there with her until she got off at her house.

All without ever saying a word.

Boys were extremely confusing.

Late Friday morning, she ran into Brook in the bathroom. Brook was tiny and seemed timid, but Denneka had seen her display more backbone than anyone would probably guess she had. Plus, she was nice. Not nice enough to actually be friends with Denneka, but nice enough to be friendly at any rate.

"Hey, Denneka," Brook said in her quiet voice after glancing around to make sure no one else was in the bathroom with them. "Are you and that new boy dating?"

"What?" Denneka gasped, blushing. "No! Why would you say that?"

"You're always together, pretty much."

"We have assigned seats next to each other."

"Yeah, but all the rest of the time, too."

"How—how could I be dating him?" Denneka sputtered. "He's only been here since Monday."

"Peter said he remembered seeing you talking to him the other day at your shop. We're all kind of assuming you knew him already."

"No, that was the first time we met."

Brook's head tilted. "Really? He seems really attached to you."

"I don't know why he's doing that. I mean, it doesn't bother me or anything." That was an understatement. Enough of one that it felt kind of like a betrayal. She didn't *not mind* Trick being around. She *liked* it. Not that she could say why, since he refused to talk to her. "Wait, what you mean 'we're all assuming'? People are talking about us?"

Brook shrugged. "You know how it is with new people. Everyone's talking about Mr. McKenzie, too."

"I haven't heard anyone talking."

She read the sudden pity in Brook's expression to mean no one was talking to *her*, which was true.

"Never mind. What are they saying about Mr. McKenzie?"

"Since he won't tell anyone anything about himself, people are mostly making stuff up for fun. Ian thinks he's in witness protection. Bobby said he's probably an undercover cop working some *Twenty-One Jump Street* style drug investigation. Amy and them think he's just messing with everyone because he thinks it's funny."

"Oh." Denneka wished she had an amusing theory to throw into the mix. Maybe she could think of one to offer later. "If anyone does figure it out, would you fill me in?"

"Sure," Brook said with a smile that made Denneka believe she actually meant it. "So there's nothing going on with you and Trick?"

"Going on? He won't even talk to me." Not even when she'd asked about the 'grave' thing again. Maybe he'd been trying to fool her or make a joke. If he'd really meant it, he would have taken it more seriously, right?

"Really? So he's not just giving the rest of us the silent treatment because he decided he hates everyone. Do you think he's shy?"

"Maybe. I haven't been able to figure out why he's not talking. I... thought I said something to make him mad, but that wouldn't make sense with him... acting how he is."

Brook gave her a reassuring pat on the shoulder. "I'm sure it's nothing. He is kinda cute, though, isn't he?"

Denneka felt heat flood her face. "Yeah. He is."

After the last bell rang, signaling the end of the school day, Mr. McKenzie said, "Patrick and Denneka, don't get up. You've got detention, remember. We all have to spend another hour together before we get to leave."

He'd said it in front of everyone, the jerk. Snickers and whispers floated toward her, but she tried not to hear him.

After everyone else had left, Mr. McKenzie closed the classroom door.

"It's just us?" Denneka asked in surprise. All week, and they were the only ones to earn detentions?

"First week lenience, I guess," said Mr. McKenzie. "And as a way of offering my own, I've decided not to make you sit in motion-less silence for an hour."

That sounded stricter than normal. Denneka would definitely try not to get another detention. "So, I can read?" Maybe this wouldn't be so bad at all.

"In a manner of speaking. I've got a project for you."

"What sort of project?"

"Come now, it can't be that hard to figure out. I'm told you're known for reading. Patrick, as we all saw on Monday, has a problem in that area. You get to spend the hour giving him some reading tutoring."

Denneka flushed, looking immediately to Trick.

He didn't appear happy.

Mr. McKenzie pulled a large box from where it had been tucked away in the back of the room. It was a good two cubic feet, and after trying to pick it up and struggling, he shuffled it toward some shelves with his foot. Opening it, he quickly removed several dozen books, setting them in piles on the floor, and pushed the empty box out of the way. "Pick any of these," he said, gesturing to the books. "Then have Patrick read it—yes, aloud, Patrick—and help him whenever he struggles with a word. Simple, yes?"

It did sound simple. She'd get to sit close to Trick again, and even though he wouldn't exactly be talking to her, she'd at least get to listen to his voice. Unless reading aloud got him to loosen up about whatever was making him not talk. Maybe getting detention first week of the year wouldn't be so bad.

"Okay." Denneka got up, went to the piles of books, and pulled out one that wasn't too difficult but also not too easy.

Mr. McKenzie motioned to a cushioned bench against the back wall, near the bookshelf. "Why don't you work on that here? You don't need a desk to read, and this way you could work closely more easily."

Denneka took a seat on one end of the bench. *There's nothing to be nervous about,* she told herself. *This isn't that different from sitting next to him on the bus.* But judging by the untethered feeling in her stomach, her body wasn't convinced.

Mr. McKenzie eyed Trick. "Get going. One hour of reading. That's not so bad, is it?"

———

One hour?! One whole hour of nothing but *reading*?! Trick had never read for an hour in his life! Even his mom hadn't forced that on him. It was bad enough sitting still for that long when he wasn't allowed to fall asleep, but at least during class he could look out the window or observe the humans. But now the teacher man was going to force him to stare at a page?!

He had half a mind to challenge the man over it. But the teacher man was bigger than him, so there was a good chance Trick would get hurt and then still have to do the reading. Growling softly, Trick got up from his desk and sat beside the familiar girl on the bench.

"Good boy," the man murmured.

"Is this one okay?" the girl asked, holding up a plain brown book with two words on it. Trick only recognized one of them: 'Travels'. He shrugged. It wasn't like it mattered. She flipped a few pages and held it open, leaning closer to him. "Start here."

Trick stared at the book in irritation before quietly beginning to read. "My father had a small estate in Not... Not..." Great. The first sentence, and already he was stuck.

"Sound it out," the girl encouraged. "It's a place name."

"Not... ing... ham... shire."

"Good. I'm not sure that's how the locals would pronounce it, because place names can be weird like that, but that's good enough. Keep going."

"I was the third of five sons." All right. That one was easy. "He sent me to Emman—"

"Emanuel."

Trick gritted his teeth. An hour. An hour of this. When all he wanted to do was run outside and chase some birds.

"It's okay. You're doing well," said the girl.

Trick kept reading. There were a lot of words he didn't know, and instead of skipping past them like he usually did, he had to sit there working them out letter by letter until he either got it right or the girl said it for him. He'd never liked to read, but he hadn't thought he was *that* bad at it. Stumbling over the words felt like a weakness, and it made his skin itch to know the teacher man was watching him stumble, sitting over there by the bookshelf, all smug as he organized the books. Trick's eyes kept wandering over to the man, checking to see how closely the man was watching him and his constant failure. Most of the time, the man appeared to barely be paying them any attention, which did make Trick feel a little better, though he still wanted to find a nice, safe hole to crawl into.

The third time he looked over to check on the man, his eyes landed on something else: that big, empty cardboard box the books had come in. The man must have moved it, because now it sat in the middle of the floor, not very far away.

It was a good size, even with Trick as big as he was now. He stared at it for a little while, ignoring the girl, who was asking him why he'd stopped reading. Then Trick got up, quietly walked to the box, and stepped into it. He sank down, sitting on the bottom with his knees pulled up to his chest and his arms wrapped around his legs, the comforting closeness of the sides of the box all around him. Yes, this was good. Maybe he could wait out the rest of detention here.

Of course, the teacher man was still in the room—smirking now and putting his phone in his pocket. Trick sank a little further down in the box. If he could get low enough that the sides of the box hid him, maybe the man would forget he was there. He was able to get pretty far down in the box by shifting around, until most of his body was hidden. He kept his head just high enough to peer over at the man, keeping an eye on him in case he moved. The man's mouth pursed, and he took his phone out and then put it away again.

"Trick?" the familiar girl asked. "Are... you okay?"

He was fine.

"Why are you hiding in a box? Do you not like reading that much?" Her voice was higher than normal. She looked over at the man.

The man said, "Maybe he was traumatized by books at some point? Patrick, you can sit—or crouch—wherever you want, but you still have to practice reading. Denneka, have a seat on the floor next to him and keep trying."

The girl came over to Trick, her movements wary, and knelt on the floor beside the box. "I think, um, I think you were here." She held the book up in his line of sight to the man.

Trick kept reading, grumbling the words under his breath.

After what had to have been five or six hours, the teacher man finally said they could go. Trick hopped out of the box, got his bag, and sprinted outside. He ran wildly around the lawn, chasing the few birds who got close enough, before finally stopping to look around. There were hardly any people. Only the familiar girl, who stood on the sidewalk near the lawn, watching him.

His mom's car wasn't here yet. He thought about running home, but she'd told him to wait because she was picking him up, and she'd get mad if he wasn't here when she got here and she had to look for him. So he lay down in a sunny spot of grass to wait.

As he looked up at the cloudy blue sky, he heard the sound of tires. A glance told him it still wasn't his mom's car, so he went back to watching the sky. Lying on his back was something it was a lot easier to do as a human. He didn't like how it exposed his belly, but he'd looked around enough to see that there didn't appear to be any threats, and he'd probably hear one coming in time to react.

Then he did hear the sound of feet in the grass, and he propped himself on his elbows to see the familiar girl coming toward him.

"Do you need a ride home?" she asked.

He looked up at her. She was probably waiting for him to say something, but he was still wary of accidentally saying something that Mom had told him not to say or otherwise getting in trouble with his words.

"You can… nod for yes or shake your head for no."

Of course. Humans had body language for that. He shook his head.

"Okay. See you Monday, I guess." She backed away a couple steps before turning and going to the car that had pulled up.

He didn't know how long he lay in the grass, but it was very relaxing. For a while, all he heard was the wind and birds and bugs. Then he heard footsteps.

The moment before he sat up to investigate the sound, he saw a shape soaring overhead. A familiar shape that made his pulse pound, all the more so as it began to descend.

Trick sat up and saw a man walking away from the school building, toward the parking lot. It wasn't any man he recognized.

Curiosity propelled him to his hands and feet, and he began stalking toward the man through the grass. But it was very awkward to move that way now that his forelimbs and hindlimbs were different lengths, so he moved onto his feet, staying in a low crouch. He followed the man across the pavement, sticking to shadows and darting behind things whenever he could, as the man disappeared around a corner of the parking lot.

And the bird disappeared behind the roof of the school building, heading in the same direction as the man.

Trick hurried forward, slowing when he came to the corner of the building to peer around it into a smaller part of the lot where each space had a sign in front of it that said 'Staff'. The sight that met him made him stop in his tracks.

The man stood in the nearly empty lot with a very familiar hawk perched on his shoulder. Trick was so scared, he almost turned and bolted away. But his curiosity won out over his fear, and he kept watching.

The man had his phone out and was holding it up to the hawk as if the bird could understand. "I even got it on camera," the man said to the hawk. His voice was warm with amusement. "I honestly didn't believe he'd take the bait, but I'm so glad he did. It was absolutely adorable. You can't imagine how hard it was to keep a straight face. That poor girl didn't have any idea what to make of him."

The hawk was working with a human? That hawk had tried to kill him! What did this mean? Was the man going to try to kill him, too?

Trick scrambled to get away, but his stupid shoe slipped on some dirt covering the pavement, making a noise.

As one, the hawk and man looked toward him, eyes locking on Trick. Fear coursed through him, freezing him in place for what turned out to be much too long.

The man smiled at him, head tilting in consideration, smile turning predatory. "Snooping? Aren't you a naughty kitty?"

Before Trick could get his footing and make his escape, the man raised a hand in the air and snapped his fingers.

A brilliant flash of light nearly blinded Trick, and he felt a painful twisting and pulling through his whole body. His vision went black. Something soft yet heavy covered him all around. He struggled and fought his way free of whatever had suddenly fallen over him, and as he did so, he found the light again.

He looked back toward the man, who hadn't moved from where he'd been but was suddenly at a much higher angle than he'd been a second ago. Trick lashed his tail in fear, claws instinctively extending, and for one single heartbeat rejoiced in somehow being back in his real body... before the man said something to the hawk, and the killer bird of prey flapped its wings, lifting off from the man's shoulder, and flew toward Trick.

With a frenzied skittering of claws on pavement, Trick ran for his life.

CHAPTER
SEVEN

Kester didn't even try to hold back his laugh as he watched Trick scramble away. The boy really did make an adorable kitten. Julia lazily flapped after Trick, letting him gain ground as she gained altitude. In moments, they were both out of sight. Kester went over and pondered the pile of clothes—as well as the shoes and bag—which Trick had left behind.

It had not been Kester's plan to re-transform Trick. At least, it hadn't until the boy had remained silent all through detention, save only for the reading aloud which he did under great duress. Part of Kester was impressed that Trick could stick to something so resolutely. But Trick's refusal to interact with anyone else, aside from following Denneka around like a lost puppy, had become stagnant and dull, so something had needed to be done.

Kester pulled the gold watch out of his pocket and put it on, feeling the tingle and tug of magic altering his appearance into that of his teacher persona. Once he had decided, while still sitting in his classroom, that the time had come to do something more drastic about Trick, he'd had to take it off. First, because there was nothing yet to gain from allowing the boy to learn of his deception. And second, because the spell he'd imbued into the watch came with the unfortunate restriction that he couldn't use his magic while wearing it.

Once again merely a simple, magicless teacher, he pulled out his phone and dialed a number.

"Hello?" said an impatient voice after the fourth ring.

"Hello, Jacqueline. It's John McKenzie," Kester said in a concerned tone. "Have you picked Trick up from school yet?"

There was a frustrated breath. "Not yet. I know I'm running behind, but I'll be there shortly. Why?"

"His detention ended about twenty minutes ago, and everyone else has already left. I had thought I was the last person to leave the school today, but... well, I've found something strange."

"Found what?" She was giving him her full attention now.

"It looks like Trick's things, but there's no sign of Trick himself. I'd assumed you'd have picked him up by now, but I can't think of any reason his bag would be on the ground outside the school. Along with... well, I don't know how to put this. His clothes."

Silence reigned for many long seconds. Then she said tersely, "I'm on my way."

———

No pesky thoughts cluttered Trick's head to distract him from his frantic flight. His small, black body was like a bullet as it raced down sidewalks, through alleys, and across yards, instinct and memory guiding him on the shortest path toward home.

Shortest, but not short.

He could practically feel the hawk's talons in his back as he ran. Every second, he was certain the bird was just one more second away from tackling him to the ground and tearing him apart. But whenever he spared a glance behind him, it was still high in the air. Following him, but not catching him.

He didn't know what that meant and didn't bother spending the time to think about it. He only knew he had to get to safety. Ducking into a handy building or under some trash might have saved him temporarily, but if the hawk waited for him to come out, he'd be trapped with no escape. He needed more than a quick hiding place. He needed freedom. Unfortunately, it was taking a long time to get home, and he was running out of energy. Being human had made him start losing his sense of distance, and riding the bus to and from his home had made it worse. With his lungs and muscles burning from his efforts, he wasn't even halfway there. If he collapsed or stopped to rest, he'd be as good as dead.

A fresh wave of terror flooded his brain. He wouldn't make it home. He was going to die.

Suddenly, a tiny, warm spark of familiarity popped through the terror, and he fully took in which part of town he was running through. Without thinking, without registering why he was doing it, his paws changed course, carrying him toward a certain blue house.

He shot up the walkway so fast that he slammed into the front door. Recovering quickly, he started scratching and yowling at it for all he was worth.

Open! Open! Open! Save me!

The door did open. As soon as there was a gap wide enough for him to get through, he darted inside, dove under the nearest large piece of furniture he saw, and crouched, panting.

"What the—?"

Trick watched the feet at the front door from the safety of his hiding spot under a love seat. Only when the door closed, ensuring that the hawk wouldn't be able to follow him in, did his thundering heart begin to slow. Socked feet padded toward him, then hands and knees were on the floor, and then a face was there, looking at him in confusion. "Hello," said the familiar girl.

———

"Stay in the car, okay?" Jacqueline said.

"Kay," Landon replied from the back seat, nose deep in *The War of the Worlds*.

There was only one other car in the junior high parking lot, with a man Jacqueline had never seen before standing nearby, so she got out and went toward it. He smiled warmly as she approached. Warmly enough that Jacqueline thought he must not be *too* concerned about Trick. Hopefully that was a good sign. "Jacqueline, I presume," he said, holding out a hand.

She shook it. "John?"

He nodded.

"You said you found Trick's things," she prompted, since he still didn't appear in much hurry to get to the point.

The pleasant expression fell from his face. "Ah, yes. Over here." He led her to the corner of the building, where a pile of clothes and a bag lay on the concrete.

She let out a sigh.

"Those are Trick's, correct?" John asked. "I didn't try to search them in case..." He let the thought trail off, but Jacqueline knew what he meant. In case they were evidence. In case the police needed to investigate.

"Yes," Jacqueline said. Her first instinct was to rifle through the clothes to check that Trick wasn't hiding under them, but she instantly quashed it. It was a stupid impulse... wasn't it? But the doubt in her gut kept prodding her even as her brain tried to work out a more rational answer.

Most likely, her brain said, Trick had been so annoyed by the detention that, in a fit of pique, he'd tossed off all the trappings of humanity and run off to do whatever it was he'd constantly been doing when he was running around as a cat. That was most likely. She could easily see him doing that, especially if John had made Trick sit quietly in one place against his will for too long. If that was what had happened, there wasn't much to worry about. Relatively speaking. Trick would either show up at home eventually or be brought home by the police after someone reported a naked teenage boy running around town. There'd be an unpleasant amount of town gossip that she'd have to deal with, and she'd give Trick a good lecture about trying to act normal, but there wouldn't be anything of any real concern to worry about. The most rational thing to do would be to pick up Trick's things, reassure John that Trick occasionally acted out in strange ways, and wait for her son to come home.

But, her gut said, the clothes didn't tell that story. Jacqueline had seen hastily discarded clothing enough times to know that it didn't normally end up in a single pile with shirt on top of pants on top of shoes. That might happen, though, if the person wearing the clothes suddenly vanished—or became much smaller.

Which was stupid. Which was irrational. The spell had ended, and she had no reason to believe it could spontaneously trigger again. And the odds of running into another witch here and now and for it to be Trick specifically who the witch decided to target were astronomical beyond consideration. Yes, there were witches in the world, but not all that many of them. It was statistically impossible.

But the clothes.

"He... acts out sometimes," she said, but her throat was too tight. "I'm sure that's all this is."

"You don't sound entirely convinced of that."

She cleared her throat. "No, I'm sure. He'll probably be home in a few hours."

"Still," John said, pulling out his phone, "maybe we should alert the police. You heard about the man who's missing, haven't you? There may be a serial kidnapper on the loose."

Something about the earnest way he said that made her eye him askance, checking to see if he was joking, but his expression betrayed nothing but concern.

Calling the police was what a normal mother would do in a situation like this, wasn't it? John's thumb was already on the screen. If she stopped him from alerting the authorities when her child was missing, wouldn't that be more likely to raise suspicion than anything?

"All right," she said reluctantly.

He dialed and spoke in a calm, controlled manner, requesting that an officer come out to take a look at a strange scene and that they thought there was a missing child involved. Then he hung up, and they stood there in silence for a few minutes.

"You don't need to stay," she assured him. If he left, she could gather up Trick's things and go home, and it would be John's problem later if the police thought he'd made a false report. His word against hers that anything strange had happened, and she could come up with something convincing to tell him about it if he pushed the issue.

"It's no trouble," John assured her. "If something did happen to him, it would be partly my fault for making him stay late."

How irritatingly conscientious. "That's very kind of you," she muttered.

The grin he gave her was so guileless, it was almost idiotic.

Another minute later, a police car drove up and a uniformed officer got out and came over to them. John obligingly showed him Trick's discarded clothes and bag, and Jacqueline confirmed her son had not come home. The officer frowned at the clothes, then got on his radio and called in some help.

Great. More people. More hassle. And John still wasn't leaving.

"Excuse us, ma'am," a man with a camera said to her later, shooing Jacqueline aside while he and a couple other officers investigated the scene. The police didn't seem particularly worried, for all Jacqueline could read them, so the photos and notes were probably a simple matter of procedure. Or maybe it was a slow day and they had nothing else to do.

"Let's give them some room," John suggested, motioning her toward his car. He propped a hip on the hood and made idle small talk with her. Something about being new to town and how she was finding things.

She didn't have time for idle small talk. She needed to get home and see about finding Trick. What if he was already home and this was a waste of everyone's time? That would mean she was needlessly drawing attention to herself and her family. But what if Trick wasn't home? She couldn't call and check. She hadn't gotten Trick a cell phone, and they didn't have a landline. Her feet were restless, itching to go back to the car and drive home to see if he was there. If he wasn't, she'd have to start searching. But would she be searching for a boy or—

"—and there's that clearing near the river that's perfect for dancing naked under the full moon."

She blinked a few times as the oddness of John's words worked through her distracted brain.

"Lots of small animals around there, too. For the blood sacrifices."

Jacqueline blinked again. "What?"

John laughed loudly. "Sorry, you were so zoned out, I couldn't help it."

He had a warm, pleasant laugh, and some of the worry that had begun to smother her faded. Something about the smile that lingered on his face was... no, not *familiar*. That couldn't be right. But... welcome. He was very average-looking, and she didn't find him the least bit attractive, but he wasn't exactly unattractive, either. More... nice and non-threatening. Comfortable. And he had a sense of humor, apparently. Maybe he *had* been teasing her earlier. But what kind of person would tease a woman whose child was missing? Despite herself, she kind of wanted to find out.

She felt the corners of her mouth curling, just a little. "So, no naked dancing and animal sacrifices?"

"Of course not," he said, then added in a low tone, "What kind of witch do you take me for?"

Alarm shot through her mind before rationality kicked in. *He's only making a joke.* But still... *Wouldn't a person normally say, "What do you take me for, a witch?"*

John's eyes locked onto something behind her. "We have company."

She turned to see Landon walking over to them from her car. He was eyeing John with wary intensity. When he reached them,

Landon pressed himself against Jacqueline's side, and she put her arm around his shoulders.

"This must be Trick's little brother," John said, giving the boy a small smile.

"Yes," Jacqueline said. "This is Landon. Landon, this is Trick's teacher, Mr. McKenzie."

Landon didn't take his eyes off of John, even when he asked, "Mom, what's taking so long?"

"Oh. Um… Well, it seems Trick may be missing."

Landon's gaze broke away from John and snapped to her.

"I'm sure it's nothing to be concerned about," she hurried to say. "But the police are making a note of it to be safe. Most likely, he's already gone home in the time we've been waiting here."

Landon didn't say anything more, but his sharp blue eyes roved from his mother to the police to John.

Likewise, John was still watching the boy. "I'm sure it'll be fine, Landon," he said. "Some boys are always running off, aren't they?"

"I guess," Landon conceded.

"That's probably all that happened, so surely he'll find his way home eventually." John was showing a more optimistic face to her child than he had to Jacqueline, but that was only to be expected.

A dark-haired officer came over to them and said, "We're all done here. You can take his things and go home. He's a teenager, so most likely he's only off being an idiot somewhere. If he's not home by midnight, though, go ahead and call it in and we can get a search started tomorrow."

Jacqueline nodded, relieved that they weren't taking this very seriously. There was no rational reason not to want the police involved if Trick was missing, but her gut told her it would be easier to deal with whatever was going on if they weren't.

She sent Landon back to the car, then gathered Trick's things and put them in the trunk. When she closed the lid, John was standing beside her.

"If you'd like, I could go home and wait with you," he offered.

Was he hitting on her? She eyed him, considering it. No. No, she wasn't getting that vibe from him. It did seem to be only a genuinely friendly gesture. "No, thanks. I'll be fine."

He accepted this answer with an easy nod. "If it's all right, I'll call you tomorrow to see if he made it home. Like I said, I can't help but feel partly responsible if he really is missing. I'm sure I'll be wracked with guilt until I know everything's fine."

Funny, he doesn't seem wracked with guilt. But maybe he hides worry with humor. After a request like that, how could she reasonably say no? "Okay. Thanks for your concern. There's no need for you to feel guilty, though. I'm sure whatever happened isn't your fault."

"Still." He stepped back and watched her get into the car. Before she closed the door, he bent down and waved. "It was nice to meet you, Landon."

"Nice to meet you, too," the boy said with reluctant, obligatory politeness.

As Jacqueline drove out of the parking lot, all thoughts of John already put out of her mind, she had to fight to keep herself from flooring the gas pedal. Instead, she thought positively, imagining as hard as she could that Trick would be waiting for them when they got home.

"Come on, little kitty," said the familiar girl. "You need to come out from under there. My parents and brother will be home soon."

It had been a little while—long enough for Trick's heaving breaths to return to normal—but he was still crouching under the love seat. He knew it didn't make any sense. The hawk was outside, he was inside, and the door was still closed. He was safe. He knew that. But he still couldn't manage to make his paws move.

"My mom hates cats," the girl said in a sorry voice. "If she finds you here, she'll throw you out, and I'll get in trouble."

How could anyone hate cats? Trick wondered. *We're amazing.* Still, he knew some people did. He'd had a broom swung at him more than once, and he was positive a car swerved *toward* him on the road one time.

If her mom throws me out, the hawk will get me. Fear rippled through him, making him ball his body up even tighter, but he forced himself to listen to his brain instead of his instincts. *If I stay here, her mom will find me. If her mom finds me, she'll throw me out, and the hawk will eat me. If I come out now, before her mom comes home, maybe the familiar girl will do something to stop that.*

His paws seemed to weigh ten times as much as usual, but one by one, he picked them up and placed them closer to the familiar girl, slinking across the hardwood floor until he was out from under the love seat.

"Good kitty," she cooed. She held out her hand, and when he didn't move away, she petted him gently on the head with her fingertips. He leaned into the touch, softly purring as his fear began to lessen. He missed having his head petted. No one ever petted his head when he was human.

"There, it's okay, see?" The familiar girl was smiling now. "You're a sweetie, aren't you?" Her hands wrapped around his body under his forelegs, and she lifted him up so they were face to face.

Her face was really big now. All of her was really big. It was weird seeing someone like this after first seeing them as a human. It made him feel a little dizzy.

You stopped petting me, he thought at her. *Why did you stop petting me?* He flicked his tail.

"Wow, your eyes are so green," she told him, as if he didn't know. "Just like..." For a second, her face turned pink, and she smiled again and kind of giggled.

Trick wasn't sure what was so funny about his having green eyes, but he was starting to wonder when she would put him down. And he was hungry. He looked around the room, wondering where the kitchen was.

"Trick," she said, catching his attention again.

What? he mentally asked her. *Wait...* Trick lashed his tail in excitement, looking with wonder at the familiar girl's face. *She figured out who I am just by my eyes? Of course, I did tell her I used to be a cat. I guess it wasn't that big a leap, after I slipped up like that. Obviously I might become a cat again. Still, that's pretty clever.*

Clearly, he'd done the right thing in coming here for help. Spending time with this girl in school had let her get to know him enough that she recognized him right away, and she would definitely help him because they were friends. He just hoped she didn't help him by taking him home. That had been where he'd wanted to go at first, but now that he'd had some time to think about it, he was sure Mom would yell at him—even though turning back into a cat hadn't been his fault at all. It had been that man in league with the hawk. Trick didn't want to get yelled at for something that wasn't his fault. Worse, though, Mom would definitely start trying to find a way to make him human again and might not even let him out of the house.

Probably better to stay here with the familiar girl for now.

She tucked him under her arm in an uncomfortable way that almost definitely meant she'd never held a cat before and carried him though a hallway and into a bedroom. Setting him down on top of a striped comforter, she knelt down to look him in the eye and said, "Okay, little Trick. Wait here. I'll get you some water and see if we have anything for you to eat."

Food. Yes. Maybe some kind of mental bond had already formed between them. Or maybe she was just super perceptive.

Trick sat there for a second or two after she left, taking in the room. It was about the size of his at home, though her bed was bigger than his. There was a small desk and three large bookcases full to bursting with all colors of books.

That was as far as he got before deciding he needed to pee, so he hopped down off the bed and went back into the hallway. As he expected, the bathroom was one of the doors off the hall. He heard her footsteps just as he flushed, and when he dismounted from the toilet, she was standing in the bathroom doorway, giving him a weird look. "You can use the toilet?"

His tail twitched. Of course he could use the toilet.

"I didn't know cats could do that."

He flicked his tail again.

"Well… good. I guess I don't need to get a litter box, then. But… I have to figure out how to keep you from being seen by my family. Hopefully you can hold it until I'm able to bring you in here now and then."

Trick had lost interest in whatever she was saying well before she finished, so he was already past her and almost back to the bedroom by the time she started following him. When they were both inside, she shut the door and set down two bowls. One was water, which Trick went straight for.

"We don't have cat food, obviously," said the familiar girl, "and I'm not sure what else cats eat, so I got you some cream. Cats eat cream, right?"

Trick had used to like milk and cream when he was a human kid, but after he'd become a cat, he'd found that dairy gave him a stomachache and sometimes made him throw up. So after the seventh or eighth time that happened, he stopped drinking it. Not that he could explain any of that to her in this form. Hopefully she'd get the hint from his ignoring the cream.

When he was done with the water, he started exploring her bedroom. It mostly smelled like the girl, but there were other smells, too: paper, other humans, a chemical smell that might have been a scented candle hiding somewhere. When he'd been human, the girl's scent had been very faint, like everyone else's. But now it was richer and stronger. Not bad. Not good, either. Just… her-ish. Trick had never really tried very hard to put scents into words. As weak as their noses were, humans didn't have enough words to say much of anything about smells.

He was exploring some cardboard boxes in her closet when he heard a rumbling sound and the familiar girl jumped to her feet. "They're home. I need you to be really quiet, okay?" She went to the bedroom door and opened it just far enough to squeeze through. Sticking her head in from the other side, she said, "Just be a good, quiet kitty, okay? I'll be back later," then turned out the light and shut the door… leaving Trick alone in a strange place with no company but her smell. Not that Trick was scared. He totally wasn't. He wasn't at all bothered by the weird noises and strange voices and total lack of any escape route. But it suddenly felt colder than it had a minute ago.

Wary of making too much noise, he stopped exploring and got onto the bed. That immediately felt too exposed, so he crawled under the blanket, then under the pillow, where it was nice and warm and cozy.

Trick woke up when the familiar girl pulled the pillow off of him and let out a big sigh. "There you are."

Trick tried to tell her with his stare to put the pillow down and let him go back to sleep.

She stared right back at him. "So… you're just sleeping there, then?"

Yes. Put the pillow back down. It's chilly.

"Okay, I guess," she said with a shrug, and his dark cocoon returned.

———

That girl needs to learn how to close her curtains better, Julia thought. *Anyone could see in. Doesn't she know men are perverts?*

As soon as the thought crossed her mind, she felt guilty for it. Some men were perverts, yes, but some weren't. And some who seemed like perverts were… well…

She would have sighed if she could have, but that wasn't really something hawks were built for. *Perversion's in the eye of the beholder, isn't it? And what's less perverted than a man being attracted to a woman?*

It was totally normal and not something to get upset about at all. So why did it keep upsetting her?

Sometimes, she really hated being on watch duty. It gave her mind too much time to wander and dwell on things she could do nothing about.

Anyway, the girl. There was a good two-inch gap between the curtains where they met in the middle. More than enough for Julia to get a view in from her perch on a tree branch in the back yard. By edging back and forth along the branch, her view widened even more. The sun was nearly down, the kitten was sleeping, and the girl was getting ready for bed, so Julia spread her wings and flew home.

———

Kester carefully plated two servings of grilled chicken and wild rice, then brought them to the dining table just as Julia emerged from her room. She was wearing a set of green flannel pajamas, and her hair was wet and tangled from her shower. Wordlessly, she came to the table and sat down.

"Right on time," he said, dropping a kiss on the top of her damp head before going back to the kitchen for their drinks.

"Smells good," she murmured. Through their bond, he could feel her distraction, though he didn't know what caused it.

He set a glass of water in front of her, then took his seat across the table. "Busy day today."

"Not really. Fly around, sit on a branch. Pretty normal."

He chuckled. "Yes, well, busy for other people, at any rate."

They ate in companionable silence for a minute or two, then Julia looked at him. "What were you expecting to happen?"

"Something interesting. And I wasn't disappointed."

"You mean the girl?"

Kester grinned broadly. "She's a delightfully unpredictable wild card. Thrown into their lives by sheer chance. I wonder, would he have gone to her if her house hadn't been on the way to his? I don't think so."

"I'm pretty sure he thought I was trying to eat him. He'd probably have collapsed from exhaustion before getting home, then I'd have had to perch somewhere and keep an eye on him while he caught his breath, and that would have made him wonder what was going on."

Kester tapped his fork lightly against his plate. "I do wonder what Jacqueline would have done if he'd made it home. Pretend he was sick and hope the change reversed itself? Immediately start looking for another witch?" He shrugged. "Who knows? But I think this is better."

Julia eyed him. "How was it? Talking to her?"

"She's an intelligent, straightforward woman. It's dreadfully amusing to watch her prevaricate."

"Be careful you don't fall for her," Julia commented. "I know that's your type."

He met her gaze, and for an instant, something passed along their bond so intensely it almost hurt. *My type, eh?* he thought in the privacy of his own mind. He cocked a roguish smile and winked. "Ah, but they're all my type." It was the truth, more or less, but it was also mere light, playful banter. Or intended as such.

Kester felt a pain like a bolt to his gut. Julia's eyes dropped to her plate, and she picked at her food.

His smile fell, and he went back to eating, wishing she would understand. Wishing he could explain without ruining everything.

"It's getting late," she said after a silence much less companionable than before. "Aren't you going out?"

Before she'd asked the question, he'd been intending to. That was his Friday night routine, after all. Go somewhere lively, find a woman, have some fun. It gave Julia some much-deserved time to herself, as well. It was good for both of them. But things weren't quite routine anymore.

"I don't suppose I can. This is a small enough city that I can't imagine there are many places to find like-minded women on a Friday night. And I'm supposed to have left town already. If Lisa saw me, she'd grow suspicious. If I went out with my disguise on and she saw me, she'd wonder why I was out alone instead of home with my girlfriend. And wearing the disguise for that sort of engagement would pose other problems, as well, not least of which is finding a woman who'd even want me." He shrugged. "I suppose there's nothing for it but to stay in tonight. Shall we watch a movie?"

Julia was staring at him with a blank expression, but he could feel her mood even out, the distraction and dull pain inside her fading. Finally, her lips curled into a tiny smile. "I'd like that, Master."

CHAPTER
EIGHT

Denneka woke to the strange feeling of something warm and soft occupying the space between her left side and arm. Confused, she looked down to see a small, furry face peeking out from under the blanket, its chin resting on her upper arm. It was absolutely adorable. How could her mom possibly hate something so cute?

Trying not to move too much, Denneka reached her other hand over to stroke the kitten's head. She was pretty sure it was a kitten. It was either a very small cat or an adolescent kitten, and something about the way it moved made her think kitten.

The kitten's head rose and turned toward her, opening those green eyes enough to look at her with a tired, half-lidded expression. She still couldn't believe how green they were and how they were the exact same shade of green as Trick's. Not that she'd been paying that much attention to Trick's eyes. It was just... they were striking and therefore memorable. It was normal to remember them. And it was also totally normal to notice how the cat's shiny fur was just as black as Trick's hair because... how many fair-skinned people had true black hair? That was unusual too, right? Totally normal to notice that kind of thing.

Although it probably was a little weird that she'd named the cat after him. But since she had to keep the cat hidden, no one had to know.

Kitten Trick yawned, stood, and crawled over her arm and out from under the blanket to land on the floor. Denneka checked the clock on her phone. It was almost eight. She'd slept in. Well, that was what Saturdays were for, right? She got up, stretched her arms, and headed for the bathroom.

When she was done, she went to the kitchen to try to find something to feed Trick. He hadn't liked the cream, so maybe he wanted meat. She didn't know when he'd eaten last, but he was probably hungry. Some of the curtains were open, so the house was filled with morning sunlight. Her parents were probably already at the shop, getting things ready for the day.

She grabbed some cereal for herself and found some canned chicken for Trick. On her way back to her room, she saw something in the hall that jolted any remaining sleepiness out of her. Jonah was standing in the hall, staring into the bathroom. Past him, Denneka could see that the door to her bedroom was open.

Crap! I forgot to close it! She hurried forward to see what Jonah was looking at, just in time to see Trick use his front paw to flush the toilet.

Her brother watched the kitten hop down and pad past them into the hallway, then looked at Denneka with a raised eyebrow.

"Please don't tell Mom!" she whispered frantically, not one hundred percent certain her parents were actually gone. "He ran into the house last night."

"You know they won't let you keep him," said Jonah.

"I know. It's only temporary. Please don't tell."

He shrugged. "I won't. But you'll have to do a better job of hiding him. Even then, I doubt you'll be able to for long."

"I know, I know." She puffed out a breath. "From the way he acts, I bet he's someone's pet. I'll... have to try to find his owner."

"You're probably right. I doubt a stray cat would know how to use the toilet," Jonah said before going into the bathroom and shutting the door.

Denneka went into her bedroom, deliberately closing the door behind her. She set the chicken on the floor by the water and sat in her desk chair, her cereal getting soggy in the bowl on her lap. Trick went straight for the chicken, which she was pleased to see. She'd have to get some proper food for him today.

But how much of it should I buy? She reached down to stroke his back as he crouched in front of the food bowl. He was so cute, and it was nice to have someone to hang out with, even if that someone wasn't human. "I know you belong somewhere else, but I really don't want to get you home yet," she said.

Despite never having been allowed to have anything bigger than a hamster, Denneka knew she was a pet person at heart. What other kind of person would talk to an animal?

———

Landon's right hand tingled. It had been that way when he'd woken up, after his shower it had tingled even more, and now it was tingling so much it was almost painful. Not quite pinpricky like when a body part fell asleep, but sort of like that, only more... buzzy.

He sat on a stool at the kitchen counter, wondering if he should tell his mom about it, but when he looked behind him into the living room, she was taking turns pacing and looking out the window. She'd been up all night, waiting for Trick to come home, but he hadn't.

Landon liked Trick—loved him, even—but sometimes he wondered what it would be like to have a normal big brother. Or a normal cat.

The second worst part of having a cat for a big brother was that Landon couldn't talk about him with anyone outside the family. If he mentioned a brother, sooner or later someone might expect to meet him. And if he mentioned how his cat helped him with his homework, the other kids would look at him funny. He watched cat videos on YouTube sometimes, trying to get an idea of how normal cats were different than Trick, but honestly, Trick did most of the things in the cat videos. So, since Landon never knew what was and wasn't normal cat behavior, he just had to keep his mouth shut about Trick around others.

The worst part of having a cat for a big brother was when he did stuff like this and made their mom worry.

While Landon was chewing some granola and wondering whether to bother his mom about his hand, he reached for his glass of juice. As soon as his fingers touched the glass, a weird blue glow lit up where his skin met the glass. Then little spidery lines of blue glow stretched out across the glass from his hand.

All of a sudden, the glass shattered and juice splattered all over the counter.

Landon stared in shock at the shards of glass and dripping juice. Some of it had gotten into his granola. "Uh... Mom," he said.

She didn't seem to hear him.

He got down from the stool, moving his fingers. His hand didn't tingle anymore. In the living room, he went to where she stood by the window and tugged on the hem of her shirt. "Mom?"

"What is it, Landon?" she asked, barely glancing at him.

"I... uh... broke the glass."

"What?" She looked toward the kitchen and saw the mess. "What happened?"

"It... was an accident."

"Well, I assume that much."

He followed her to the kitchen. "No, I mean... with my hand." Surprise at the strangeness of it had made his brain go foggy. He couldn't manage to explain it right.

"You dropped it? There must have been a weakness in the glass to shatter like that." She got a rag from the sink and started mopping up the juice. "Oh, no. You've gotten it on your clothes. You'd better go change."

He showed her his totally normal-looking hand. "But, Mom, my... my hand..."

Even now, he could see she wanted to be back at the window.

Her movements were clumsy and short, and she barely looked at him. "Did you cut yourself on the glass?"

"No. But..."

"It's okay, Landon. I'll clean this up. You go change. There's my good boy."

'Good boy'. Yes, he was her good boy. She needed him to be her good boy, the one she didn't have to worry about. She'd told him who-knows-how-many times that she loved how well he behaved and took care of himself.

Trick was causing her enough trouble. Landon didn't want to add to it. He washed the juice off his hand, then went to his room and changed his clothes.

Really, he didn't know why he'd even tried to tell her about it. He'd been doing weird stuff for a while now, and he thought he was dealing with it fine. It wasn't like there was anything Mom could do about it anyway.

———

Ever since sunrise, Jacqueline had been wondering whether or not to pick up whenever John called and what to tell him if she did. He'd told her he'd call to see if Trick came home, and Trick hadn't come home.

By two a.m., Jacqueline had been seriously considering going out with a flashlight and combing the streets for her son. But first, that would mean leaving Landon home alone, and she didn't know anyone in this town to ask to babysit—much less in the middle of the night—and second, even a small town could be dangerous at night for a woman out alone.

But it could be dangerous for a naked teen boy, too. Or a small cat.

She grazed her finger on one of the shards of the glass that Landon had managed to break, enough to scrape but not really cut.

If Trick was still human, the fact that he hadn't been found and brought home by now meant that he was almost certainly in some kind of trouble that meant he *couldn't* be found or come home on his own. Which pretty much meant he'd either gotten hit by a car and was lying dead behind a bush somewhere, fallen down a well and broken his leg, or been kidnapped by child traffickers.

Or, if he had somehow gotten turned back into a cat, he could have still gotten hit by a car, fallen down a well, or kidnapped by criminals, but he also could have been taken in by a nice person wanting to help out a stray cat, or taken to the pound, or he could be running around all carefree and happy to be a cat again, and it just hadn't occurred to him that she'd be worrying.

She'd never have thought she'd hope Trick was a cat again, but here she was.

The pound was a worrying thought, though. She stopped cleaning up the mess, looked up the number for the nearest pet shelter, and called it.

"Thank goodness," she breathed when someone answered. As early as it was, she hadn't been sure someone would pick up. "Have you gotten a black cat in within the last twenty-four hours? He's a kitten, actually. Around six to eight months old?"

"Let me check."

Jacqueline held her breath.

"No, we haven't gotten anything like that in the past day. Is your pet missing?"

"Y-yes. Will you tell me if someone brings him in?"

"Sure. Let me get your info."

Jacqueline gave the lady her contact info as well as a description of what Trick looked like as a cat. *But what if he doesn't look like that this time?* she thought. *What if he's not a cat at all? What if he turned into a hedgehog? Or a rat?*

"Ma'am? Are you okay?"

Jacqueline realized she was beginning to hyperventilate and worked to calm herself. "Yes. I'm just... very worried. You don't put animals down, do you?"

"Well, we're not a no-kill shelter, but the only reason we'd put an animal down right away is if it were so injured or sick that it was beyond help."

'Beyond help'. Jacqueline's chest tightened. If someone found a wounded human Trick, unless he was completely dead, he'd be taken to a hospital and she'd be contacted. But what constituted 'beyond help' for a cat?

The woman continued. "Otherwise, it would be at least thirty days. And even then, we always put the oldest or worst-tempered animals down first. Assuming the kitten isn't totally feral, he'd almost certainly get adopted before it got to that point."

'Isn't totally feral'. Trick had never been trapped in a cage before, at least not that Jacqueline knew of. She'd had to transport him in a crate sometimes, but actually trapped? By people who didn't know he was really human? She desperately hoped he'd have the good sense to not flip out on them.

"But you really shouldn't worry," the woman said cheerfully. "I've got all your info, so I'll make sure everyone here keeps a sharp eye out for a cat that matches his description, and we'll let you know right away if he comes in. We do get a lot of black cats in. Sadly, they get dumped or end up being the ones left unchosen in a litter because people think they're too plain or associate them with bad luck. So I'm always happy to hear someone so passionate about taking good care of their black cat. Don't you worry, ma'am. If your little boy comes in, I'll personally make sure he gets back to you safe and sound."

The woman sounded so sincere and reassuring, Jacqueline actually calmed down a little. "Thank you. I can't tell you how much I appreciate that."

"My pleasure, ma—"

Jacqueline's phone beeped.

She looked at the screen. John was calling.

Before she could decide whether to answer, the shelter lady hung up, and Jacqueline heard John's voice say, "Hello?"

Since when do phones auto-answer like that?!

Never mind. It was inevitable anyway, she supposed. "Um, hello, John."

"Good morning, Jacqueline. Just checking in like I said I would. Has Trick come home?"

She tried to think of some way that 'yes' made sense as an answer, but trying to find a way to convince people she had a son that she currently couldn't actually produce was a bad sitcom waiting to happen. And she probably would need some kind of help to find him.

"No. He hasn't."

"Oh, dear. I'm coming over."

"What?"

"I told you, Jacqueline. I feel responsible. I already got your address from the school. I'm coming over to help look for Trick. You should call the police, too. They did say to call if he didn't turn up."

If Trick was a cat, the police wouldn't be much help. It wasn't as if Jacqueline could tell them a boy had gone missing but they should look for a cat. But if he was injured somewhere... or taken... "All right."

———

Lisa VanBuren settled into her chaise longue with her second cup of coffee and a scone, an ankle-length silk nightgown wrapping her bare skin in luxury. She sipped contentedly, enjoying the hillside view from her living room window and the peaceful quiet of morning.

The quiet was broken by heavy footsteps and the sound of a belt being buckled, both coming from the direction of her bedroom.

"You're up early, Marcus," she said, turning to greet her guest. "It usually takes you until almost noon to get your butt out of my house."

"Always a charmer, Lisa," Marcus said as he worked on the buttons of his shirt. "That's what I love about you."

She *could* be charming when she wanted to, but she'd known

Marcus long enough that she didn't see the point in bothering. "Really? I thought what you love about me is how I let you—"

"Please stop talking," he begged. "You're gonna make me want things I don't have time for right now. I gotta be at the station in half an hour, and I still have to get home and change."

Lisa sat up straighter. "I thought you had today off. Is something wrong?"

"I just got a call. That kid that went missing yesterday still isn't home, so the chief's calling us in."

Lisa stood and walked over to him, all playfulness and humor gone. "Kid? What kid?"

He stopped pulling on his jacket. "You haven't heard? I thought for sure the teacher would have called you."

"No one's told me anything. What happened?"

"One of your students went missing from outside the school yesterday evening. We came out and took pictures, but we figured he was just being a teen boy and would be home later."

"Pictures of what? If you thought he'd be home later, what made anyone think he was missing?"

"Well, it's weird, but… his clothes were there. Undies, shoes, and all."

A fiery anger came to life inside Lisa's chest. "What teacher was there who you thought would inform me of this?"

"I didn't recognize him, but I think his name was Mick something?"

"McKenzie?"

"Yeah, probably."

She clenched her fists. "And who's the missing student?"

Marcus shifted his feet uncomfortably under her glare. He'd never been very good with remembering details. "I don't have my notepad, but I think his last name was Saint something."

Patrick St. Andrew. The new boy. At least it wasn't one of the students from families who'd be breathing down her neck about it and threatening lawsuits until he was found, but that was very small comfort.

She poked Marcus hard in the chest. "You keep me in the loop about this. Personally."

"You got it, Lisa."

"Good," she said and stormed to her bedroom to get dressed.

——————

John was the first one to show up. Jacqueline wondered what that meant. She hadn't seen a wedding ring, so he was probably single— or at least unmarried—and being able to leave on such short notice on a Saturday morning likely meant he didn't have any kids. So maybe he really was trying to hit on her? Having some help finding Trick might be nice, but it wasn't worth the irritation of staving off advances from a man she wasn't interested in.

"Good morning," he called pleasantly, coming from his car to where she stood in the front doorway. As he got closer, his expression fell into a frown. "You didn't sleep at all, did you?"

"Would you?"

He shrugged. "To be honest, I have no idea. I don't have kids. Well, none that live with me."

So, she was partly right. Maybe he was divorced.

"Have you called the police yet?" he asked.

She nodded. "They said someone will be out soon."

"Have you eaten breakfast?"

Jacqueline blinked in surprise. The word 'breakfast' sounded like a foreign language right now, with her son missing. She'd cleaned up the mess Landon had made of his, but had she even fixed the food for him? No, he'd probably made it himself.

John tsked at her. "If you're not going to get sleep, you need to at least feed yourself." He moved past her into her house without the slightest pause. "You'll be no good to Trick if you faint before you can find him."

Suddenly unsure what exactly was happening, Jacqueline closed the front door and followed John into the kitchen. "I'm not going to faint. I don't have time to eat."

"There's always time to eat." He was already standing at her fridge, inspecting the contents.

Someone knocked on the front door.

"That's probably the police," John said. "You'd better go talk to them. I'll take care of the food."

Jacqueline wanted to tell him not to bother, that it wasn't important, but a second knock spurred her toward the door. The sooner the police started looking for Trick, the sooner they'd find him. Hopefully. If he was still human.

She opened the door to a woman in a pencil skirt and red blouse with her hair in tight bun. The third car in Jacqueline's driveway wasn't a police cruiser or unmarked sedan but a red convertible.

"Ms. St. Andrew?" the woman asked.

"You're not the cops, are you?"

"No, though the police did alert me to your son going missing. I'm Lisa VanBuren, the principal of Trick's school."

"Oh." Jacqueline panicked for a moment while her brain tried to figure out if this was a good or bad development. Several seconds passed before she realized that for the time being, it didn't matter, and she needed to roll with it. "Please call me Jacqueline. Yes, Trick's been missing since yesterday evening, though I'm not sure why the police bothered to tell you."

"May I come in?" It was more of an order than a request.

Jacqueline stood aside to let the woman in but pressed, "I appreciate the concern, but why are you here? No offense, but this doesn't have anything to do with Trick's school."

"A student disappeared from a school I'm responsible for. I'd certainly say that makes it my business."

They'd stepped into the living room, and from there Jacqueline could look across into the kitchen, where John was busying himself on the other side of the kitchen island. The odd man really was cooking something.

Lisa followed Jacqueline's gaze and gave a start. "You!"

John jerked, looking up in surprise, his eyes darting from Lisa to Jacqueline and back.

Lisa strode over to him, not stopping until she was inside his personal space. "I heard from the police that you were the one to discover that one of our students went missing. Care to tell me why you didn't bother to inform me?"

After carefully setting down the large bowl he was stirring, John cleared his throat. "Good morning, Lisa. I'm surprised to see you."

No kidding, Jacqueline thought.

Lisa frowned and glanced around the room. "Why are you here?"

John straightened his shirt. "I came to see if I could help Jacqueline look for Trick. I didn't tell you because at the time, no one was sure he was really missing and not simply being stupid and rebellious. I checked in with Jacqueline this morning to discover he hadn't returned home and came right over. I was going to call you after I saw to it that Jacqueline got some food in her. As you can see, she's had a rough night."

Lisa took a step back from him, her lips pressed together, but it seemed his explanation had drained most of her temper. "Fine. But in the future, if you see anything suspicious on school grounds, especially anything involving a student, I want you to notify me immediately, even if it does turn out to be a false alarm."

"Absolutely," John said. "I'm making waffles, if you want any."

Lisa huffed like she'd had enough of him and went back to Jacqueline. "I wasn't aware you two knew each other."

"We didn't until yesterday. You're his boss?"

Lisa nodded.

Jacqueline led her back into the living room and spoke softly. "He says he wants to help because he feels responsible, since Trick was at school late because John gave him detention. But..."

"What is it?"

"Well, you're a woman, and you know him better than I do. Do you think he might be doing this to hit on me?"

Lisa's eyes widened at that. "I certainly hope not. He has a girlfriend he lives with, so I assume it's relatively serious. Why? Has he been inappropriate?"

Jacqueline let out a small sigh. "Not at all. The whole situation is just so weird, and you can never tell with men, you know?"

For the first time, Lisa's face softened. "I'm single, too. Believe me, I know."

"And you're sure he has a girlfriend?"

"I've met her. Briefly. She definitely exists."

"Good. Then that's one thing I don't have to worry about. Wait, how did you know I'm single?"

"You're the only emergency contact listed for Trick," Lisa told her. "There's only one car in your driveway, other than mine and what I assume is John's. Call it an educated guess."

Someone knocked on the door, and all the fear and anxiety that had briefly been nudged to the side came crashing back around Jacqueline.

"I can talk to the police with you if you want," Lisa offered. "I know most of them. Small town and all."

Jacqueline didn't think she'd be saying anything to the police that she wouldn't be willing to tell the school principal, and it sounded like Lisa might find everything out later from them anyway, so she said, "Okay. Thank you."

There were two officers, both men. "Good morning, Ms. St. Andrew," the dark-haired one said. "I'm Officer Smith. This is Officer—"

"Lisa?" blurted the blond one.

Guess she wasn't kidding about knowing the cops, Jacqueline thought.

"Yes," Lisa answered. "I came to offer my help. Is that a problem?"

"Uh, no."

Smith elbowed his partner.

The blond one suddenly focused on his notepad as if checking something. It was an obvious attempt to stall for time as he schooled the surprise off his face.

"This is Officer Parkes," said Smith. "We're here about your missing son."

Jacqueline stepped aside for them to enter. "Thank you. Come in."

The blond cop glanced at her as he did so—and then looked again. So his partner elbowed him again. Jacqueline always enjoyed a good appreciative double-take from a man, but in this case, she wasn't sure the double-take hadn't been because she looked *that bad* after staying up all night worrying. Not that it mattered. She couldn't spare the mental energy to care either way.

———

The smell of waffles hit Landon's nose all at once, like it had been wafting into his room for minutes before finally building up enough to break through his focus on the novel he was reading. Even though he'd already had breakfast—or half of breakfast—he got up right away and went to the kitchen.

Instead of his mom, he found the strange man from yesterday. Trick's teacher. "What are you doing here?" he asked the man.

The man—Mr. McKenzie, Landon remembered—looked up from the waffle iron and gave him a smile. It was charming, that smile. It made Landon suspicious. "Good morning, little one. Would you like a waffle?"

Landon got up onto the bar stool and pulled a plate off the stack on the counter. "My name's Landon."

Mr. McKenzie chuckled and put a waffle onto Landon's plate, sliding the butter and syrup over. "I know."

"Why are you here?" Landon asked again, this time around a mouthful of waffle.

"To make breakfast," said Mr. McKenzie. "And then to see what I can do to help find your brother."

Landon eyed him. Most likely, Trick was a cat again. That was what it had looked like to Landon, anyway. He didn't know how that would have happened, but if it had happened once, it could happen again. And Mom had always been very firm on the idea of never telling anyone about Trick being a boy who'd been turned into a cat by magic. So unless she planned on telling this teacher about that, how did he expect to help find Trick?

That was Mom's problem to worry about, Landon decided. His problem was to keep an eye on this strange man to make sure he didn't mean to do anything bad.

Landon looked over his shoulder and saw his mom talking to two men in uniforms and a lady. "Police again?" he said, not really meaning it as a question, but Mr. McKenzie answered it anyway.

"Most of them. I doubt they'll be here long. There isn't much new information since yesterday. Unless... there's anything relevant that she wouldn't have told them then?"

He definitely meant that as a question. Landon could hear it in his tone. "Like what?"

"Anything at all." Mr. McKenzie was grinning, all innocent like. It had to mean he was up to something.

Landon met his eyes and said in a low voice, "I'm watching you. So don't do anything to my mom."

"Like what?" Mr. McKenzie asked.

"Anything at all," Landon said in a voice like a growl.

Mr. McKenzie's grin only got bigger, like he thought Landon was funny. Like he thought he didn't need to take him seriously because he was just a kid. It was starting to make Landon really mad.

So Landon zapped him. Only a little. Just a stinging shock to the back of Mr. McKenzie's hand that made him drop the spatula he'd started stirring the waffle batter with.

But instead of freaking out, Mr. McKenzie only smiled even bigger, and his eyes lit up. Who was this guy?

Mr. McKenzie glanced over Landon's head toward the living room, then leaned in so their faces were inches apart and said very quietly, "I'm not your enemy, Landon. I promise." Then he winked and stood straight and asked, "How did it go?"

"Fine, I guess," Mom said, and Landon turned to see her standing behind him. The other three people were already gone. "Wow, you... really did make breakfast. How are they, Landon?"

"Good," Landon reluctantly admitted. They were the best waffles he'd ever had.

Mom slid onto the stool next to him, and Mr. McKenzie passed her a waffle. She dug in, letting out pleased hums. It was good to see her eating, especially after she hadn't had dinner last night.

"A man who can cook," she said. "Your girlfriend must love you."

Mr. McKenzie smiled again, but it wasn't charming or innocent. This time, it actually looked real. "I do spoil her. But she deserves it."

Mom's shoulders relaxed, and she dug into her waffle again.

Mr. McKenzie finished cooking the last waffle, and then made a plate up for himself and came partway around the island. "Mind if I sit?" he asked, nodding at the empty third stool beside Mom.

"After you cooked breakfast for us, it would be rude to say no, wouldn't it?" she answered.

He sat and started eating.

"So, what were you two talking about before I got here?" she asked.

"Landon was warning me not to, quote, 'do anything' to you," said Mr. McKenzie.

Heat rose to Landon's cheeks, and his mom gave him a look that made it worse. "Sorry," she said to Mr. McKenzie. "Boys can be protective, even little ones who shouldn't be worrying about things like that."

Mr. McKenzie laughed. "It's fine. After how I was a bit harsh on Trick in class, I doubt he would like me being here any better."

Really? Landon wondered. Trick often had a weird view of things. Landon wasn't sure if Trick not liking Mr. McKenzie was a point for or against the teacher.

Mom was quiet for a minute, then she said, "The police are making this their main priority, so… I'm not sure what else we'll be able to do."

"I see," said Mr. McKenzie.

"But I can't just sit here and wait. I'll go crazy."

"Understandable."

She was quiet for a while again, pushing the last bite of waffle around the syrup left on her plate. "When we got home last night, I was so distracted, our cat got out, and he hasn't come back home yet either."

"I see," said Mr. McKenzie. "That's unfortunate."

"He's mostly Trick's cat, and Trick will be devastated if the cat's still missing when he gets home."

So that was how she was going to play it.

The man's mouth twitched like he was fighting a smile. What kind of person smiled that much, especially at a time like this?

"Well, then," said Mr. McKenzie. "I guess we'd better find Trick's cat."

"You don't need to come," Mom said. "You didn't agree to help—"

"Nonsense. Of course I'll help. The cat went missing because of what happened with Trick, so I'm partly responsible for that as well. I'm at your disposal."

"Thank you. I do appreciate it."

"Of course. By the way, what's the cat's name?"

CHAPTER
NINE

"What's the cat's name?" asked the receptionist.

The word 'Trick' got caught in Denneka's throat. It was one thing to name a cat after a boy she liked when it was only her and the cat hearing it. The idea of someone else hearing what she'd named him, even if that person didn't know her, made her face start to burn with embarrassment. "He doesn't have one," she told the receptionist. "He's just a stray I found. He's not mine, so—so it wouldn't make sense to give him a name, would it?"

"All right," said the receptionist. "Can you give me your name?"

"I—I'm not in your system. I don't have any pets, so I haven't been here before."

The receptionist let out a breath and tried to hand her a form. "Fill this out and we can get you set up."

Denneka froze up with indecision. She was supposed to be at the shop, starting work. Not at a vet on the other side of town, taking a cat she wasn't allowed to have for a checkup. If her mom found out from the receptionist's brother's neighbor or something (small towns were the worst for sneaking around), Denneka would be in trouble and Trick would be kicked out onto the street. She thought about turning and walking out before anyone she knew saw her, but

Jonah's words came back to her: "You better hope he doesn't have fleas."

Jonah had come into her room to say something to her and had seen Trick playing on her bed. Denneka hadn't even considered that the kitten might have fleas, but as soon as Jonah said it, it was as if she could feel fleas already on her. He was a stray cat—or at least one who'd been outside for some period of time. Of course he might have fleas. Why hadn't she thought of that? So even though she'd searched through the fur on his back and belly and couldn't find any fleas, she was afraid she'd missed some. She wouldn't be able to sleep in her bed until she was reassured little Trick didn't have fleas.

"Look, I—I don't really want to be set up as a client or anything," she told the receptionist. "Like I said, I don't have pets. I'm just holding onto this kitten until I can find its owner, and I thought I should get it checked for fleas and, you know, general health stuff. Just for safety. I can pay cash." She hoped she had enough left from her salary for the last month to cover it.

The receptionist was still holding the form toward her. "We need to get you set up in our system anyway."

Denneka took a step backward. Maybe another vet would be more reasonable. Or maybe she could buy some flea shampoo and—

"It's fine, Mallory," said a woman who stepped up behind the receptionist. "We're not busy right now. I can give the cat a quick exam, on the house. That way you won't have to figure out how to get it in the system." She gave Denneka an understanding smile. "What do you say?"

"Thank you!" Denneka blurted. "That sounds great."

The vet looked at where Trick was sitting calmly on the reception counter. "But if you need to bring him back later, please have him in a carrier. Cardboard ones are pretty cheap and will do the trick. It's for his own safety."

"Oh. Right." Denneka hadn't even thought about a carrier. She'd carried Trick in her arms partway here, but when he'd gotten tired of that and squirmed to get down, he'd kept walking along beside her like a well-trained dog. She wasn't sure how confining him would be for his own safety, but she couldn't really buy a carrier anyway. If her mom spotted it...

"Around the corner," the vet directed, and Denneka picked up Trick and met the vet going into an exam room. "Put him on the table there." Once Denneka did so, the vet gently combed him a bit, looking at his fur. "Let me guess, hiding it from your parents? It's okay. But if you're allowed to keep him once they find out, you will need to have one of them set up a patient account with us, if you plan to keep bringing him here. I can't give him any shots for free, but a physical exam is no problem. Do you have any particular concerns?"

"I just wanted to make sure he doesn't have fleas."

The vet hummed and kept checking Trick with the comb. "Good news. I don't see any sign of fleas."

"Oh, good."

The vet went through the steps of the checkup, and as she did so, little Trick got increasingly tired of being handled. He didn't fight back, but he squirmed and tried to get away more and more.

"His ears and mouth look good," said the vet. "His lungs are good, and everything feels fine in his abdomen. Let's get a weight and temperature, then we should be done."

Denneka had to help stop Trick from walking off the scale, and then she had to hold his shoulders while the vet took his temperature. He yowled when she stuck the thermometer in and turned his head like he really might try to bite the vet.

"I know, I know," Denneka said with sympathy, "but it's the only way for her to get your temperature." As if a cat could understand her explanation.

When that step was done, Trick slunk to the edge of the table and jumped down.

"It's fine; we're done anyway," said the vet. "He looks perfectly healthy. Everything is within normal parameters. The only things I'd suggest are the usual shots and getting him neutered. You should really consider the neutering even if you don't keep him. He's old enough to have it done now."

Denneka hadn't even thought of that. She actually hadn't even been totally sure Trick was a boy cat. "Oh. Is that... urgent?"

"Not exactly. But with stray cats, especially if you're not allowed to keep him and can't find an owner, it's highly recommended in order to keep the stray cat population managed. There are programs that will pay for it, so it wouldn't necessarily cost you anything."

Denneka looked at Trick, who was sitting in the corner, furiously grooming himself. "I'll keep it in mind. Thanks again for checking him."

"Not a problem. He's a nice cat. He's still young, so it's possible he's a stray, but you might see about finding his owner if he's got one. You could check with the shelter to see if anyone's looking for a missing black kitten."

"Oh, yeah, that's..." Denneka cleared her throat. "That's a good idea."

It *was* a good idea, and she knew she *should* do it. But... later. There was no rush, right?

"You should get him a collar, too," said the vet. "Even if you don't get a tag, if he gets out, it'll let people know that he's not feral, and most of them have reflective strips that will make him much more visible at night. We've got some in the lobby."

Denneka picked up Trick, then went to the front desk and bought him a bright yellow collar. He kept ducking away when she tried to put it on him. "Calm down. It's just a collar. It's for your own good. You don't want a car hitting you if you get out at night, do you?" There she went again, talking to the cat. But the receptionist didn't bat an eye, so maybe that really was normal with pet people. Eventually, she got the safety snap closed without catching any fur in it. Trick shook his head and pawed at it, but it stayed in place. She picked him up and carried him out of the vet clinic. As soon as they were back out in the sunlight, Trick squirmed until she set him down on the sidewalk.

He immediately ran away down the street, too fast for her to follow.

———

For several hours, Kester drove creeping circles around the streets of Agreste with Jacqueline beside him and Landon sitting silently in the back seat. The woman had been hesitant to accept his offer to chauffeur her on their search, but she'd quickly seen the sense in it. Not having to pay attention to driving allowed her to scrape her gaze across the passing scenery in a manner both speedy and thorough. For Landon's part, he only read a book and occasionally glanced at Kester.

It was well past lunchtime now, but Kester didn't mention it. He kept to his own task of making sure they didn't hit another car or accidentally run over the kitten. This would have been much more relaxing if the blasted child hadn't escaped his handler. While they waited at a stoplight, he focused his attention on what Julia saw. Trick was frolicking in some grass at a fast food restaurant a mile away, oblivious to the hawk who, so far, was keeping well enough out of his sight.

Kester disengaged the connection with Julia and turned left when the light turned green to put a little more distance between Trick and themselves.

"Mom, I'm hungry," Landon said.

Jacqueline checked the dash display. "It's two o'clock already," she said in a tired, restless voice. "I'm sorry, Landon. John, would you mind stopping somewhere to eat?"

"Happily, if it means we can get out of the car for a while. My legs aren't used to sitting this long at a stretch."

"I'm sorry, John. You don't have to stay. You've already done more than enough to help."

He raised both hands in apology before quickly placing one back on the steering wheel. "I didn't mean that. I'm happy to help, and I have nothing better to do. I honestly only mean that my legs are getting sore and could use a break."

"Oh. Thanks." She fiddled with her hands in her lap—an action out-of-character enough to catch his full attention. "I'm not used to getting help from anyone. I don't want to take advantage."

To Kester's great surprise, a sharp pang of remorse and sympathy struck him. But it was gone almost immediately. "It must be very difficult to be a single mother."

"Difficult, yes. But better than the alternative."

"Were the boys' fathers so horrible?"

Jacqueline shot a glance over her shoulder at Landon. Maybe Kester shouldn't have said anything while the boy was in the car. "Horrible, no," she said in a tight, quiet voice. "But frivolous, selfish, and irresponsible. Hardly the type of men who could ever make good fathers. Or husbands, for that matter."

Kester wanted to press her, to remind her what Trick had said about a 'sperm donor' and ask how she could know what sort of person said donor was. But it was clear she wouldn't say any more while Landon was present.

She sighed. "Why don't we grab something quick and go home; that way I can make some calls while we eat. Landon, how do tacos sound?"

Before the boy could answer, Kester said, "If it's not too much trouble, I actually have a craving for some fried chicken," because the only taco place in town was the one where Trick was currently sunbathing on an outdoor table.

"I want a chicken sandwich," Landon said in a mild tone. Kester didn't fool himself to think that the boy was warming up to him, but at least he wasn't one of those children who were contrary for the sake of being contrary.

When they returned to the St. Andrew residence, they settled in at the dining table, and Jacqueline made phone calls with one hand and ate fries with the other. It didn't take long for her to hang up the first call with a grim expression. "The police haven't found anything yet."

"I'm sure he'll turn up," Kester said. He'd finished the fried chicken, so he started peeling the wrapper off his crispy chicken sandwich.

"You're awfully calm about this," Jacqueline accused.

"I prefer to think optimistically." He laid the sandwich on the wrapper and took off the top bun. "I truly believe that Trick will be returned to you, safe and sound. Sooner or later."

Jacqueline stabbed a fry into the small tub of ranch dressing forcefully enough that it broke and she had to dig it out with her fingers. "Didn't you say you had kids that don't live with you?"

Had he said that? "They don't just not live with me. I'm not in their lives at all."

It was obvious she wanted to ask for details about what he meant, but all she said was, "If you were, maybe you wouldn't take this so lightly."

Kester picked out a packet of hot sauce and a second packet of mustard, then applied them both to his sandwich. "Perhaps. Does the worry help you focus? Is it some sort of magical force, bending reality to your will?"

She blinked at him. "No. Never mind." Then she dialed another number.

While she talked on her phone, Kester put the bun back on his sandwich and took a bite, savoring the flavor. He noticed that Landon was watching him with intense concentration. When their eyes met, Landon picked up two packets and replicated Kester's application on his own child-sized sandwich. He took a bite, brow still furrowed as he considered it.

"Good?" Kester asked him.

Landon nodded and kept eating.

Kester leaned closer to him and said, quietly enough that Jacqueline wouldn't hear over her phone conversation, "I know many secrets, small one."

Jacqueline dropped her phone onto the table in frustration. "And the shelter hasn't seen anything of Tr—uh, Charcoal either."

"What about vets?" Landon suggested.

Blast him.

"Landon, you're brilliant! Why didn't I think of that?" Jacqueline tapped and swiped quickly on her phone. "There are two in town. Let's try them."

As she called, Kester ate the rest of his sandwich in a sullen mood. Julia hadn't been able to actually get inside the veterinary office, so he had no idea what information the girl had or hadn't given them. That was the problem with wild cards. They could make things much more exciting, but they could also end the game prematurely if one wasn't careful.

―――――

Late in the afternoon, Denneka stood in the women's section of her family's shop, glumly folding sweaters. After little Trick had run away, there hadn't been much else to do other than go to work. She'd tried to find him at first, but it had been no use. It wasn't so much that he was gone—well, it was, but she'd always known she couldn't keep him. But the fact that he'd run away from her like that hurt.

She'd have thought she'd be used to rejection by now. How pathetic was she that even rejection by a cat could sting so much?

A hushed voice nearby broke through her depression. "At least it wasn't one of ours."

Two women around her mom's age had strolled closer to Denneka while they browsed. The short-haired one lightly back-handed the long-haired woman on the arm. "Lucy, that's awful!"

"I know, I know," said Lucy, still nearly whispering. "But I mean, aren't you glad? I know it's terrible that any kid got abducted, but if it had to happen, at least it was the new kid no one even knew."

Denneka forgot how to breathe.

"But what about next time?" the short-haired one asked Lucy. "First the teacher, then one of the students? What if they're connected? What if there will be more? My son's almost in sixth grade."

Denneka couldn't hold back anymore. "Excuse me," she said, moving close to the women so quickly that they both jumped. "Who was abducted? What are you talking about?"

They looked at her with pity and hesitated before the short-haired one finally spoke. "I'm sure you'll hear about it sooner or later. It's not like they can hide it for long. It sounds like one of the students from the junior high got kidnapped from school last night."

All the blood drained from Denneka's face.

"Oh, no," said Lucy. "That's your school, isn't it? You look the right age. Don't worry, I'm sure it wasn't anyone you know. They say it was a new boy who just moved into town and didn't have any friends."

"Are—are you sure that happened?" Denneka asked.

"I heard it from my brother, who's the school secretary," said the short-haired lady. "The police are all searching. I'm sure if they don't find him, they'll let everyone know on Monday anyway."

Denneka forced her lungs to expand and contract.

Lucy laid a hand on her shoulder. "I'm sure you'll be fine. Just be extra careful and try to stay in groups. We're all really worried about what this means, but it won't help to panic about it."

Too stunned to say any more, Denneka wandered away from the women and toward the back of the store. Alex stopped her before she got there. "Denneka, are you okay? What did those women say to you? You look like you've seen a ghost."

"Tr-Trick's been abducted."

"Who? Never mind. Come on."

He took her arm, led her back to the break room, and guided her into a seat. Which was good because Denneka was wobbly and, once they had arrived, couldn't remember getting there. She stared at a spot on the floor for a long time.

How had this happened? *What* had happened? Who would want to abduct Trick?

It was her fault.

She fought back the urge to throw up.

She should have insisted on giving Trick a ride home. Or at least stayed with him until his mom came to get him. Why had she left him just lying in the grass like a helpless target?

What if he was sold to a pimp or cut up for parts? What if he'd been taken by a serial killer?

Her vision started to get blurry.

"Honey, what's wrong?" asked her mom.

Denneka blinked away the blurriness to see Mom kneeling in front of her. Alex stood there, too. They both looked really worried.

"Trick—Trick's gone," she said. Her voice squeaked, and it was hard to push the words out at all.

"She was talking to some customers, then she looked like this," Alex said.

"See if they're still here," Mom told him. "If they are, find out what they told her."

Alex left, and Mom took Denneka's hand. "You're not hurt, are you?"

Denneka shook her head and squeezed her mom's hand.

Alex came back and told Mom the news.

Mom gasped. "What? That's horrible!" Then her tone softened and she said to Denneka, "You know the boy, don't you?"

Denneka nodded.

"Is he… a friend?"

Denneka wasn't sure how to answer that. "K-kind of."

Mom stood and came around the chair to wrap an arm around Denneka's shoulder, holding her close. "Why don't you go home for the day? It's still light out, but be careful. I'll see if I can find out any more news about what happened."

Taking the help that her mom offered, Denneka got up and gathered her things, then started the two-block walk back to their house.

On the second block, something fast-moving intercepted her.

———

By the time the sun started getting low, Trick had almost forgotten what he'd been angry about.

Almost.

Things had been going well with the familiar girl. She'd fed him (sort of) and given him a place to hide and a nice, warm bed to sleep in. But then she'd taken him to the vet, and the doctor kept poking him and then had stuck something hard in an *extremely* uncomfortable place.

He couldn't be blamed for getting mad about that. Anyone would.

Then the girl had put a collar on him. A collar!

He remembered, after he'd calmed down, how his mom had kept trying to put collars on him, saying it was for his own good. The girl had said something like that, too.

Mom had taken him to vets for checkups, too. The girl was… probably… he guessed… just trying to look after him.

He stood in the middle of a sidewalk somewhere and wondered what to do now. He'd played a lot, he'd taken a nap, and he was starting to get hungry. He'd tried to catch a bird, but that time as a human must have dulled his hunting ability. Or maybe they saw him coming more easily now that he had a bright yellow collar around his neck.

It wasn't all that uncomfortable, now that he'd gotten used to it. And it did remind him of the girl and how she tried, in her own way, to take care of him.

A car drove by, so much bigger than he'd gotten used to them being, and it scared him.

He needed to be with the familiar girl again. That would make him feel better.

Trick knew the town pretty well by now, and it didn't take him long to reach the girl's blue house. As he approached, he ran past someone walking the same direction. Her scent hit him as he passed, and he tumbled to a stop and spun around. The familiar girl was right there, so he ran back to meet her, ran between her legs, and then swept around in front to make sure she noticed him.

She nearly tripped over him, though—he'd forgotten how clumsy humans could be—and cried out.

"Tr-Trick?" she asked, looking at him strangely. She picked him up and held him out in front of her. "You're back."

Then she buried him in her shirt, squeezing him too tightly in her arms, and her body shook as she made crying sounds.

Sheesh, I wasn't gone that long, he thought. He squeaked softly in protest, but when she didn't put him down, he decided to let her hold him a little longer. Even if it was too tight, it was kinda nice to have been missed. And to not be scolded like his mom would do.

The crying stopped after a few minutes, and she moved him into a more gentle hold. "I'm so glad you're back," she told him. "But—but Trick..." Her face shifted expression, and her voice had a faraway sound. "What happened... There must be a connection.... Trick... and Mr. Haug."

Haug. Trick remembered seeing that name before. He tried to visualize it, and finally it came to him. That was the word on the poster in the school hallway.

Was she asking him about seeing the man's body? She'd asked him about it again after that day, but it hadn't felt safe to risk speaking in order to tell her. For some reason, she wanted to know now. She seemed upset, and if it would make her feel better, he guessed could at least show her.

Trick squirmed until she put him down and then headed off in the direction of the cemetery.

"Hey, wait!" she cried, and he stopped and turned, waiting for her to catch up. She sure was a slow human. She didn't even start moving toward him right away. But eventually she did, so he ran off a little farther.

He had to check and make sure she was still following him a bunch of times, but eventually they both made it to the cemetery on the hill, and he ran through the rows of headstones, looking for the right one. What had been that long name he'd seen written on it?

"Trick, hang on!" the familiar girl called. "It's nearly dark! I shouldn't be out this late! Get back here, will you?"

Trick glanced at the sky, nearly full dark now. Maybe that was why the girl had such a hard time keeping up. It had taken a while to get here on foot, and it was harder for humans to move in the dark.

Never mind; they were here now. If he could just find that grave he'd seen the man's body in, then they could go back to her home.

He closed his eyes and tried to visualize where the gravestone was and what had been written on it. It had been... over there, on the right side of the graveyard, a little way from the tree line. And the name... the name had been...

Right. There it was. He loped over to the grave, which had been filled in. The dirt didn't smell super fresh, but there wasn't anything growing on it yet. He jumped up on top of the gravestone and sat waiting for the familiar girl to come over.

She stumbled around a lot but eventually made it. She was panting hard. "My goodness, Trick, why did you run? Is this where you've been living?"

Trick cocked his head at the question. *Who lives in a graveyard?* True, she would always get off the bus before it got to his house, so he didn't expect her to know exactly where he lived, but she had to be able to see there were no houses around here.

Maybe she was making a joke. He didn't get humor a lot of the time.

She pulled out her phone, not even looking at the grave. "Oh no, the shop closes in fifteen minutes. Then Mom and Dad will be home in thirty. If I don't get back by then, they'll be really worried."

Why wasn't she even looking at the grave after they'd come all this way? Maybe she'd only been curious about it for a minute and now she didn't care.

Whatever. He hopped down and went over to her. He was even more hungry than before. If they could get back to her place without her parents seeing her, she could get him something to—

A flash of something caught Trick's eye, and he stopped in his tracks, head swiveling toward it.

He froze still as a statue as he searched for what had made that flash, and spotted it. In the tree line, partially hidden behind one of the first trees, a big man stood with something held to his face. Another flash of light, and Trick realized they were binoculars.

"Trick?" the girl asked. "What's wrong?"

Trick didn't take his eyes off the man. After a short while, the man lowered the binoculars enough that Trick could see his face.

His fur stood on end all the way from his neck to his tail.

It was the man who'd buried the body. The one who'd chased him off. He was still here, and he was watching them.

Trick didn't understand what was going on, why the man was here, or what he was watching for. But his instincts told him to be very afraid.

Trick bolted down the hill as fast as his paws could take him, ignoring the cry of the girl behind him. He stopped to wait for her when he reached the front gate, but she wasn't running. She was only halfheartedly jogging to catch up to him.

She didn't see him, Trick realized with horror. *She doesn't know there's danger.*

Trick ran back to her, darting around her feet to urge her on, meowing as loudly and desperately as he could, wishing he could form the word 'Run!' with his cat mouth.

"What's wrong with you all of a sudden?" she asked him. But she sped up. Maybe even if her brain didn't know what was going on, her instincts were finally kicking in.

He hurried her along, out of the graveyard, not slowing until they reached the end of the street, where it intersected with another street and there started to be more buildings and streetlights. The girl stopped to catch her breath, and Trick watched carefully behind them.

The big man wasn't following. They'd escaped.

The girl took out her phone, dialed, and started talking. "Jonah, are you home?... Okay, good, can you pick me up?... Out by the cemetery, but I'll be walking back to meet you, so just keep an eye out for me…. It's kind of a long story…. Yes, it's stupid. I'll tell you on the way back, but please don't tell Mom and Dad."

Then she put the phone in her pocket and picked Trick up. He was still wired and tense, but she started moving away from the cemetery again, so Trick decided to let her carry him. After a minute, his limbs felt like jelly, and he fell asleep in her arms.

chapter TEN

Denneka awoke Monday morning with kitty Trick curled up in the crook of her bent knees. For such an independent cat, he sure was clingy when he slept. He always burrowed under the blanket some time during the night, too. She got up slowly, trying not to wake him, and went to the bathroom.

By the time she got back, Trick hadn't moved. He'd slept a lot yesterday, too. Maybe he was still worn out from whatever he'd done on Saturday after running away from her. Considering she wouldn't be able to let him loose in the rest of the house, she really hoped he wouldn't get restless enough to make noise and get found by her parents. She would have let him keep sleeping all morning, but he needed to use the potty before she left for school or she'd have a mess to clean up when she got home. Fortunately, both her parents were already at the shop, so she was able to wake him up and carry him to the bathroom so he could do his business while she brushed her teeth.

"Be good while I'm at school," she told him when she put him back in her room. He hopped on the bed and went right back to sleep.

The bus ride was lonely without Trick—the real Trick. She hadn't heard any news of him, not that she was anywhere on the list of

e who'd be alerted to news of him. Yesterday, she'd been so
and worried, her Mom had told her to stay home instead of
king in the shop. She'd only barely managed to get her home-
rk done, and she'd probably messed most of it up because she
ouldn't concentrate.

She sat staring out the school bus window, the empty seat beside
her making her feel like she was sitting on the edge of the Grand
Canyon.

At school, there was more buzz of conversation than normal. The
Sunday paper had carried news of the missing student, and several
kids had copies and were sharing them around. Denneka tried to
put it from her mind, but she couldn't avoid hearing the wild speculations as she walked into the school building and down the hall.

"Do you think there's a serial killer?"

"He was pretty weird. He probably finally snapped, and that's
why his clothes were left. Then he wandered out into the woods and
went feral. Do you think the police have checked the woods yet?"

"Didn't he say his dad didn't live with them? Maybe it was some
family thing and his dad came and kidnapped him."

Denneka wasn't sure who'd said that last one, but she clung to
the idea. Every possibility that had gone through her mind so far
was of the 'shallow grave' or 'sold into human trafficking' variety.
The idea that maybe his dad had come and gotten him because of
some domestic dispute with his mom was actually really encourag-
ing, because at least then he probably would still be alive and might
even come back once they found him.

She didn't *think* Trick would have gone feral. Though there was
that whole bird-chasing thing. *Maybe the police should check the woods,
just in case.*

Denneka went to homeroom with her head down, but that didn't
help. As soon as she entered the classroom, a taunting voice asked,
"What happened, weirdo?"

She kept her head down and took a few more steps toward her
desk. *Not today. Will you just leave me alone?*

But Amy couldn't resist landing the second blow. "Your

boyfriend get so sick of you that he completely disappeared from existence to get away from you?"

Denneka stopped to glare. Amy, Trevor, and Flora were congregated around Amy's desk, all of them laughing at her. Mr. McKenzie sat at his desk at the front, reading a book and paying no attention to any of them. Denneka tried to think of a good comeback, but she couldn't come up with anything adequate. Simply telling them to shut up would only lead to more taunting. So she tried to ignore them and made her way to her desk. Thankfully, that seemed to pacify them enough that they didn't continue their assault.

As the last few minutes before the bell counted down and more kids came in, Denneka could see people looking at her and people pointedly *not* looking at her. She pretended to be reading, and no one actually spoke to her again.

Then class started, and Mr. McKenzie put down his book and stood in front of them. "Before we begin, Principal VanBuren asked all the teachers to make an announcement. In case you haven't already heard, a student from this school has gone missing."

There was actually a surprised, "What?" from one kid in the back.

"Yes. Patrick went missing some time Friday evening." Mr. McKenzie sounded bored *and* he was still calling Trick the wrong name. Did he really not care at all? "The principal wants to assure everyone that the police are on it and there's no reason to think anyone else is likely to go missing, though she urges you all to be cautious."

That was it? Denneka's jaw clenched, and she raised her hand.

Mr. McKenzie ignored it. "If you want more information about that and haven't read yesterday's paper, I suggest you do so. Now, get out your homework and pass it forward."

"Mr. McKenzie!" Denneka blurted, hand still in the air. "Aren't you worried about him at all? He disappeared from school. Because *you* kept him here late. That doesn't bother you?"

Mr. McKenzie cast her an annoyed glance. "I see that detention did nothing to teach you not to speak out of turn, Denneka. Trying for another?"

Several kids laughed or at least snickered. "I raised my hand!" she protested.

"Just as knocking does not grant you leave to enter a room uninvited, raising your hand does not grant you leave to speak without being given permission." He sat on the edge of his desk and folded his arms. "But I will be lenient this once, due to what is most certainly your unstable emotional state. If it will calm you enough to stop disrupting my class, I'll tell you that I have offered my help in locating Patrick. As it happens, there isn't much I can do, being neither a police officer, private detective, FBI agent, nor psychic."

More snickers from around the room.

"Does that sufficiently satisfy your righteous indignation?"

Denneka lowered her hand. "Yes, sir." If he had offered his help, even if he couldn't do anything, there wasn't much else she could try to get out of him. An actual apology obviously wasn't going to happen. She ducked her head and held still, waiting for everyone to stop looking at her.

The rest of the class proceeded without incident. Worried that Amy and the other cool kids might ambush her in the hallway to mock her some more, when the time came to switch classrooms, Denneka waited until most everyone else had gone out, trailing back at the end of the group.

She jumped a little when she heard Mr. McKenzie's soft voice as she passed by his desk, where he was sitting with his head already bowed toward his book. "Denneka." When she stopped and took a step closer, he looked up just enough for their eyes to meet. Was that *amusement* she saw? "The reason I don't appear concerned about your friend isn't because I don't care that he's missing. It's because I believe that wherever he is, someone is looking after him."

"What?" she gasped. "Have you heard something? Do you know anything? Do you have any evidence of that?"

He gave a small shrug and looked down at his book. "I suppose I'm simply an optimist by nature."

Denneka stared at him for another couple seconds as he went back to reading, then she huffed and left him to his groundless delusions. He was probably mocking her. But even if he wasn't totally heartless, if he dealt with any guilt he was feeling by telling himself empty, stupid, naïve lies to make himself feel better, then what good was he?

Still, she did hope he was right.

───────

Trick woke up when he heard the bedroom door open. He raised his head to watch through sleepy eyes as the familiar girl came in, dropped her backpack, and fell into her desk chair with a loud breath. Trick uncurled himself from his napping spot in the middle of her bed and had a good stretch and yawn.

Based on the way the sunlight was coming through the curtains, it was mid-afternoon, so she must have come straight home after school. Had he really slept through the whole day? His mom never let him sleep that long. Whenever he'd tried to sleep all day, she'd always ended up waking him partway through to try to teach him more reading or math or some other stupid human thing.

He hopped down from the bed and went to the girl, brushing against her shin with his body until she reached down a hand to stroke his back.

"You probably need to go potty, don't you?" she asked him.

Now that she mentioned it, he did, and he meowed to tell her so.

"Okay." She sounded tired. After she got up and pulled off her jacket, she opened the bedroom door. "Mom and Dad are still at the shop, so it's safe to go out."

Getting to the bathroom on his own was easy when the coast was clear, so he took care of his business and then came out to find her in the kitchen. She opened a can, and a fishy smell zipped across his nose. Sudden hunger made him impatient enough to jump onto the counter, even though he knew he wasn't supposed to do that—at least, Mom never tolerated it—and sure enough, the familiar girl shooed him off immediately. So he meowed at her to hurry until she set a plate down in front of him.

"I figured it would be suspicious to have cat food around in case my mom ever found it somehow," the girl told him. "So I bought some canned tuna and salmon instead. I hope it's true about cats liking fish." After a pause, she said, "Well, you're scarfing that down, so I guess so."

It wasn't as tasty as a fresh bird or even the cooked meat dishes his mom used to make him, but it tasted all right and filled his stomach, so it was okay by Trick.

When he finished eating, he looked up to see her standing there, staring at him. He wasn't very good at reading the way human faces changed to express their emotions, but something about her stillness and the breath she let out when she squatted to pick up the dish made him think she was unhappy. He didn't want her to be unhappy. She'd kept him hidden and safe, hadn't even tried to take him home, and hadn't stopped being nice to him just because he'd turned into a cat.

"Come on, Trick," she said after she washed out the dish. "You probably shouldn't spend too long out here, just in case Mom or Dad come home suddenly or something."

He went with her back into her bedroom. She sat on her bed to take her shoes off. Before she could get back up, he jumped onto her lap and laid down. *Don't be sad*, he thought, wishing he could say it out loud. There were maybe—*maybe*—times when being able to speak would be useful. She wasn't telling him what was wrong, and he couldn't ask her, but whenever his mom or brother had been unhappy about something, Trick had found that getting on their laps and letting them pet him seemed to help. Plus, it was warm.

The girl stroked his head and scratched his ears, which felt so nice he started to purr.

Soft, gentle hands scooped him up under his chest and moved him onto the mattress. The girl pulled some books out of her backpack and started reading. Trick recognized the one she chose first as their math textbook.

Trick wanted to run. He wanted to chase something. B[t] bedroom door was closed. Trick walked over the bed to the win[w] right behind it and pawed the curtains apart enough to jump onto the windowsill. Maybe the girl had left the window crack[e] and he could go outside.

Nope. She hadn't. Trick pawed at the edge of the window and meowed.

"Do you want to go outside?" the girl asked. She was so smart. "Sorry, Trick, I don't think I should let you out. It's... it's not safe out there."

Not safe? What was she talking about? He'd spent lots of time out—

He froze. At her words, he'd started scanning the area for danger, and it didn't take him long to find it.

The hawk was watching him. Right there in the tree. Barely hidden by the branches, the hawk was just sitting there, staring at him. Waiting for him to step a paw outside so it could kill and eat him.

Trick scrambled out of the window and landed on the floor with a thump. His heart raced, and his paws weren't much slower as he bolted for the open closet door and threw himself into a pile of laundry, burrowing as deeply into it as he could get.

The girl was right. It wasn't safe out there. But it was safe in here. There were solid walls and windows and doors around him. It was warm, and there was food and water. And the familiar girl was here to watch out for him.

When he calmed down from that scare, he dug himself out of the laundry and poked around the closet. The bedroom itself was mostly clean and tidy, but the closet had lots of things to investigate. He nosed around, then pulled a stuffed animal off of a shelf and wrestled with it. Which was fun, but there wasn't a lot of satisfaction in subduing a stuffed animal. Next to the door of the closet, he found an open box half-filled with magazines. It was a good box. Big enough but not too big. He carefully put one paw in, then

r, then slid his body in to see how much of the space he could
.p.

.he sudden silence grabbed his attention, and only now did he
.lize the scratch of pencil on paper had been going on in the back-
round for a while. He looked up, peeking over the edge of the box
just enough to see the girl sitting on her bed. She was watching him,
her head tilted, and then her face contorted and tears fell down her
cheeks.

Why was she suddenly sad again? He thought he'd taken care of
that.

Trick leapt out of the box and went to her. As soon as he was
near, she scooped him into her arms and held him close, pressing
her face into his fur and breathing in shallow gasps. It was uncomfortable, but he stayed still because the longer she held him, the
more even her breathing got. It wasn't very long before she set him
down and petted his head. "Good boy."

It felt like a warm balloon inflated inside his chest when he
heard that. His little brother was always the one his mom had called
'good boy'. Not him. He got 'silly boy' or 'brave boy' or 'troublemaker', but never 'good boy'. To his surprise, it felt really nice to be
someone's good boy.

Trick lay down beside the familiar girl and watched her do
homework. She was on history now. Her textbook was laid out on
the bed in front of her folded legs, and she had another book on her
lap to use as a writing surface. It was some kind of short-answer
quiz she was working on. After steadily going through a cycle of
flipping pages, reading, and scribbling, she got stuck in a loop of
flipping pages.

"What was the reason for the Boston Tea Party?" she read from
the paper she was filling out.

Trick remembered that one. Well, not the actual answer, but he
remembered reading about that. He knew what part of the book it
was in and could picture the big painting that had been on that
page. The girl was looking in the wrong place.

When she started flipping pages going the wrong direction, Trick got up and lay down on that side of the book so she'd stop going the wrong way. With one of his forepaws, he pawed at the corner of the pages, eventually getting them to turn. He kept turning pages with his paws. He couldn't turn them all the way, since he was still lying on the other side of the book, but he'd do that once he found the right page. Until then, he was holding the pages in place with his other forepaw.

He was so focused on finding the right page for her that he didn't notice she was laughing until the bed started bouncing.

"Trick, come on," she said between laughs. "That's not a toy. I'm trying to do my homework."

He knew that. He was helping. Did she not see that?

Apparently not, since she picked him up off her book. All the pages he'd tried to turn flopped back where they'd been. She set him down beside her and petted him.

Trick didn't purr now. The end of his tail flapped against the bed in agitation. She thought he was playing? He knew he wasn't very book smart, but every so often, he did know what he was doing. Her rejection of his help stung.

But even as she went back to flipping the wrong pages, she was smiling. He'd made her laugh. And that was more important than homework.

———

The look on Jacqueline's face when she walked into the restaurant was well worth whatever the lunch would cost. Kester smiled and waved to her from a table situated near the decorative stone waterfall covering most of the back wall. She dodged past the hostess, moved much too quickly through the tables, and stood over him with a wide-eyed scowl of disapproval.

"John!" she whispered. "I had no idea this place was so fancy! Why did you ask to meet here?"

"Jacqueline, please, calm yourself and have a seat." He gestured across from him. "I asked you here because it's one of the few places in town with excellent food, and I was tired of eating sack lunches."

After a moment's pause, she acquiesced, set down her purse, and picked up the menu. "I know you said you wanted to treat me, but I can't let you. This restaurant is too fancy. It would be inappropriate." She perused the menu selection, and her jaw dropped. "These are the *lunch* prices?"

"I'm not a teacher because I need the money," he explained.

She was frowning at the menu. "I guess... Ugh, even the salads are expensive."

"Order whatever you want. I said it's my treat. After all the stress you've been under, you deserve it."

"How does Julia feel about you taking another woman to eat at a place like this?"

"She didn't object." Because she was his familiar and he was her master. Julia had never objected to anything Kester had ever done. Not in so many words, at least. But he could feel her... unhappiness about it deep in his core.

"Oh," said Jacqueline, clearly interpreting his words to mean Julia had given her approval. "Fine, then. But just this once."

A young waiter approached. He was tall and very handsome (in the most generic possible way). Likely he hadn't been a waiter here for long, because Kester could detect a faint reaction in his eyes when he approached the two of them. It was a reaction that said, *What is a guy like him doing with a woman like her?* Kester still wasn't used to other men perceiving him as a non-threat, and that look which questioned whether he was even allowed to associate with beautiful women was even more strange. He didn't care for it.

"We're ready to order," Kester told the waiter, his tone slightly more biting than perhaps it should have been. He ordered first. It was always more polite for the gentleman to order first if he was paying so that the lady worried less about the cost of what she wished to order. If he ordered the second most expensive dish on the menu—which he did—then she wouldn't wring her hands over ordering something in the middle range of prices.

To his satisfaction, Jacqueline took him at his word and ordered a respectable entree rather than trying to soothe her sense of propriety by ordering soup and salad.

The waiter took their menus and left but circled back very quickly with water and bread.

Kester helped himself to a slice of bread, dipping it in oil and vinegar. "I don't expect a single mother to be flush with cash, but if you don't mind my asking, what is it you do for a living?"

"I'm a writer."

"Oh? What do you write?" He already knew, but 'John' hadn't asked, and it might come up later, so he wanted to be prepared.

"Romance novels. I'm indie, so I do all the publishing stuff myself."

"That must be a lot of work."

"It is, yes. But it allows a lot of flexibility, and I love it."

"You don't seem like the romance novel type."

"A lot of us don't."

"But working for yourself means if you don't work, you don't get paid, am I right? No paid health insurance. No paid leave."

"I still make money from the books I already have out, but you're mostly right."

"How much have you been able to work since you moved here?"

"Not much, what with getting unpacked, getting the boys ready for school, and now Trick."

Kester took another piece of bread. How much savings did she have? How long could she go without having time to work?

And why was he thinking about any of that?

"Have you heard anything more from the police?" he asked.

She was tearing her bread into small pieces with her fingers and eating them in tiny bites. "I call them every day to ask for an update, but so far they haven't had anything to tell me. I feel kinda bad for them. It must be frustrating to put all that work into something and get nowhere."

"I'm amazed you have room for sympathy for them around all the worry about Trick."

"I am still worried, of course! In fact, I wonder how long they'll stick with it without finding anything."

Kester nodded. "That does seem like a real danger. But rest assured, even if the police give up, I'll still help you however I can."

"Thank you. Speaking of helping, did you ask your students about our cat?"

"I did," he lied. Jacqueline had learned from one of the veterinary clinics that a girl had brought in a cat matching Trick's description. The girl—bless her—hadn't given the vet any information about herself, so all they could tell Jacqueline was her approximate age. Deducing from this that she probably went to Trick's school, Jacqueline had asked 'John' if he might make an announcement or two that if anyone had picked up a stray cat recently, they should contact her. "No one came forward."

Jacqueline sighed. "Maybe she's shy. Or"—she swallowed— "maybe she wants to keep Charcoal for herself. Still, at least if he's with a girl who cares enough about animals to take him to get checked out at a vet, he's probably not in much danger. I still want him back, though. I've printed out some lost cat posters. Would you put some up around the school?"

"Of course. I'd be happy to."

She pulled a small stack from her purse and handed them to him. "Thank you."

The poster had a clear, full-color picture of the black kitten boy with the words, "Lost Cat – $1,000 reward."

"One thousand dollars?" Kester asked in surprise.

She looked away. "We're very attached to him."

This won't do, Kester thought.

As soon as they finished lunch, Kester drove back toward the school. *Julia, meet me now.* He sent the message through their bond, along with a mental image of the park located between the restaurant and the school. She broke off her surveillance of Trick (he was still sleeping) and was already overhead by the time Kester pulled the car into the parking lot. There were some small children with their parents by the playground and some adults playing ball in a field farther away, but no one close enough to se strange.

He got out, taking the posters with him, and dropped al into a large waste bin as he went to the nearest large tre moment, Julia swooped down and landed on his shoulder balance precise so she didn't dig into him with her talons. stroked her head with one finger while showing her the poster.

"Jacqueline is going to start putting these up around town. don't want you to leave the kitten boy for long enough for him to get himself in trouble, but if you could find some time to tear as many of these down as you find, my dear, things will go easier. We wouldn't want Denneka to see one and be tempted by such a bounty."

He felt the mental nudge of Julia's acknowledgment, and she flapped off into the sky.

It probably would have been more expedient to give her that command through their bond. As he watched her fly away, he wondered why he hadn't. It hadn't been a conscious choice. After the lunch date with Jacqueline, he'd simply felt the need to see Julia in person.

He took a breath, focusing on the familiar feel of their bond. She wasn't so unhappy anymore.

———

Nobody cared. It was only Wednesday—less than a week after Trick disappeared—and nobody at school was even talking about him. Denneka should have been happy that they weren't mocking her about him anymore or loudly speculating on what terrible things might have happened to him. But at least when they were doing that, it was clear they actually noticed he was gone. Now, it was just like it had been before he'd come. Like he'd never even been here.

How could everyone forget about someone—even someone who was new and never talked—that quickly?

As the school day wore on, Denneka stopped feeling hurt about

...etermined. She would not forget him. More than that,
...not give up on him. It hadn't been that long. If no one
...ere he was, how could anyone know he was gone for
...Maybe she'd be able to find some clues to what had
...ned to him.

...fter school, she went to the library and pulled out the newspa-
...s from the past few days. With a notebook in her hand, she read
...d re-read the initial article telling what had happened. It was
mostly official statements from the police and the principal, but it
basically only said that a teacher (name not given) had found Trick's
clothes and bag on school grounds and that he hadn't come home
after school.

The teacher had to be Mr. McKenzie. When she'd left school, it
hadn't looked like there was anyone left except for him and Trick.
They probably left his name out of the paper because they didn't
want people bothering him about it. Or maybe even speculating that
he'd had something to do with it. Small towns could be pretty
unwelcoming to newcomers sometimes. One whisper of accusation
from the right person, and he could have been in a lot of trouble.
Still could, if anyone were to go around asking all the other teachers
if they were the one who found Trick. Which someone was probably
in the process of doing.

Did Mr. McKenzie know what kind of storm could ensue if it got
out that he was the one who found Trick's things? Especially
considering—

Denneka stopped sketching out notes and momentarily froze
into a statue. *Especially since he took Mr. Haug's job.*

It was almost certainly a coincidence. It had to be. But it was the
kind of connection that bored reporters and busybodies would latch
onto, and they could make his life really unpleasant. Maybe even
get the police to actually investigate him, even though the police
surely already knew all of those facts.

Knowing that the police obviously knew about that potential
connection and (as far as Denneka could tell) weren't investigating
Mr. McKenzie calmed that small, niggling part of her that wondered

if he did have something to do with Trick's and Mr. Haug's disappearances.

A memory surfaced all of a sudden, and she sucked in a breath.

What if the connection didn't involve Mr. McKenzie and Trick and Mr. Haug, but it did involve Trick and Mr. Haug? Trick had said he'd seen Mr. Haug's body when no one else knew where he was or if he was dead. And now Trick was gone.

Denneka launched herself at the newspaper rack, riffling through the past couple weeks' worth until she found any that mentioned Mr. Haug's disappearance. There were only a few articles, and only the first one had any real information. Just like with Trick, the follow-up articles only said the case was ongoing and urged anyone who knew anything to come forward.

The facts of Mr. Haug's case were similar to Trick's but not identical. He was unmarried and lived alone, so no one else had been there when it had happened, but a neighbor had heard noises and come by at some point that night to find the door open. There had been enough signs of a struggle that it looked like foul play. He had gone missing suddenly and without anyone having any idea why it might have happened, but there'd been no pile of clothes and he'd disappeared from his home.

And then, according to Trick, he'd ended up in a grave. If that was true, how had Trick seen it? Where? When? Trick had only just arrived in town.

Unless Trick's arrival had something to do with Mr. Haug's disappearance?

Denneka shook her head. That didn't make any sense. She had too many questions, and the newspaper didn't have enough answers. She could ask Mr. McKenzie if there was anything else about Trick's disappearance to tell, but given how mean he was to her, she doubted he'd cooperate. For about two seconds, she considered blackmailing him into telling her—threaten to start some unpleasant rumors. But she knew she wouldn't do that. She wasn't like Amy and the others.

But the police had to have information they weren't letting in the paper, and maybe they'd share some of it with her if she told them what Trick had said about Mr. Haug. It wasn't much, and they might not think it was anything at all, but it was all she had. And if it could help get Trick back, she had to tell someone.

The police station was only a ten minute walk from the school, so on the way she called her mom to tell her what she was doing.

"That's terrific, Denneka," Mom told her. "How responsible of you. I hope whatever information you have does help the police find your friend. Be careful on the street, though."

"It's only three-thirty, Mom."

"That doesn't seem to mean much. I'm going to send Jonah to the station to give you a ride home."

Hopefully her brother wasn't getting sick of playing taxi for her. But she was glad for the ride.

The police station was a small, one-storey building with tan paint and a sign that needed to be replaced a couple decades ago. Denneka went through the big glass doors to the reception desk.

"How can I help you, miss?" the receptionist asked.

"I—I might have some information about Trick. The boy who went missing. He was my—my friend, and I—"

"You have information? Fantastic!" He picked up the phone and said, "Marcus, I'm sending a girl back. She says she has information about the missing boy." Then he pressed a button and the door buzzed. "Go on in, straight back." He handed her a visitor's badge and waved her through.

She'd never been in the part of the police station that the actual cops worked in before. It looked a lot like what she imagined most offices to look like, except there weren't cubicles, just desks pressed up against each other in pairs: four pairs, not counting reception or the walled-off office with big windows on the left.

None of the desks were occupied, though. She hoped that meant they were all out looking for Trick.

A tall, blond man in a police uniform strode toward her from the back of the room as she came in. He didn't smile in greeting but looked like he was analyzing her. Did cops have some sort of internal trouble meter that they weighed everyone on as soon as they met them? She looked away instinctively from his direct gaze and clutched the straps of her backpack.

"I'm Officer Parkes," he said, offering a handshake. His hand was big, warm, and solid. "Please come this way." He led her to what must have been his desk, since he sat down at it and gestured to the guest chair beside it. "Have a seat and tell me your name."

She sat, holding her backpack in her lap. "Denneka Sparrow."

He nodded. "Ah, right. The clothing store."

"Yes."

He took out a notepad and wrote on it. "So, you have information?"

"Have you found anything more about Trick?" She couldn't hold the question in any longer.

"We can't really talk about ongoing investigations too much. Is he a friend of yours?"

"Y-yes. I think so."

"You think so?"

"I've never really… had friends… so I'm not sure."

Kindness and pity softened his expression. "Ah. You care about him, though?"

"Yes." Tears started forming in her eyes, but she fought them back. "Yes, I do. But no one else seems to."

"Other people care," he assured her. "We've been working our butts off for days to find him. I know his family's worried. And even your principal is."

"Really?" So the adults cared, at least. Some of them.

"Yep. Look, I can see you're his friend by how worried you are for him, so I'll tell you this, and don't spread it around. We're working hard to find him, but we're not getting anywhere. We've got no leads to follow. So if you have anything—anything at all— I'm all ears."

Denneka's heart sank. She'd hoped the cops had some leads they were working on that they hadn't shared with the press yet. "I don't have much. I only just remembered something Trick said once, though. It was weird, but I got distracted right after he said it, and he never explained what he meant, even when I tried to ask later."

"What did he say?"

"It was when he saw the missing poster for Mr. Haug. Even though he's brand new to town, he said he'd seen Mr. Haug before. When I asked him where, he said..." She hesitated. Was this a good idea? Would it implicate Trick in something? What if it implicated her for not reporting it sooner?

"Go on."

Too late for cold feet. "He said, 'In a grave.'"

Officer Parkes's eyes went wide and he froze, staring at her. "He said, 'In a grave'? Those were his exact words?"

She nodded.

He let out a long breath. "He didn't say anything about where or how he saw this?"

She shook her head.

He wrote on his paper again, then set it aside. "Thank you, Denneka. I'll look into this."

"Do you believe me?"

"You haven't given me any reason not to."

"And you'll really investigate it? You don't... think it's stupid?"

"Are you kidding? You've given us the first real lead we've had on two high-priority cases. Yes, Denneka, I'll definitely investigate this, and it's not stupid at all. You were right to bring this information to us. Is there any other information you can think of? Anything else Trick might have said or done that was out of place or strange?"

He chased a bird once. But she couldn't imagine how that was relevant, and she didn't really want that getting around. She didn't want people having more to tease him for when he definitely came back. "I don't think so. The past week or so, he hadn't been speaking at all."

"At all? That's odd."

"Only when the teachers made him."

Officer Parkes flipped a page in his notepad and wrote something down, but he was frowning. "I'm not sure what that could mean, but I'll keep it in mind. Anything else?"

She shook her head.

"All right." He handed her a business card. "If you do think of anything, be sure to let me know right away, okay?"

———

Marcus watched the mousy girl leave, impressed that a shy kid like that had gotten up the nerve to come to the police on her own. Could it be that she and Trick were more than friends, or that she hoped they might be? She was a sweet, pathetic girl; he wanted to root for her. But to do that, he first had to make sure Trick came home safe and sound.

He picked up the phone and called the mortuary. "Hi, Sally. It's Marcus. Can you get me a list of any burials that have happened within the past month?

CHAPTER
ELEVEN

"Lisa, there's a police officer here to see you."

Lisa looked up from the volleyball team's financial paperwork to see the school secretary poking his head into the open doorway. She dropped the papers immediately and stood. "Please show them in, Michael."

Michael stood aside and, to her surprise, Marcus entered. She didn't particularly like seeing him here. It muddied things too much. But the look on his face brushed all that from her mind.

"Hi, Lisa. Got a minute?"

"Yes. A few. Please hold my calls, Michael," she said, smoothly closing the door. "Is there news on the case?"

"Yes and no. And on both cases, potentially."

"Make sense, Marcus."

"I need your help with something."

She crossed her arms. "What's going on?"

Marcus began to pace as he talked. "One of your students came to us with a lead. Barely a lead, but since it was all we had, I followed it. Her name's"—he pulled out his notepad—"Denneka Sparrow."

"Really?"

"She said that the missing boy, Trick, once said something about seeing Haug."

"That doesn't make sense. When would he have?"

"I don't know. But it's not *that* he saw him that's the really weird thing. It's *where* he said he saw him."

"And where's that?"

"In a grave."

Coldness flowed through Lisa's body in a rush. "So... he is dead?"

"We haven't confirmed it yet. That's what I need your help with. See, I checked, and there have only been two burials in the last month. Two recent graves, that is."

"This is beginning to sound a bit crazy."

"I know. That's what the chief said. He denied my request to exhume the bodies and check it out."

"I'm not surprised."

"But if Bradley Haug is in one of those graves, as much of a long shot as that is, then not only would it give us more to go on in finding who killed him, it might lead to some kind of information on Trick."

Was he invoking her student's name on purpose? She pursed her lips. "So what do you need my help with?"

He looked at her like he thought she was kidding. "The chief's your uncle. Convince him to let us dig up the graves."

She'd been afraid that was what he wanted. "I wouldn't want him to come in here and tell me how to run my school. I doubt he'd want me to tell him how to run the police."

Marcus grasped her hand. "Lisa, please. This is literally all we have to go on right now. I want to get that kid home safe. I know you do too."

She pulled her hand away quickly lest anyone happen by the window and see them, then let out a breath. Part of her didn't want the lead to pan out because it would mean Brad was dead, not just missing. But a greater part of her wanted to seize any lead they could get on finding her student. "Okay. I'll try."

"Thank you." Marcus turned to leave, but Lisa couldn't help voicing the worry that suddenly shot into her mind.

"Marcus. There are two graves?"

"Yes."

"What if they both have an extra body in them?"

"I've considered that, but I don't believe it."

"Why not?"

"Because I can't. Not yet." He looked over his shoulder at her, his brown eyes as firm and reassuring as the earth. "We start treating these like homicides too soon, we might forget there's a boy out there who could need saving."

Sometimes Lisa wished she were the marrying type.

———

On Saturday morning, Kester woke up earlier than he'd woken up on any Saturday that he could remember. So early that it was still dark and Julia was still sleeping in her room. *Surveillance duty isn't exciting, but it can be tiring for her*, he thought as he dressed. *Fighting the urge to sleep is exhausting.*

Though how adorable she had been when she'd fallen asleep on his shoulder while they watched a movie last night. He smiled as the memory crossed his mind. When she slept, her face relaxed, and she looked almost like the child she'd been when they'd first met.

Halfway through making the two of them breakfast, Kester realized that he hadn't even considered trying to go out to find a woman on Friday night. He shrugged the thought off. No doubt he would catch up once this diversion was past and he was back to his normal habits.

After he'd eaten, donned his disguise, and put his jacket on to leave, he went into Julia's room. She lay on her side, curled up, having kicked her blankets off during the night. Her pajama pants had ridden up, leaving her legs bare to the knee. Kester gently picked up the blanket and laid it over her up to her shoulder. Then with a light touch, he brushed a lock of oak-brown hair from her face and kissed her forehead.

"Mmm," she hummed, waking.

"I'm going out," he whispered. "It's nearly dawn. Breakfast is in the kitchen."

She sat up and rubbed her eyes. "Thank you, Master. What will you need me to do today?"

"I'll let you know when I decide."

Kester made one stop on the way to Jacqueline's house, then sat outside in his car, watching for signs of movement inside. He probably hadn't needed to come over so early, but one never knew what a woman like Jacqueline would take it in her head to do, and he didn't want to risk missing his opportunity by being late.

Half an hour after dawn, the living room curtains were thrown open to reveal Jacqueline in a bathrobe. She spotted him at once. He waved and got out of the car, and she met him in the doorway.

"John!" She pulled the robe tighter around herself, which made him smirk. "When did you get here?"

"Just now." He held up a box. "And I brought cinnamon rolls."

The desire to tell him to go away and come back later flashed across her face, but then her eyes lingered on the cinnamon rolls, and she nodded him inside. "Thank you. Put them on the counter."

He went to the kitchen while she hurried back to (he presumed) her bedroom. The boy was not yet in evidence, so Kester took his time finding an adequate plate—she really needed to get some better flatware—and removed the cinnamon rolls from the box to arrange them more artfully.

When Jacqueline returned, she was in jeans and a sweater with her auburn hair tied up in a ponytail. "Don't you have anything better to do today?"

"Has Trick been found yet? Or your cat?"

"No and no." She was frowning, but she still moved around him to pour a glass of milk and plate a cinnamon roll. After putting it in the microwave, she turned to him. "But you must have your own life."

"I do," he said with a nod. The kitchen was not large, and he hadn't left when she'd come into it. She was within easy reach of him and they were alone, yet she wasn't moving away and did not appear nervous at all. Had he finally gained her trust? "But helping you is part of that. And I have no more pressing issues today."

The microwave beeped, and she sat at the island to eat her meal. "Well, I'm grateful, but I feel like you're doing too much."

"Not at all. Is that all you're having?"

"I don't have time to fix anything else. I was planning on skipping breakfast, so it was helpful that you brought this."

Kester *tsk*ed at her and opened the refrigerator. "Where are you in a hurry to get to?"

"I haven't found anything about Charcoal all week. No one's called with information, and I think someone's tearing down my posters. Why would someone do that?"

He pulled out some bread and lettuce. "How awful."

"So I thought I'd try going door to door and asking if anyone knows anything."

"Oh? And where do you plan to start?" he asked, choosing a sauce and cheese next.

"On the west side, up by Seventeenth. I thought I'd work my way inward from there."

That would not do. If she did that, she'd reach Denneka's house by mid-afternoon. Kester washed the lettuce and said casually, "If that's your plan, you should start on the east side, near Lincoln. If you're looking for a girl around Trick's age, your odds are better starting there. For some reason, an unusually large number of our students are clustered around that area."

"How do you know that?"

"I made sure to familiarize myself with the school records before I started." It was not a very good lie. Hopefully that area was not unusually dense with the elderly, at least.

"All right. I'll start there, then."

"Good." Kester efficiently assembled the sandwich and wrapped it in a paper towel. He opened several drawers looking for sandwich bags.

Instead of telling him to stop snooping, Jacqueline pointed to one and said, "The bags are in there." She had accepted him in her kitchen. How far did that trust extend?

"Have you found someone to watch Landon?"

"I haven't had time to try. I'll just have to take him with me."

"And let the poor boy sit in a car all day? None of that. I'll watch him."

Jacqueline eyed him. "Why would you do that? I might be gone all day."

"Jacqueline, do I really have to go over this? I started helping you because I felt guilty about Trick going missing. Even though it's only been a week, I'd like to think we've become something like friends. I care about your well-being and that of your boys. I have no other plans for the day, and you need a babysitter. Besides, Landon is a well-behaved child. I don't foresee any issues."

The protective gaze of the mother bear sized him up. Finally, she said, "All right. Thank you. I'll go tell him."

She left the room, and Kester didn't try to fight the victorious smile that took over his face.

A few minutes later, Jacqueline came back alone. "He'll probably go back to sleep for a while. I've told him to call me to check in every couple hours."

So, not *complete* trust, then. That was all right. "Are there any special instructions? Anything I should see that he does?"

"No. He knows what he needs to do. If he needs anything from you, he'll ask for it." She donned her jacket and put the sandwich in a pocket.

Kester should have asked more about Trick by now. With a tentative tone, as if he'd held off because he was worried about the answer and not because he'd forgotten, he asked, "Jacqueline, have the police given you any news of Trick?"

"They've got a lead, but they're still looking into it. The officer who told me about it didn't sound like he believed it would go anywhere, but after I'd been badgering them every day, I think he felt like he had to give me something."

Kester's spine went rigid with interest. "What lead?" How could they possibly have any lead?

"It has to do with that teacher who disappeared. Apparently, Trick told a girl at school that he'd seen the teacher. Or, from the sound of it, the teacher's dead body."

Kester could feel his eyes lighting up and immediately tamped down on his reaction. "Oh? And where did he see him?"

For some reason, Jacqueline hesitated and then said, "I probably shouldn't say until the police have verified it. If they do. Anyway, I'll be off. I have my phone if you need anything at all." She left the house before Kester could press her for more information.

Kester grinned and stroked his chin, delighting in this unexpected new twist. *The police have a lead on a missing persons case where the person isn't actually missing. What does a corpse have to do with a kitten?*

An interrogative prod from his familiar interrupted his pondering. He sent Julia's instructions for the day over their bond. *Resume watch on Trick, but keep an eye out along the road. Jacqueline's going door to door.* A brief pulse of acknowledgment was the response.

A missing teacher, a corpse, and a curious kitten boy who had somehow gotten himself involved. Where on earth would this lead?

———

When Landon came in for breakfast, that weird man Mr. McKenzie was standing in the middle of the kitchen with a creepy grin on his face.

"What are you happy about?" Landon asked him.

He hadn't been trying to be sneaky, but the man jumped. Then Mr. McKenzie grinned even bigger. "Life, small one. Life makes me happy."

Landon didn't see what there was to be so happy about. "Mom said to call her if you try to touch me or anything."

That seemed to actually hurt the man's feelings. He was practically pouting now. "Did she actually say that?"

"She mostly did."

Mr. McKenzie narrowed his eyes. "You don't like me much, do you?"

"Why should I like you?"

Now his mouth slid into a smirk. Sheesh, this guy's face never sat still. "Why indeed, little Landon?"

"Yeah, that was my question."

Landon wasn't tall enough to see on top of the counter, but Mr. McKenzie started shuffling things around up there, so Landon got up on a bar stool. But by then the man had moved to the counter against the wall and was messing with the fridge and microwave. A minute later, Mr. McKenzie set a glass of milk and a cinnamon roll in front of Landon. "Is this enough to buy any goodwill?"

The cinnamon roll smelled delicious, so Landon took the fork the man offered and started eating. "Does this count as taking candy from strangers?" he asked himself around a mouthful of pastry.

"Would your mom have left you with a stranger?" Mr. McKenzie asked.

No. Mom wasn't stupid or reckless. She always took good care of Landon. Even when she was really worried about Trick, she didn't totally forget about Landon. He didn't think she was doing it now.

When he didn't answer, Mr. McKenzie turned toward the stove. "Would you like an egg with that?"

"Yes, please."

Just as Landon finished his cinnamon roll, Mr. McKenzie set something weird in front of him.

"What's that?" The thing on the plate was a squishy lump covered in yellowish… he wanted to say 'sauce'?

"You've never had eggs Benedict before?"

"What is it?"

"Nothing abnormal. Try it." Mr. McKenzie handed him a fresh fork and a knife.

This looked like some kind of trick, but Landon cut into the weird thing. Bright yellow egg yolk poured out of the squishy lump. He poked it. It was an egg, but he'd never seen one cooked that way before. And underneath was only a normal English muffin. Maybe not a trick, then. Landon cut off a piece, fighting to keep the layers together, and tried it.

"What do you think?" Mr. McKenzie asked, leaning on the counter to watch him.

"It's good." It was amazing, actually. Better than anything Jacqueline ever made him for breakfast. "You're a man. Why do you cook so well?"

Mr. McKenzie laughed. "When I was a boy, I didn't have a mother to cook for me, so I had to learn. And when you have to cook for yourself, you have a great deal of incentive to learn to do it well. Besides, I enjoy it." He came around the island to sit on the stool beside Landon. In a quieter voice, like he was telling a secret, he said, "Life is uncertain. That's what makes it interesting. But that's also what makes self-sufficiency important. From the way your mom talks about you, you're well on your way, but you've a long way yet to go. Cooking is one of many things a man needs to learn to do for himself. Have you ever cooked anything?"

"I'm six. Mom doesn't let me use the stove."

"While I have no doubt your brother at six might have burnt the house down, you appear more competent than that to me."

'Competent'. Landon knew that word, didn't he? It meant... able to do things. More able than his brother, even at the same age. He wouldn't want to say so himself, but yeah, he probably was.

And that wasn't counting the things he could do that Trick couldn't do at *any* age.

"Do you want to try?" asked Mr. McKenzie.

"Try... cooking?"

The man nodded.

"Why?"

"We've got all day. Why not?"

Landon had been planning to spend most of his time reading, but he guessed this was fine, too. "Okay."

"Excellent. Finish your breakfast, then change into something more comfortable."

Landon looked down at his slacks and button-up shirt. "But I like this. It looks nice."

"Indeed it does. And that's precisely why you shouldn't be wearing it when doing something which may get messy. Don't you have a t-shirt and jeans?"

"Yeah. I guess that makes sense."

When he came back into the kitchen after changing, Mr. McKenzie was wearing Mom's blue apron. He handed the smaller checkered apron to Landon. "This won't be as necessary as you get better, but for now, put it on."

Landon slipped the neck loop over his head, but he had trouble figuring out how to tie the thing at the waist.

"Here," Mr. McKenzie said, reaching behind Landon for the tie strips.

Landon backed away. "I've got it." He didn't need help doing something so simple. If he couldn't work it out with his fingers, all he had to do was... There. Just focus on making the ties do what he wanted and it was done.

Mr. McKenzie was looking at him strangely again and wearing one of those weird smiles. Then he clapped his hands together and said, "Let's start with eggs. There are many ways to cook eggs, but one of the easiest is scrambled."

Two hours later, the phone in Landon's back pocket rang. He washed the egg off his hands and answered it before it could go to voicemail. "Hi, Mom."

"Landon, everything okay?"

"Yeah. Sorry I forgot to call."

"What are you up to?"

"Mr. McKenzie's teaching me how to cook."

"Really? Cook what?"

"Eggs. First we did scrambled, then soft-boiled and hard-boiled, then poached, and now we're working on fried. Oh, and we're out of eggs now, so you might want to get some while you're out."

She gave a small laugh. "Just keep the ones that came out edible in the fridge and we should be fine for a few days."

"You're not mad that I used the stove?"

"As long as an adult is supervising you, it's fine. I didn't know you wanted to learn to cook."

"I didn't, but Mr. McKenzie said it's something a man should know how to do."

She laughed again, louder. "Well, he's right. I guess I should have offered to teach you already. I'm sorry about that, Landon."

"It's okay. I know Trick keeps you busy."

"He does, but that's no excuse."

"Have you found anything?"

"Nothing yet, but it's still early."

"Okay. I'll remember to call in a couple hours."

"Thanks, sweetie. Love you."

"Love you too, Mom." He hung up and saw Mr. McKenzie watching him, leaning with his elbows on the island counter. He looked kind of… sad and happy at the same time.

"Must be nice having a mother," the man said.

"It is." Landon fiddled with the edge of his apron. "Did you… have a dad?"

Mr. McKenzie stood straight. "Not since I was a little older than you."

"Oh. Do you… remember what it was like?"

"Not really, other than that he was angry at me a majority of the time." He squatted down to look up at Landon. "What do you know about your father?"

Landon shook his head. "Not much. Only that he looked like me. Mom doesn't ever talk about him. I asked one time, but she… she looked hurt that I'd asked, so I didn't do it again. I mostly pretend I don't have one."

"How do you know you do?"

That was such a dumb question, Landon rolled his eyes. "I've… read some of Mom's books. She didn't actually say I couldn't," he wanted to make clear, "only put them on a high shelf. So I know it takes two people to make a baby."

Mr. McKenzie's eyes widened, then he laughed. "So it does. Then what do you think he's like?"

Landon shrugged. "I don't know."

"What do you hope he's like?"

"Does it matter? I'm never going to find out. There's no point guessing. Makes more sense to spend the time learning to take care of myself. Like you said."

Mr. McKenzie stood and put a hand lightly on Landon's head, and for some reason Landon didn't care enough to step away from it. "Yes," Mr. McKenzie said softly. "Like I said."

"What was he like?" Julia asked as she worked on applying her makeup. She didn't do it very often, so she kept it light; that way the mistakes wouldn't show up as much.

Behind her, Kester was brushing her hair. She was perfectly capable of brushing her own hair, but he enjoyed touching it. He'd always had a thing for women's hair. Long, short, curly, straight, dark, light—it didn't matter. As long as it was healthy and full, he liked it. And taking joy in touching hers seemed to be the only concession he made to acknowledging Julia as a woman.

Or maybe when it came to her, it was more like petting a cat. She could never really tell.

"Very cynical for one so young," Kester replied, easing the brush through gentle strokes. "But intelligent, curious, and talented. He's more gifted than I'm sure he realizes."

"He did magic in front of you?"

"A few times, though I think he believed he was hiding it. Or perhaps he doesn't see it as something that needs to be hidden yet. I'm not certain."

"What are you going to do about it?"

He hummed thoughtfully. "I haven't decided yet." He set the brush on the counter and stepped back. "You are beautiful, dearest."

Julia compared their reflections in the mirror. The gold dress he'd bought her was lovely, her makeup was adequate, and her hair looked okay. But she knew she wasn't beautiful. Not like him. He had to disguise himself when he went out now, but here at home, he could be himself. His gorgeous, radiant self: bright, blue eyes; silky, blond hair that just touched his shoulders; and the sort of face that made artists' hands restless. In his jacket and tie, he looked like a prince beside the commoner that was her.

He put the gold watch on and changed before her eyes. Now they made sense. This dull, average-looking version of him made sense beside her. She liked the real Kester better, but this version made her feel less like a dog whose master had dressed it in human clothes.

They arrived at Jacqueline's house a few minutes after the agreed-upon time. Since Kester had refused pay for babysitting Landon all day, Jacqueline had insisted on cooking dinner for them instead.

Jacqueline answered the door in a blouse and black trousers, not at all looking like she'd just spent an hour slaving in the kitchen. "Oh good, John, you're here. And you must be Julia." The woman sounded genuinely pleased and even went in for a hug instead of a handshake. Would she have been so friendly if she'd known how Julia had spent so much time stalking her on Kester's behalf? "It's good to see you actually exist," Jacqueline added with a wink.

"Of course I exist," Julia said, confused. "Why wouldn't I?"

Kester leaned close and whispered, "Maybe Jacqueline believed I'd made you up to gain her trust." He could have told her that without saying it verbally, which meant he'd intended Jacqueline to hear it, which she clearly did. He confirmed this by winking at their hostess. "Is that it?"

Jacqueline had the good manners to look slightly embarrassed. "It had crossed my mind once or twice."

Since Jacqueline had initiated a friendly physical contact

between them, Julia felt okay taking her hand and giving it a squeeze. "You're gorgeous. Of course you'd be suspicious. I'm sure men can be quite a nuisance to you sometimes."

Jacqueline returned the squeeze before pulling her hand away. "You're right about that. About men, I mean. Not about me being gorgeous."

"I was only stating a fact," Julia said, "not complimenting you, so there's no need to be modest."

Jacqueline laughed. "All right. You win." She ushered them into the living room and took their coats. "You look quite lovely in that dress, by the way."

"Thank you. I don't get many chances to wear it."

"Oh? What do you do for work, anyway? I've never heard."

I stalk you, your son, or anyone else my master tells me to watch. "I'm... sort of a private investigator. Not like the movies or anything. Mostly just checking into people for perfectly boring reasons."

"Like for an insurance company?" Jacqueline asked.

"Yes, something like that."

"Landon, come say hello." Jacqueline waved a small boy over from the dining table. He was dressed in a blue button-up shirt, gray tie, and black slacks and jacket. His blond hair was neatly combed. Overall, it gave the impression that a CEO had been shrunk in the wash. When he arrived at Jacqueline's side, she said, "Landon, this is Mr. McKenzie's lady friend, Ms...." She looked to Julia. "I'm sorry, what's your last name?"

Julia waved the question away. "Some long Norwegian thing I don't even like. He can call me Ms. Julia."

"Hello, Ms. Julia," Landon said.

"Hello, Landon. What a polite boy you are."

"Thank you."

Julia had been watching this boy for his entire life—off and on at first, then nearly all the time. It was strange to finally meet him. Both pleasant and unpleasant.

"I was very sorry to hear about your son," she told Jacqueline, because it had to be said sooner rather than later. "I'm sure he'll be recovered safe and sound."

Something heavy weighed Jacqueline down with those words. "I... believe so. I just wish it would be soon."

"And I hear your cat's missing as well. That's awful."

"Yes, John's been helping me look. It sounds like he might have been taken in by someone, so I have hope I'll find him all right as well."

"I feel certain you will," Julia told her.

Some of the weight seemed to lift off of Jacqueline, and she managed a smile. "Thank you. Now, let's eat before it gets cold."

Dinner was lasagna, salad, garlic bread, and red potatoes.

"Jacqueline is a vegetarian," Kester told Julia as if she hadn't already known it.

Jacqueline nodded. "I don't have anything against meat on an ethical level. I just think it's disgusting, so I don't like cooking or eating it. You're not a vegetarian, are you, Julia?"

She had to smirk at that, thinking of the mouse she'd caught herself for lunch that day. "No. More the opposite, if anything."

"What's the opposite of vegetarianism?"

"I'm not a big vegetable eater. Though this is mostly grains and starches, so it's fine," she said before Jacqueline started to apologize for cooking a meal for them.

Jacqueline drew back a little in surprise. "But you're so slim and toned."

"Am I?"

"Don't you have a mirror? Look, Julia, if I have to own up to being beautiful, you have to own up to your amazingly fit body."

Julia blinked, not sure how to answer that. She always thought of herself as being too muscular and not curvy enough. Not womanly enough. To hear a woman as overtly feminine as Jacqueline talk about Julia's body as if she envied it was... She just didn't know what to say.

Kester chuckled. "You see, I told you. You're beautiful."

"I think Ms. Julia's very pretty, too," said Landon.

Julia narrowed her eyes at him. "Are you just sucking up, kid?"

"What's 'sucking up'?"

Julia pointed at him and told Jacqueline, "You'd better watch out for that one."

Having been mid-drink when she'd said that, Jacqueline nearly choked. "Watch out for Landon? He's the well-behaved one."

"The lady-killers often seem that way."

Julia had been dead serious, even if she'd said it in a lighthearted tone, but Jacqueline broke out into laughter like that was the funniest thing she'd heard all week.

After they finished eating, Landon asked to be excused to his room to read, and Kester said, "Allow me to clean up."

Jacqueline put up token protest but soon relented. She did look pretty exhausted and worn-down.

Try to get her to talk about the boys' fathers, Kester instructed Julia as he cleared the table.

Julia poured herself a glass of the wine that had been on the table all night and barely touched, then poured a second and offered it to Jacqueline. "Want to go sit and chat a bit?"

Taking the wine, Jacqueline led her into the living room and took a seat on the couch. Instead of taking the chair opposite, Julia sat beside her. Smaller spaces were better for sharing confidences.

They made small talk for a while, but Julia knew her time was limited to however long Kester could stretch out the cleaning up, so when it seemed like Jacqueline was feeling relaxed and comfortable with her, she brought the conversation around to the topic she'd been instructed to. "I know this is a very personal question, and if you don't want to answer it just say so, but would you mind telling me... what's the deal with the boys' fathers?" That surprised Jacqueline, but she didn't outright refuse to answer, so Julia went on. "John told me that Trick said they have different fathers and neither is in the picture now. Call it the nosiness of an unmarried, childless woman who doesn't understand why anyone would want such a complicated life, but I can't help but wonder how that happened."

It took Jacqueline a while to decide to answer, and she made sure to check that neither of the males were in hearing range, but finally she lowered her voice and said, "You know, I don't think I've ever talked to anyone about this. I've never really had anyone to tell. So, okay." She heaved a heavy sigh and took a deep draught of wine. "Trick's father was my college boyfriend. When I was young, I was... a foolish romantic. Kept waiting for Prince Charming to sweep me off my feet and give me a happily ever after. My parents were pretty liberal, so I never had any plan to save myself for marriage. I thought that when I loved a boy enough, however things naturally progressed would be fine. I was certain that a boy would feel the same, that he wouldn't want to go that far with me if he didn't really love me, too."

"Ouch."

"I was painfully foolish. I kept falling for boys, giving them what they wanted, and being an absolute wreck when they broke up with me. Somehow I kept thinking that the way to get a guy was to fall in love with him, give it all to him, and magically he'd love me and want to marry me and be with me forever."

"And I take it things never worked out that way," Julia offered.

"Do they ever? But I kept trying. Time and time and time again, and I kept getting my heart broken. When I met Chad in college, I thought I'd really found the one this time. We were together for a year and a half, our senior year and a bit after. I didn't mean to get pregnant—though looking back, I'm a little surprised it didn't occur to me to try it as a further way of hooking him. It was a happy accident for me, but as soon as Chad found out, he ran for the hills."

Julia nodded in understanding. "He didn't want the commitment."

"Until then, I didn't see how immature and selfish he was. He didn't even offer to help me out or anything. Just broke up with me, changed his phone number, and moved to a different state."

"What a piece of garbage."

Surprisingly, Jacqueline shook her head. "He wasn't a bad guy. Not really. He just wasn't the husband-and-father kind of guy, and it was my fault for not seeing that sooner. I actually feel ɛ grateful to him. First, because he gave me Trick. And sec because he finally knocked some sense into my head. Because him, I finally realized that there is no Prince Charming and happily ever after. Not in real life. That's all fantasy."

"But John told me you write romance novels."

Jacqueline smiled wistfully. "Because I still love the fantasy. The unbelievably handsome man who falls for a woman with all his heart, treats her right, and commits to be with her forever."

"You still want that," Julia realized, apprehension twisting her stomach.

"Don't we all? Don't you?"

Breaking eye contact, Julia looked into her half-empty glass of wine. "I do. But you're right. It's just a fantasy."

"You don't think John's the one?"

An answer sprang to Julia's mind, and it almost stayed there. But in that moment, she realized that she wanted someone to talk to, too. Even if it was Jacqueline. Even if Kester could hear it if he was tapped into her senses—which he probably was. She was sure he knew how she felt already, though. That was the way their bond worked. So she gave her thoughts voice. "I do. But I know I'm not his."

Jacqueline laid her hand over Julia's and squeezed it. "I like you, Julia. I hope you'll stay around, because I think we could be good friends. And John's a decent guy. I admit I don't know either of you very well, but I think you may not be giving him enough credit. I could be wrong about that, but I hope I'm not."

Julia swallowed the lump that had suddenly formed in her throat. She wasn't finished with her task. She needed to get back on track. "So, what about Landon's father?"

Releasing Julia's hand, Jacqueline downed the last of her wine and laid her head back on the couch. "That's another matter. When Trick was five, I decided I wanted another child. Motherhood is really great, you know. You should try it some time."

Julia seriously doubted the opportunity would ever arise.

, she wasn't her own person. She belonged to Kester. How
she raise a child?

cqueline didn't see her discomfort at that comment and was
ng on. "I could have adopted, but I liked having a child of my
vn blood. Maybe that's selfish, but I know I'm not alone in feeling
nat way. And I could have gone to a sperm bank, but there are a lot
of costs involved in that sort of thing, and I didn't have much
money. And the long and short of it is: I've never had trouble
getting the attention of men. So, I went hunting. I'd go out, meet an
attractive man who seemed like a decent person, take him home,
and see if I could get pregnant. You'd be surprised how few men
insist on protection when the woman says she doesn't want to
use it."

"You didn't worry about diseases?"

"I tried to be careful in who I picked, and if they had anything
visible, I'd send them packing. But yeah, I knew I was taking a risk.
Having another child was worth it to me, and I got lucky that I
never caught anything."

"When you got pregnant, how did you know which man was
the father?"

"I always waited long enough between men. When I was sure I
wasn't pregnant, only then did I go find another man. I timed my
cycle and everything. It took over a year before one of them
managed to knock me up, but I'm not a floozy by nature. I wanted
to at least know which man was my child's father."

"Did you ever tell him?"

"Why would I tell him? He had some fun, which was all he'd
wanted out of the encounter. I had what I wanted, a second child of
my own. Win-win. No need to complicate things. Besides, he didn't
even offer to use protection, so I didn't bring it up. He had to know
pregnancy was a possibility and obviously didn't care. When I said I
wanted to know who my child's father was, I mean in a general
sense for my own sake: which encounter it had been, what the man
had been like. We didn't exchange life stories first. I didn't even

184

catch his last name. So I couldn't have contacted him afterward even if I'd wanted to."

Julia knew she should leave it there. She could hear Kester's footsteps coming closer, preparing to interrupt them. He'd gotten all the information he'd wanted. But something inside her just couldn't quite let it go. "Do you have any feelings for him?"

Jacqueline snorted a laugh. "Feelings? Why would I have feelings for a man I met once? We had some fun, I got a wonderful child out of it, but that's it. There's nothing to have feelings about. And even if I did, my boys come first, and the type of man who'd go around sleeping with total strangers isn't the type of man I want being a father to my children."

"Isn't that a little... hypocritical?" Julia asked.

"I was doing it because I wanted to have a child. He was doing it to get his rocks off. It's not the same at all."

"I see you ladies have been getting along," Kester said as he came into the room. "Not gossiping about me, I hope."

Jacqueline raised her empty glass as if toasting with it. "What else could we have to talk about?"

Julia rose from the couch and said, "Jacqueline, it was very nice to meet you. I had a great time."

Getting up, Jacqueline helped them retrieve their coats. "Likewise, Julia. I'd love to get together sometime, if you want to."

"As friends?" she asked, glancing uncertainly at Kester. He smiled encouragingly. "Okay."

"Great. Can I get your phone number?" Jacqueline was going over to get her phone from an end table.

"Oh! Uh, I don't have one."

"You don't have a phone? Don't you need one for your job?"

"That's, um, a company phone, and the company doesn't like me to use it for personal things." Julia hoped that was a plausible enough reason. She didn't have any actual experience as an employee of anything.

But Jacqueline accepted it easily enough. "How can I reach you?"

Just look for the bird stalking your cat son. "Just talk to John and he can relay anything to me."

That did sound weird to Jacqueline, but she accepted it too after a moment.

After they got in the car, Kester asked Julia, "What did you think of him?"

"He's a lot like her. And too much like you."

Kester smirked. "I have no idea what you mean."

"Liar."

He started the car and got them onto the road. They drove for a while in silence, and then he said, "You like her, don't you?"

Julia took a deep, bracing breath. "Yeah. I do."

The two gravediggers were working fast, but it was well past nine p.m. and they still hadn't gotten to the bottom of the first grave. Marcus hated doing this at night. It made him feel like he had something to hide. Which he didn't. The request for exhumation had finally been approved, but it had taken until well into Saturday for it to happen, and then they'd had to organize things.

"Hey, take it easy!" he shouted to one of the gravediggers, who was sticking his shovel into the dirt with what Marcus considered way too much force. "If there is anything in there other than a coffin, you're gonna damage it!"

The gravedigger hunched his shoulders to his work and went with a little more care, though Marcus could hear him mutter, "Are we digging up a grave or excavating a fossil?"

The two other people who'd come with him were busy on their phones. Marcus's partner, David, had made it clear he thought this was a wild goose chase. Their what-passed-for-a-CSI-guy, Kevin, was frowning as he scrolled through something on his phone screen.

The mortician stood a little way back, making sure the floodlights didn't short out and the cops didn't destroy more of the cemetery than they absolutely had to.

After another half hour, the shovels met something hard with a thunk. Marcus watched as the gravediggers removed the dirt from on top of a coffin. There was nothing else. Not yet.

"All right. Get the winch," he instructed.

They did, but there turned out to not be anything under the coffin or anything inside the coffin other than the partially-decomposed old woman that was supposed to be there.

"Oh for one," David said, still distracted by his phone.

Marcus felt a weight lift off his chest, but a different one settled in his gut. They hadn't found a boy's body, which was excellent. But if there was nothing in the second grave either, that would mean their only lead was a bust, Marcus would look like a fool, and Lisa would probably kick him in the balls for making her stick her neck out for nothing.

Okay, she wouldn't actually do that, but she'd definitely want to.

He waved the gravediggers into action. "Lower the coffin back in, then dig up the next one. You can fill them in after we see what's inside."

Marcus stood, silent and still, as they worked. Hoping they'd find something and kinda hating himself for it. David kept staring at his phone. Kevin paced around, clearly past the point of boredom. The mortician was hard to see since the old man was outside the range of the floodlights, but he seemed to be circling the area.

The steady *shuf-shuf* of dirt being moved was suddenly interrupted with a wet, too-solid squelch.

"What did I say?!" Marcus shouted, rushing forward to see into the grave.

The floodlights didn't reach that far down the hole, so Marcus took the flashlight from his belt and shone it in.

"Holy hell," David muttered beside him. "Is that blood?"

"Looks like it," Marcus said, watching dark liquid ooze out of the ground around the shovel, permeating the surrounding soil. "Probably some other liquids, too."

The gravedigger who'd hit whatever it was left his shovel sticking in there and bent to brush dirt away with his gloved hand.

First he revealed a lump that looked like a torso, then an arm, then finally a face—and all the while the stench of rot got worse and worse.

Kevin moved beside Marcus to watch. "You were right." He started getting equipment out of his bag.

Marcus moved the light to examine the corpse's face. "Hard to tell through all of that, but it sure looks like Haug to me."

David nodded. "I'll call the chief."

"Get that body up here so we can get it to the morgue," Marcus ordered. Then the stench got to him and he had to step away. He walked far enough that he left the area illuminated by the floodlights and took a deep breath of crisp night air.

Movement in the corner of his eye made him turn and aim his flashlight at the edge of the nearby woods, his hand on his side arm just in case. For a split second, he caught a glimpse of a face, but it was a few dozen yards away, and then the man—he was sure it was a man—darted out of sight.

"David, I see someone!" he called back toward the group. "Come on!"

His partner was by his side in moments, and together they ran for the tree line, but by the time they got there, there was no sign of which way the man had gone.

"Keep an eye out," Marcus told David, then he shone his flashlight around the area where he was pretty sure the man had been standing. "Footprints."

David nodded. "Gotta say, this night turned out a lot more interesting than I expected."

"No kidding. When Kevin's done with the corpse, tell him to come see what he can find over there. Have you called the chief yet?"

"Was just about to." David took out his phone.

Marcus looked around, searching for any more clues or any sign that the man was still nearby. "Looks like we're finally catching a break on this one."

———

Julia kicked her feet up and held a hot chocolate in both hands. She was glad to be out of the dress and heels, back in her comfy pajamas, and sitting in front of the fire with Kester. "You don't resent the fact that she used you?"

Wrapped in a paisley robe, he peered at her over the top of his mug. "On the contrary. I think it was quite clever. In fact, it reminds me of a Bible story." His shining sapphire eyes twinkled in a way that begged her to ask him to elaborate.

He'd tell it anyway, so she said, "I have a hard time believing you ever went to Sunday school."

"I did not. I doubt this is a story they would teach to children, anyway. It was about Tamar, the daughter-in-law of Judah—as in 'the tribe of'. In those days, if a married man died without children, it was his brother's duty to marry the widow and give her a child. So Tamar's husband died before managing to impregnate her. His brother married her and duplicitously refused to impregnate her— for which he died. Judah had another son, but one too young to marry yet, so Judah told Tamar to wait until the third son was older. So Tamar waited. Eventually, Judah's wife died, and by this time, his youngest son had grown and still not been given to Tamar so that she could have a child. Judah didn't ever actually intend to give him to her, afraid that his third son would die also. Well, clever woman that she was, she dressed herself up in disguise as a prostitute and put herself in the path of Judah himself. It was entirely his own doing that he saw this strange woman and not only didn't recognize her as his daughter-in-law but also initiated an illicit liaison with her. And so, finally, she got what she was owed."

"A baby."

"Two, in fact. And in the process also managed to situate herself in the direct lineage of Jesus, thus securing her place in history."

"I didn't realize you knew so much about the Bible."

"You know I'm well-read. And I happen to have a fantastic memory when it comes to anything involving magic or interesting scandals. My point is, men very commonly use women to get what they want—and yes, I am self-aware enough to include myself in that—and so I have nothing but respect and admiration for any woman who can use a man by leveraging his own attempt to use her."

"I can't decide whether that attitude is despicably prehistoric or refreshingly enlightened. You know it would be better for everyone if men would just stop using women in the first place."

"You may as well wish for the moon, my dearest."

Julia sighed and shook her head. "Anyway, did you find out what you wanted to know?"

Kester slouched lower in his seat. "I had hoped the story of Trick's paternity would be more interesting. College boyfriend who was scared of commitment. How dull. All those years of wondering, and that's all I get?"

"Not everyone can be a secret witch child," she pointed out.

"I suppose that's true. Speaking of Trick, he appears to have settled in well with young Denneka."

"I don't think she's even letting him outside, though he doesn't seem to be fighting it." Julia tapped her fingers on the side of her mug as she sipped. "That might be because of me. He saw me watching. I'm sorry about that."

"I'm sure it couldn't be helped. Jacqueline has put us into a bit of a time crunch, though. If she's as set on searching the city house by house as she appears to be, it's only a matter of time until she reaches Denneka's. And though the girl may not be eager to find an unknown owner of a lost kitten, I don't think she's naughty enough to outright lie when said owner shows up asking about said kitten."

"So, what now?"

His mouth spread into a wide, foxy grin that meant someone was going to have an interesting morning. "Poor Denneka has been so lost and lonely without her companion boy this week. I think I'll give him back to her."

———

It had been a perfectly good dream about butterflies that tasted like fish when all of a sudden the butterflies turned into snakes and tried to rip him limb from limb.

Trick woke up all at once, his body aching. But he was fine. He was safe. He was in the familiar girl's room, on the foot of her bed. She was sleeping soundly. Everything was fine.

Except he was human again.

Trick wanted to cry out at the unfairness of it. Why had this happened again? What had caused it this time? But there wasn't anyone else around that he could blame, and the jolt of energy he'd felt on waking was already gone, and he was crashing again.

He was so tired. And his fur was gone, so now he was cold too.

With no immediate target for his anger, it leaked away, and all he felt was depressed, chilly, and sleepy. He crawled under the blankets and curled up against the warmth of the girl's body. Maybe, in the morning, she'd know what to do.

CHAPTER
TWELVE

It was taking Denneka a long time to crawl out of unconsciousness this morning. That happened sometimes. It could be frightening, when her mom was trying to wake her up and she could hear her but not respond. When Mom kept saying, "Denneka, get up," over and over in more and more annoying tones and Denneka just wanted to say, "I'm trying! Give me a minute!" but she couldn't.

This morning, though, no one was trying to wake her up. Her last dream had faded enough that she didn't remember what it was, and some part of her mind was conscious enough to know it was Sunday, so no one would be barging in to tell her she was late for school.

Sensations from the real world gradually worked through into her awareness: the soft mattress under her side, the softer pillow under her head and gripped in her hands, the warmth of Trick's body curled up against the backs of her bent legs. That last one had taken her a few days to get used to. The kitten wasn't always there. Sometimes he was against her side or lying on top of her. But no matter where he started the night, by morning he was always touching her somewhere. She'd learned to be careful on waking up so she didn't kick him off the bed inadvertently or trap him in blankets.

Finally, she had enough control of her body to take a deep breath, and the rush of oxygen brought her fully into wakefulness. She rubbed her eyes with one hand and propped up on an elbow, preparing to slide out of the bed without disturbing the sleeping kitten beside her.

She looked at the lump in the blankets behind her knees. That was way bigger than a kitten. Adrenaline and directionless panic coursed through her, and a faint notion of *What is that?!* flashed through her brain as she grabbed the edge of the covers and flung them all back, clearing the bed in one go.

Only when she saw human skin did she realize she'd been afraid that Trick had turned into some sort of monster cat or something, so for the tiniest instant she was relieved. Until she realized that there was another person in her bed with her.

She scrambled out of bed and grabbed the first thing that came to hand—a large book. With this as her defense, she began to creep around the bed toward the door, never taking her eyes off the person in her bed. All she saw at first was a curved back—someone was curled up in a ball with their back to her and their head at the foot of the bed. She couldn't see anything besides the back and head, but from the unfamiliar curves of the person's waist and hips, she guessed it was a boy.

Clearly she'd been reading too many fantasy novels because the first thought that came into her mind at that point was that Trick had transformed into a human. Obviously she hadn't sufficiently woken up yet. She glanced around the room, looking for the kitten, but she couldn't find him. Maybe he'd run into hiding when this strange person had entered the room.

This guy was probably some freak who'd snuck in while she slept. She kept inching her way toward the door. Her phone was on the other side of her bed, so it was a clearer path to get to the landline in the kitchen.

As she crept closer around the intruder, she noticed that the boy wasn't just wearing skimpy clothes that she couldn't see. He wasn't wearing any clothes at all.

A squeak of surprise jumped out of her.

The naked boy stirred and raised his head to look at her over his shoulder.

Grass green eyes. She knew those eyes. She'd started thinking she'd never see them again. "Trick?" she whispered.

His only response was a slow, sleepy blink.

The energy electrifying her body and the confused spinning in her head made her sure that she wasn't dreaming. But maybe she'd gone crazy and was hallucinating?

Setting the book down, she put one knee on the bed to get a closer look at him. "Trick?"

"Hm?" It wasn't a word—was barely even a sound—but his voice sounded sweeter than anything.

"Are you really here?"

"Yeeesss." He drew the word out like it was a stupid question and he wasn't sure why she was asking it. Then, still lying on his side, he stretched his arms and legs out in front of him with a moan and rolled over to kneel facing her on the bed, sitting on his heels.

"Why?" she asked. But then her stupid eyes caught the sight of all that bare skin and moved down to check it out. All the blood in her body flooded into her face, and she clapped her hands over her eyes. But it was too late. She'd seen everything. "Why are you naked?!"

She couldn't see Trick's expression, but his tone told her she was still asking stupid questions. "Because I'm not wearing clothes."

"That's not a reason! That's a definition!" She peeked through her fingers, careful to look only at his face, and saw that he was cocking his head at her but hadn't made any attempt to cover himself. "Would you put the blanket over you or something?"

She covered her eyes as he moved so she wouldn't see anything. When she heard him stop moving, she put her hands down.

He was sitting just as he had been, now with the blanket draped over his head and shoulders, covering him entirely down to mid-chest but nothing below that. "Why?" he asked, voice muffled by the blanket.

"I meant your lap!" She grabbed the blanket off his head and pulled it down so it pooled over his lap instead. Finally, she could breathe again.

"You're acting weird today," he said.

"I'm acting weird? *I'm* acting weird?! You've been missing for over a week and suddenly you show up naked in my bed?!"

"I haven't been missing. I've been here. And you haven't cared about me being naked in your bed before. Why are you weird now?" Something jingled as he shifted into a cross-legged sitting position. Luckily, the blanket stayed in place.

"Been here? Here where? What do you mean?" she asked. Then she saw what Trick had picked up and started to play with.

It was the collar she'd put on kitty Trick. Human Trick played with it absently, snapping it closed and then pulling it open. She glanced around the room. Kitty Trick was still nowhere to be seen.

No...

"What's that?" she asked Trick carefully.

"You don't know? You gave it to me." He snapped it open and murmured, "Guess it came off when I turned human again." Remembering her, he asked, "How did you forget that? Are you sick?"

Turned human again? "Trick," she said very slowly, "are you telling me that... you were the kitten I took in?"

He cocked his head and gave her the most feline look of *I can't believe you're asking me something so idiotic* yet. "Yeah. You knew that."

"No, I didn't! How could I possibly know that?!"

His expression shifted into uncertainty. "You... knew that."

"How could I have known that? What rational person would see a kitten and think, 'I bet that's that guy I know from school'?"

"But... you called me by my name."

The heat in her cheeks had begun to subside a bit, but now it came back. "I... I named the kitten after you. Because his eyes reminded me of you."

Even to her, that sounded like some kind of love confession. It was hard to talk positively about a boy's eyes and not have it sound cheesy. But he didn't seem to notice. He pointed at his own eyes. "That's because they're mine. Isn't that how you recognized me?"

"How is this possible? People don't just turn into cats and back. There's no rational reason why you're here, but you having been a cat is still less rational than other explanations." She started counting off reasons on her fingers as she thought of them. "Like, maybe you got kidnapped, then escaped, and in the process you lost your clothes, and you ended up here because it was closer than your house. Except why would you come to my house? It's not like I'm anyone special to you. You have no reason to—"

"You're special."

Her head snapped up as something inside her chest lurched. "What?"

"You're special to me. I like you." Trick said it in a totally matter-of-fact way.

How could she be special to him? How could she be special to anyone other than her parents, who were kind of obligated to think she was special? She was just a nerdy girl no one liked or paid much attention to. She wasn't someone that got to be special to cute boys with gorgeous eyes and nice, lean—

She cleared her throat. "Still, Trick, it doesn't make sense. How can you expect me to believe you were my cat?"

"Because... I was?"

The sound of footsteps in the hallway stopped any response she might have attempted. *Oh, no!* Her parents were away at a day conference, but her brother was still around. And if he found a boy in her room—much less a naked boy...

"Can I have breakfast yet?" Trick asked.

Denneka shushed him, but it was too late. She heard the footsteps coming closer. "Come here!" she hissed, leaping off of the bed. Grabbing him by the arm, she dragged him from the bed and shoved him into her closet. His eyes were suddenly wild with panic and fear, and he tried to come back out of the closet immediately. She had to press a hand to his chest to hold him inside. Beneath her palm, she felt heat, firm muscle, and a racing heartbeat. "Stay quiet. My brother's coming. If he catches you, we're both dead!" If anything, the fear she saw in his eyes got worse, but he became very still, and she was able to close the door just in time.

"Denneka?" Jonah asked from outside the door. He knocked once, which gave her enough time to find a spot to stand other than right in front of her closet door, then he barged in. "Are you talking to someone?"

"What? No. Who would I be talking to?"

Her brother gave her a look that was both doubtful and suspicious. "I thought a heard a boy's voice."

She laughed a little too wildly. "What? A boy? You think I have a boy in my room? That's crazy."

After a second, Jonah chuckled and leaned against her dresser, crossing his arms. "Yeah, it is. That was the joke. Anyway, Mom left a note for you on the counter. Wants you to do something at the shop today while they're gone."

"Oh. Okay." She hoped it wasn't urgent, but she went out to check. She'd barely left her room when a muffled thumping came from the closet.

Her eyes went wide with panic, and she knew the last thing she should have done was look at her brother, but her eyes just weren't obeying her at all today. All she could do was watch in frozen horror as her brother raised an eyebrow at her, then walked over to the closet door and opened it.

But he didn't shout or drag Trick out by the neck. He bent down and reached for something, his body blocking Denneka's view, then stood up and said, "You still have that cat? I thought you were gonna try to find its owner." He came back to her, and past him she could see the small form of a black kitten sitting on the floor of her closet.

"Yeah," she said mechanically. "I'm working on it."

"You shouldn't keep it in the closet, though," Jonah said as he passed. "Unless you want your stuff all messed up."

Denneka was so stunned that she stared at Trick from outside her room for at least a minute. Long enough for Jonah to go back to his own room at the other end of the hall. Then, quietly, she stepped into her room and closed the door.

Trick padded a few of his small steps over to her. A fraction of a second later, human Trick crouched there on all fours, groaning in discomfort. The transformation had been too quick for her to even see properly.

"It's true," Denneka breathed. Suddenly lightheaded, she lowered herself to the floor so she didn't pass out.

———

Trick panted a few times, then the tight pulling feeling stopped and he could relax.

"Does it hurt?" the familiar girl asked. She was on the floor now, and her eyes didn't focus right. Was she sick? Had she hit her head when he wasn't looking?

"Not really," he said. "But it doesn't feel good." Still on his hands and knees, he crouched and tightened in on himself. Without his fur, the air felt too cold. After scanning the room for options, he crawled onto the bed and wrapped the blanket around himself so only his face stuck out.

The girl's mouth hung open as she looked up at him. "You… can turn into a cat?"

"If I could, I would." Being a human was such a pain.

"But you did. Just now."

"That wasn't me."

She shook her head with her eyes pinched closed. "The cat wasn't you? But you said it was. And I saw you."

Why couldn't she understand what he was saying? She probably had hit her head. "I didn't change myself."

"So… you are the cat."

"Of course I am."

"But… you can't control the transformation."

Now she was getting it. He tried to flick his tail, realized he couldn't, and remembered to nod.

"Then how?"

"A witch."

The familiar girl groaned and rubbed her hands over her face. "A witch? You mean magic?"

"I guess."

"A witch cursed you?"

"Not a curse. I like being a cat."

"Okay, Trick, I really appreciate that you're talking to me again after giving me the silent treatment for a week, but—"

"I couldn't help it. Cats can't talk."

"I mean before that."

"Oh." He thought back. "I wasn't supposed to tell you about when I was a cat. I almost did, so I was trying not to slip again. But now you know, so it doesn't matter."

She leaned her back against the door. "I guess that makes sense. So it wasn't... me?"

"What wasn't you?"

"I was afraid I'd made you mad and you didn't... like me anymore... or whatever."

"Not that." He'd stayed close to her all the time while they were at school and on the bus. How could he have made it any clearer that he liked her?

Her fingers fiddled with the leg of her pajama pants. Trick watched with concern as her face started to turn pink. "So, does that mean that... you do like me?"

Was the girl blind and deaf? Maybe he needed to say it again. He slipped off the side of the bed, landing on all fours. She was already on the floor, so he crept over to her, not minding the sudden chill as the blanket fell away from him. This was more important than his comfort right now. The familiar girl froze up as he got closer, like she was afraid he'd attack her. What a weird girl. But he supposed he was a lot bigger now than he was as a cat. So he got a little lower to the ground to try to stop scaring her. She pulled her knees up, so he couldn't crawl into her lap—not that he'd fit now anyway. The best he could do was sit beside her on the floor and mirror her posture, pressing his side against hers. Even then, she was still pretty stiff, so he rubbed his head against hers affectionately.

If that didn't say *I really like you*, he didn't know what would.

When he turned his face to hers, her eyes were wide and her skin had gone really red. Something seemed to be very wrong with her. Sometimes when his mom or brother were sick, he could smell the sickness on them, but when he leaned close to her face and sniffed, he couldn't smell anything. With his weak human nose, though, that didn't mean she wasn't sick.

Maybe petting him would make her feel better. He leaned down enough to bump her shoulder with his head. Usually she petted his head right away when he did that, but it took her a long time to get the hint now. Finally, he felt her gentle hand lightly stroking his head. It didn't feel quite as nice as when he was a cat, but still good. He really wanted to purr but couldn't figure out how to make his lungs do it.

"Trick," the girl said in a soft voice, "are you a cat or a human?"

"Cat," he answered without thinking.

Her hand stopped moving. "You were born a cat?"

"Born human," he said, nudging her hand until she resumed petting him. "Cat now."

Her legs relaxed, becoming not as tightly curled against her chest. "You mean you feel more yourself as a cat than as a human. I can kinda get that."

When her legs straightened all the way in front of her, Trick let his body fall over, only his top half fitting onto her lap.

Then her hand was gone from his head and she slid away from him quickly. He looked up at her, annoyed and hurt. Why was she running from him? Why did she look scared again? He glanced at his own body, at what she saw, and then he could understand. "You don't want to cuddle with me because I'm big and awkward now and I don't have fur anymore," he said sadly.

"No, it's not that!" she insisted, then immediately corrected herself. "It's a little that."

He rolled onto his back and stared at the ceiling. "You don't like me anymore."

"It's not that!" she said again, and this time didn't correct herself.

In order to look at her, he had to crane his head back like he was looking straight up. She seemed to be upside down now, but he could still tell that she was covering her eyes with her hands. "I'm not cute anymore. You can't look at me."

"It's not that!" Her tone was a shouty whisper. "It's that you're naked!"

He sat up and faced her. Maybe if he had a direct view he could figure out what she was saying. "I've been naked the whole time," he reminded her.

"But you're a boy now! It's different!"

His mom had tried to tell him something like that. He hadn't quite figured out what she'd meant, either. "How?"

"Because cats are meant to be naked. People aren't."

"Why not? It's not always cold."

She lowered her hands and gaped at him. "It's not about being cold. It's about—about decency. Boys don't go around naked where girls can see them."

"Why not?"

"Because—" Her gaze dropped lower for an instant. Whenever she was looking at him, her eyes kept flicking to his boy parts before quickly away, but every time it happened, her face pulsed redder. "Because they don't."

"It's my boy parts, isn't it?" he asked, pointing to make himself clear. "Sorry. I told you before they get in the way."

"That's not the point! I shouldn't—I haven't—I've never seen that before and now you're just sitting there and you're not even trying to cover yourself and it's really freaking me out!"

That didn't make much sense. Why should his boy parts freak her out? Sure, they weren't cute, but he didn't think they were *scary*.

Something occurred to him. The thing Mom had explained to him a while ago. He'd been a cat at the time, and even then the idea of what she described had seemed pretty scary. He'd seen animals doing it sometimes, and it was different from what Mom had described, but similar enough that it still looked a lot like fighting. And the female usually looked like she was losing. *Ahh. Now I get it.* "You're... afraid I'm going to try to mate with you?"

The familiar girl lifted her shirt collar up to bury her face in it and let out a muffled sound somewhere between a squeal and a groan.

"I won't," he assured her. "I wouldn't ever hurt you."

Her face still half-buried in the top of her pajama shirt, she jerked suddenly as if realizing something. Her face was red as a tomato and her brown eyes round as golf balls. "You've seen me naked, too." Her words were so soft, they were hard to hear through her shirt.

"No, I haven't."

"You lived in my room for a week!"

"But you always change clothes in the bathroom after you shower at night, and in the morning you're always dressed by the time I wake up."

Her wild look calmed a little. "You're... you're right."

"Why does it matter? I don't care if you're naked."

"That's... that's not the point, Trick."

He crawled closer until he was kneeling in front of her. "Is that why you're sick? Does seeing my body make you sick?"

"I'm not sick. I'm—I'm embarrassed."

He'd heard of embarrassment, though it seemed to rely a lot on caring what other humans thought, so he didn't think he'd ever experienced it. "Why are you embarrassed about my body?"

"I... I don't know. It's just how it is."

This whole embarrassment thing seemed kinda sketchy to Trick. "I still think you're sick. You're very red. That isn't normal."

"You're right. I'll get it checked out." She shot to her her feet and went to her dresser. "In the mean time, would you just humor me and put something on?"

He was still kind of cold, so he said, "Okay."

The familiar girl dug through her drawer and tossed something at him. "I think these should fit." Turning her back to him, she waved in his general direction. "Could you hurry and put them on, please?"

Fortunately, it was a simple t-shirt and sweatpants, and he'd gotten the hang of dressing himself while he'd been human. It hadn't been so long since then that he'd forgotten completely.

"Done," he said after a few minutes, already warmer.

Hesitantly, she turned, then let out a breath, and the redness in her face got much better. "Good. Thank you." Ignoring him completely, she carefully made up her bed, straightening the sheets and blanket, and then sat cross-legged in the middle of it. When Trick moved to sit beside her, she pointed forcefully at her desk chair and said, "Could you sit over there, please?"

He tried not to let that hurt too much, reminding himself that she wasn't feeling well. He could sit in a chair if she needed him to. Even if he did think she'd feel better if she went back to petting him. "Can I have breakfast yet?"

Apparently that hadn't been something she'd expected. Her mouth was already open to say something, and she sort of halted a few times before saying, "Okay. Sure. Stay here. My brother's still in the house, I think."

She got up and left, and Trick obediently stayed in the chair. Except shortly after she closed the door, that uncomfortable pulling in his body happened again, and then he was sitting on the chair in a pile of fabric. Carefully stepping out of the pile, he hopped from the chair to the bed. It felt so good to be a cat again, and he had his fur back so he was warm and the girl wouldn't yell at him to wear clothes because for some reason she was okay with him being naked when he was a cat. She seemed to like him a lot better as a cat, which he was okay with. He liked himself better that way, too. So he curled up on the bed and waited for her to come back with food. She'd be so pleased to see him back to his normal self.

As long as he didn't suddenly transform back like last—

A few seconds before the door opened again, Trick felt the tight pulling thing. Then he was a boy, still sitting on the girl's bed only without the clothes she'd made him put on, and she was in the doorway holding a plate of food that she almost dropped.

"I didn't do it on purpose," said Trick.

She turned her back, exited the room, and closed the door. Not wanting to get yelled at, Trick scrambled back into the clothes she'd given him and sat in the chair.

After a minute, the door slowly opened a crack, and she peeked around the edge of it to see him behaving himself.

Please still let me have my food. Please still let me have my food, he thought to her. As if she could read his mind, she came in and handed him the plate. Breakfast was eggs and bacon, and it tasted almost as good as raw finch.

Finally, Denneka thought. Trick was sitting at her desk, dressed and looking normal enough that if Jonah came in again he might not immediately murder Trick. Adrenaline no longer suffused every inch of Denneka's body, and her brain was working well enough to form thoughts again. "As I was trying to say," she started. When had that been? Like, fifty years ago? She'd been trying to focus their conversation when Trick had suddenly come up all close to her and shorted out her brain. Between trying not to pass out from embarrassment and trying to make her eyes behave, she hadn't had any room left inside her for thought. It wasn't like she'd *wanted* to see all of that; she just hadn't been able to stop looking.

Trick watched her as he ate, waiting for her to continue. Those green eyes were more distracting than anything else about him, in their own way.

"What I meant was, while I'm glad you're talking to me again, you haven't told me much about this whole"—she waved a hand at him—"situation. Can you start at the beginning with the witch thing? You can finish eating first."

It didn't take him long to set the empty plate aside. "When my mom was pregnant with my brother, he was sick, and she was afraid he wouldn't be born. Doctors couldn't help. So she made a deal with an old witch. If I was the witch's familiar for seven years, she'd save my brother. The witch died after a year, so I went back home. The seven years just ended, and I turned back into a human even though the witch isn't around anymore."

A bargain with a witch. Wasn't that the sort of thing that only happened in fairy tales? "Okay... but if the witch is gone, why are you changing now?"

"Another witch."

Naturally, I guess. "Did your mom make another deal?"

"I don't think so. She doesn't want me to be a cat."

Denneka remembered when she'd briefly met Trick's mom. Jacqueline had seemed normal. Not like the kind of woman who'd trade her son away to a witch. Even if she didn't want Trick to be a cat—and who could blame her?—that didn't necessarily mean she hadn't made another deal. If she'd done it once, she might have done it twice. "Do you know anything about this... other witch?"

"It's a man. I didn't know him."

"You saw... him?" Weren't male witches called warlocks? Whatever. Semantics weren't important right now.

"He was at school. I followed him because I saw the hawk, and he caught me and changed me."

"Why would a witch be at school?"

"I don't know why. To attack me, probably."

"Why would he want to?"

Trick jerked his shoulders in what was probably meant to be a shrug.

"What do you mean 'the hawk'?"

"A hawk's been stalking me."

That sounded a little paranoid. "You think you're being stalked by a bird?"

"I am. See?" He got up and reached to the window behind the head of the bed. When he pulled back the curtain, they both jumped in fright.

A small hawk was perched right on the windowsill, like some peeper who'd been watching and listening to them the whole time.

Trick yelped and dove behind the end of the bed for cover, but Denneka watched in amazement as the hawk took off and flew into the branches of the big tree in the back yard—and then kept watching them.

Denneka swiftly pulled the curtains closed. "That... is super creepy."

"It was so close!" Trick whined. "Normally it's in the tree. It wants to eat me."

"Trick, you're like twenty-plus times the size of that bird. I don't think it can eat you."

Trick peeked over the end of the bed at her. "I'm not always."

"I don't know. Even as a cat, I think you're bigger than it. I don't think hawks usually prey on animals bigger than they are." Though she wouldn't swear to it.

"Why else would it be following me?"

Denneka considered that very valid question. An idea began to put itself together in her head. "When you said the agreement was for you to be the old witch's familiar, what did you mean by that?"

"She made me a cat. I stayed with her. I could hear her voice in my head sometimes." He ducked back behind the bed and crouched, hugging his knees. "It was a long time ago. I don't remember much."

Denneka crawled to the end of the bed and looked down at him. "Is it normal for witches to turn humans into animals to be their familiars?"

He tried to shrug again.

"But you said this hawk was with the male witch who turned you back into a cat?"

Slowly, his head turned toward her. "You think... the hawk is the witch's familiar?"

"I don't know much about all this, and I kinda can't believe I'm even having this conversation right now, but... what do you think?"

His eyes lit up. "I think you're very smart."

.pliment made her so warm, she had to look
.ack to the window, pulled the curtain open, anc
.wk in the tree. It was watching them. It was too fa.
st well, and she couldn't exactly read bird expressions,
thought there might have been intelligence in those small,
eyes.

"Then it's not trying to eat me," Trick said excitedly. "I can
outside!"

"What? Wait!" She spun to stop him, but he'd already thrown
open the door and taken off down the hallway.

Before he reached the bathroom door, he vanished, his clothes
crumpling to the floor, and a small, black kitten tumbled around in
them before finding his way out. This didn't stop him from running
to the front door and pawing at it, meowing to be let out.

"Trick!" Denneka whisper-shouted at him. But as she followed,
collecting his dropped clothes, she saw that the door to her brother's
bedroom was open. She peeked inside. He wasn't there. Maybe he'd
left the house? She went into the living room, but as she approached
Trick, he abruptly turned back into a human. When he got over the
discomfort of the change and reached for the door handle, she ran at
him and grabbed his forearm. "Trick, stop!"

Surprisingly, he did, only to pull his arm forcefully out of her
grip and back away from her in fright. Had she *scared* him?

She shoved the clothes into his chest and turned her face away
from him so she wouldn't see too much. "You can't go out like that.
Just wait for now. Hurry and put these back on."

With a wary look, he took the clothes.

"I... I'll check to see if my brother's still here. If he is, we're both
gonna be in big trouble soon."

She looked out the window to see that Jonah's car wasn't in the
driveway anymore, but just to be sure, she decided to give Trick
some privacy while she checked the rest of the house. Her brother
was nowhere to be seen, fortunately. When she returned to the
living room, Trick was standing in the middle of the room, still
naked, with the clothes in a pile by his feet.

my fault," he protested, sounding quite falsely-accused.
ing it, but as soon as you left, I became a cat again, and
rned human right when you came back."

turned her back. "Okay. Just put them on now, please."
thing was starting to come together in a way she did not at all
. When she stopped hearing sounds of movement, she turned to
e him fully dressed but standing there with a stance and expression that clearly said he thought she'd wronged him. "I—I'm sorry,"
she said, coming closer. "I see that it's not your fault." He didn't
look at her, and she had the strangest urge to try petting his head.
Her hand was half-reached out to do so. *What am I doing? He's not
really a cat. But... he does seem to act like one.* Very slowly, she kept
reaching until her fingers touched soft, black hair. Immediately, he
pressed his head into her hand, so she stroked it gently a few times.
Finally, he looked at her again, and his expression wasn't angry
anymore. "You keep changing, and you can't control it," she said,
making clear that she understood he wasn't doing it on purpose. "It
may not be random, though. I want to test something. Please come
this way."

With Trick right behind her, Denneka went to the laundry room
and found a measuring tape. Then she led him to the hallway.

"Hold onto this." She handed him one end of the measuring
tape. "I'll stand here. You walk as far as you can that way. Don't let
go of the tape."

The slight cock of his head said he didn't understand what she
was doing, but he didn't question her. He just started walking. She
watched the tape as it unrolled in her hands. It went slack at the ten-
foot mark. Kitten Trick sat on the floor of the hallway. As soon as he
started to return to her, he transformed back into a human.

She covered her eyes. "You don't have to put your clothes on yet.
I want to test this a few more times."

After four more trials in various places in the house, Trick
groaned, "Can we stop? I'm getting sore."

"I'm sorry. Yeah, we can stop. If you need to use the bathroom, you should probably do it now, while no one else is home." She moved to wait in the hall just outside the bathroom while Trick used the facilities and got dressed. When he came out, she said, "I know what triggers your transformation. It... it looks like you can't get more than ten feet away from me without changing back into a cat. Or closer than that without changing into a human."

Denneka didn't know what kind of response to that revelation she was expecting, but she should have known to expect the blank stare that Trick deemed it worthy of.

"Did you hear me?"

"Yes," he said. "Can we go outside now?"

"Um..." She wasn't sure that was a good idea. Her parents were away for the day, but she didn't know where her brother had gone or who else might be around. Would it be a problem if someone saw Trick at her home alone with her? Especially if anyone realized he was the boy everyone thought was missing?

He moved down the hall toward the main part of the house, his shoulder rubbing against hers as he passed. After a couple steps, he stopped and looked back at her expectantly.

Was he... waiting for her? Assuming she'd agree? She couldn't figure it out.

He came back to where she was and turned so that his shoulder rubbed against hers even harder as he moved toward the door again. "Outside?" he said in a tone so close to the plaintive mew he sometimes used in his kitten form that all her resistance crumbled.

What is this crazy boy doing? "All right. I guess we could go into the back yard," she conceded against her better judgment. As soon as she opened the sliding glass door, Trick rushed out. She had to run to keep up so he wouldn't transform back into a cat out in the open. He ran a few laps around the yard, then stopped suddenly and made a bee-line to the tree.

"Hey!" he shouted at it.

No—at the hawk. Denneka could see the small bird of prey still perched on one of the lower branches, watching Trick.

"Why are you watching me?" Trick yelled to the hawk. "Go away! Go back to your witch!"

Denneka cast a worried look around the yard. They had a six-foot wooden fence and no neighbors that could easily see over it, but it was hardly a properly enclosed space, and she didn't know who might be standing on the other side, listening even if they couldn't see. "Trick. Stop yelling at the bird."

The hawk didn't respond to him at all, which only made him angrier. "You think you're so scary. You're just a bird. I eat birds. I don't need to be afraid of you."

Maybe it knew that he'd been quite afraid of it until just recently, because the hawk didn't do anything but continue watching him.

"You think I'm afraid of you?" Trick taunted it. "I'm not afraid. I'll show you." He spun and turned a burning gaze on Denneka, then stormed toward her.

She backed up in a hurry. "What? What are you doing?"

Once he'd gotten her back a good twelve feet, he stopped, turned, and raced full-speed at the tree. Realizing too late what he was about, Denneka could only watch as he transformed into a cat mid-run, tumbled around in the fallen clothes, then crawled his way out and scrambled up the tree trunk. Denneka had never seen a cat run up a tree so fast, his claws giving him the kind of grip she thought only belonged to squirrels and chipmunks.

Far from being concerned, the hawk waited until he'd made it to the base of the branch it was sitting on, then casually flapped to a higher branch. With a skitter of claws on bark, Trick grabbed the next higher branch in his front paws, then clawed at it with his hind legs until he pulled himself up. This time the hawk waited until he was a hairsbreadth away from it before flapping up to a higher branch.

"Trick, stop!" Denneka yelled—but not too loudly in case anyone was nearby to hear. Maybe the hawk wouldn't eat him, but that didn't mean it wouldn't defend itself if attacked, even if it was a human familiar in animal form.

Unsurprisingly, Trick didn't listen to her. He chased the hawk up the tree until it spread its wings to leave the tree entirely, landing on the edge of the roof where Trick didn't have a hope of reaching it. Denneka expected Trick to descend the tree as easily as he'd ascended, but apparently cats really did get stuck in trees. He tried to find a footing and nearly fell several times before Denneka came closer to help him down.

For a moment there, she'd forgotten about the transformation issue. Instead of a cat stuck in a tree, Trick was suddenly a naked boy stuck in a tree. And he was high enough that anyone looking from the other side of the fence could probably see him. "Trick!" she hissed. "Come down!"

With his much, much longer limbs and body, he was able to lower himself down the branches and land unharmed on the grass.

"Trick, clothes!"

He looked at them and then totally ignored them, choosing instead to flop onto the grass and stare up at the bird sulkily.

Denneka resigned herself to being stuck out here until he got his fill of sunshine, turning to examine the hawk perched on the edge of the roof. It was a pretty red-tailed hawk, and it was now watching her with what looked like curiosity. A regular hawk wouldn't still be hanging around by this point. It would either have attacked Trick when he was a cat or been driven away from the yard.

"I'm right, aren't I?" Denneka asked it. "You're a familiar, like Trick was. You're with that witch that he saw, the one who changed him back into a cat."

The hawk gave a slow nod.

Wow. Even believing it was true, it was totally surreal to get a human response from a bird like that. "What does he want with Trick? What connection does he have to him?"

The bird didn't respond. Not that it could actually have said anything. Maybe it would give her 'yes' or 'no' answers, but since the bird couldn't speak, anything more than that was likely impossible.

So, how much information *could* Denneka get out of it? "Can you change back into a human, too?"

The bird nodded.

"Can you do it now?"

A slow, subtle shake of its head.

"Are there any other familiars or witches around, other than you and your witch?"

No answer.

"Are there any others *that you know of?*"

The bird shook its head.

This was the weirdest game of twenty questions Denneka had ever played. She wondered how much the bird would be willing to tell her. "I'm right about what causes Trick to transform, aren't I? That it has to do with how close he is to me?"

A nod.

"But why?" she blurted. "What's the point of that?"

No answer. Of course.

She sighed. "Do you or your witch mean any harm to Trick or me?"

For a second, the bird didn't respond, but then it slowly shook its head. Denneka sighed. If she could believe what it told her, then that was a good thing. It didn't tell her what the witch did want, but she really hoped they didn't have cause to be afraid of him. Given how reluctant the hawk had been about its last answer, Denneka thought she might be at the limit of what it would say.

Confirming her suspicion, the hawk flew back to a branch high in the tree.

Trick was spread-eagle on the grass, eyes closed like he was soaking up the sun. Denneka groaned, picked up the clothes he'd dropped, and tossed them at him, aiming for the area that most needed covering. "Trick, please get dressed now. You need to go home."

He did not like that idea. Like a sleeping cat startled by a vacuum, he jumped up into a crouch, his green eyes huge and pleading. "Can't I stay?"

"What? Why?"

"I like it here."

The fluttery feeling that statement caused in Denneka's chest was unhelpful to the situation. "But your mom's worried. And the police are looking for you. Everyone thinks you've been kidnapped. It's a whole big thing."

"I don't care."

Well, that was straightforward. "You should go home to your mom."

"If I do, I'll get in trouble."

"How could you? She knows about witches, right? You can explain what happened. She couldn't possibly be angry at you for getting changed by force."

"She'll be mad that I didn't come home anyway. She'll know I could have."

Denneka considered him. "Why didn't you, then? If you could have left, why did you stay? You did escape from me once, and— Oh." The memory of the vet asking if she wanted to have Trick neutered flashed through her mind. If he hadn't noticed that or known what the word meant, it was probably best not to bring it up now. "I mean, you could have gone home then, but you came back to me. Why?"

"I like it here," he said again. He crawled over to crouch in front of her, gazing up at her with wide, puppy-dog eyes. "Don't make me leave. Please."

"You—you can't stay here. If you get caught—"

"I won't. I'll be careful."

"But the police—"

He shot to his feet and leaned forward to rub the side of his head against hers. "Please. Let me stay."

He was so cute and pitiful. And he wanted to be with her more than going home. Of all the people he knew, even his own family, he wanted to be with her the most.

"Okay," she breathed.

He hummed happily and rubbed his head on hers even harder. "Thank you."

"But please put some clothes on. We need to at least go inside so

one sees or hears you out here. Then I need to go to the shop and
o something for Mom. I'll see if I can find you any boys' clothes
while I'm there."

Trick didn't push his luck but obediently dressed and followed
her back into the house.

CHAPTER
THIRTEEN

One more, then I'd better eat lunch, Jacqueline told herself. The day was bright and beginning to get hot, but she wouldn't stop searching until either she found her son or it got so late that people stopped answering the door. Agreste was a small town, though, and she'd already covered more than half of it, so she felt certain that if Trick was a cat and some girl had taken him in, she'd find him soon. The tip John had given her about most students living on the east side of town not only hadn't given her any edge in finding the girl the vet had mentioned, she wondered if John was sure he'd remembered the part of town correctly. As far as she'd been able to tell, there'd been no more kids there than in any other area.

The next house on the block was pale blue with a partial stone façade and a small front porch. There weren't any cars in the driveway. Hopefully someone was home and she wouldn't have to add it to the list of houses to circle back to. Jacqueline walked up to the front door and raised her fist to knock.

Before she could, the door opened, and someone with a lot of brown hair almost ran smack into her.

"Ah!" The girl staggered back a step into the house.

"Sorry," said Jacqueline. There was something familiar about the girl. "Have we met?"

"What? No! I mean, maybe." She wasn't getting over being startled quickly.

"I didn't mean to scare you," Jacqueline said. "I was just about to knock when you came out. My name's Jacqueline. I'm looking for my lost cat. You haven't seen a black kitten around, have you?"

"No! I mean, I—I don't think so."

Jacqueline looked the girl over. She was pretty nondescript. Cute if not exactly pretty, with brown hair and wide, chestnut eyes. "Denneka, isn't it?"

"What?" the girl cheeped, her eyes getting even wider.

"You work at the clothing shop. We met once when I was in there with my sons."

"Oh. Right. You—you remembered?"

"I'm pretty good with faces. And with names, if I see them written down, like with your name tag."

"Oh. Good." Denneka's mouth split open in what it took Jacqueline a second to realize was meant to be a smile.

"Are you sure you haven't seen a black kitten or small black cat?" Jacqueline asked. The girl looked like she was the right age, and the vet had mentioned that the girl was brunette.

"I... don't see a lot of cats around here," Denneka said. "And Mom hates cats, so she'll chase them off our yard if she sees them."

"Well... okay." Jacqueline wanted to push, but she had no real reason to. If the girl was acting oddly, it might have only been from the surprise of suddenly finding a strange woman standing unexpectedly right outside her front door. Jacqueline reached into her purse and pulled out one of the extra fliers she'd printed off. "Here's a picture of him and my phone number. Please call if you do see anything."

The girl took it without looking. "Okay. Will do!"

Jacqueline's instincts told her to push her way into the house and search the place, but then the girl would probably call the cops. Even if Trick was there, Jacqueline was pretty sure that was no defense for trespassing. And if the girl was hiding Trick in the house, it meant he was probably safe.

She was most likely only being paranoid and suspicious because she was reaching the end of her rope. She wanted Trick home, and she was running out of ideas for how to find him.

Going back to her car, Jacqueline pulled out the sandwich John had made her and ate as she drove to the next area. But she made a note of the blue house and the girl Denneka. Just in case.

———

Trick lay curled up in a ball on the familiar girl's bed, right up against her pillow where it smelled most like her, settling in for a good, long nap while she was out. Then he heard her footsteps pounding toward him a second before magic pulled and stretched his body like taffy. Groaning, he sat up to watch her blow into the room and shut the door in a hurry.

"Trick, your—" Her wild look suddenly became angry, and she pointed accusingly at his boy parts. "Would you cover that, please?" The words were a polite request, but her tone was an order. Trick wasn't sure which of those she meant.

He slid his body out so he was lying across the bed on his stomach, propping up on his elbows enough to still look at her.

She put a hand to her forehead. "That's... not much better." Then she let out a huff. "Never mind that for now. Trick, your mom was just at the door."

Trick's body went stiff with fear, his fight or flight response activated, but there was no one to fight and nowhere to run except the closet.

"She's gone now," the girl said, and Trick relaxed. "She said she was looking for her black cat." The girl thrust a piece of paper in his face. It had a picture of him on it—real him, not human him—and the only phone number he knew. "She knows you're a cat again, and she's looking for you."

Trick watched her, waiting for her to explain why she had come back to the room when she'd been meaning to go to her shop.

217

"I had to lie!" she said, her tone going high at the end. "I hate lying! Trick, if you hadn't convinced me to let you stay…"

"You… didn't tell her I'm here?" Trick offered, trying to help her get to the point.

"If I still thought you were a cat, I would have. I… was being selfish, keeping you instead of looking for your owner."

"Selfish?" That was doing things you wanted to do, right? Why did everyone always say that word like it was a bad thing?

"I… I liked having you here, so I kept putting off trying to find where you belonged."

"I like being here," Trick said. He didn't see the problem. He'd thought she had already known where his home was and that he didn't want to go there, and that was why she was keeping him. But if she hadn't known he was a cat before, then he must have been wrong about that. "Can I nap now?"

"Trick! Aren't you worried? Your mom almost found you. Do you see why you shouldn't go outside unless you want to be found out?"

Trick curled up in the spot by her pillow and waited for her to go away.

———

It took Landon all morning to get his homework done, mostly because he spent half the time watching Mr. McKenzie.

Yesterday, they'd spent so much time in the kitchen that Landon hadn't gotten to his homework at all, but Mom hadn't been upset about it. Before she left this morning, though, she'd told Landon that he needed to get it all done before doing anything else. So he'd sat at the dining table with all of his school stuff and worked on it while Mr. McKenzie sat in the living room with a book.

Even though Landon could see straight through the archway from his spot at the dining table to where Mr. McKenzie sat, it took him a while to notice how weird the man was acting. It looked like Mr. McKenzie was reading a book. A paperback with an old painting for a cover with the words 'Don Juan' and 'Lord Byron' in big letters. Landon wasn't sure which of those was the title and which was the author. He kept hearing laughter while he worked. A lot of laughter. Like it was the funniest book ever. So Landon watched Mr. McKenzie a little, wondering if he should ask to read the book next. That was when he noticed that Mr. McKenzie didn't turn the page very often. Even when a book had a lot of words on each page, Landon usually turned the page at least every few minutes while reading. Mr. McKenzie turned a page maybe once every half hour, for a good three hours. But he kept laughing and chuckling and muttering under his breath. And his eyes would go in and out of focus, like he was looking through the book instead of at it. Landon didn't notice that right away, not until he was watching and suddenly saw Mr. McKenzie's eyes snap into focus on the book, and he only then realized they hadn't been focused for a long time before.

If he's not reading that book, Landon wondered, *then what is he laughing at?*

Pretending like he was still focused on his homework, Landon waited until he saw Mr. McKenzie stare through the book again. Then he asked in a normal tone, "Mr. McKenzie? Can you help me with this?"

Mr. McKenzie didn't respond.

"Mr. McKenzie?" he asked a little louder.

Nothing.

"Mr. McKenzie?" he said again, nearly shouting.

The teacher's face snapped to him, and he smiled. "What is it, small one?"

"Can you... help me with this question?" Why had it been so hard to get his attention?

Mr. McKenzie came over and helped Landon with a question on his history homework which he didn't really need help with, then hurried back to his book. Or to whatever it was he was paying attention to while pretending to read.

By lunch time, Landon had finished the homework that would

normally have only taken a couple hours, but he kept sitting at the dining table, watching Mr. McKenzie over in the living room.

Suddenly, Mr. McKenzie took a deep breath and set the book aside. "Well then," he said cheerfully, "what time is it?" He looked at the wall clock and said, "Time for lunch. Excellent." He headed for the kitchen like everything was normal, pausing to examine Landon's pile of books and notebooks. "Have you finished?"

Landon nodded.

"Good. Do you want to help me with lunch?"

"Mr. McKenzie," Landon said carefully, "what were you doing all that time?"

"Just reading. Why?"

"No, you weren't."

A surprised blink wiped the happy expression off Mr. McKenzie's face. "Wasn't I?"

Maybe Landon shouldn't have said anything. He didn't really know Mr. McKenzie or what kind of person he was. But he'd told Landon he wasn't his enemy and he'd been really nice yesterday, so Landon was starting to believe him. "No. You weren't."

Mr. McKenzie's mouth widened into a grin that Landon couldn't understand. It wasn't evil, but it was... evil*ish*. But happy, too. It was weird. His brown eyes pierced Landon so sharply, Landon had to look away. "You really are the cleverest boy, aren't you?" Mr. McKenzie said in a voice that gave Landon the creeping feeling that the man wanted to put him in a bag and carry him off.

"Never mind," Landon said quietly, still not able to look at the man. "You don't have to tell me. I just wondered."

There was a really loud silence, and then Mr. McKenzie went into the kitchen. "Clear your things off the table, please."

Landon hurried to gather his school stuff and take it all to his room. He was still weirded out from Mr. McKenzie's reaction, so he stayed in his room and read until Mr. McKenzie knocked on the closed bedroom door.

"Don't you want to eat at the table?" Mr. McKenzie said through the door.

Landon considered saying he wasn't hungry, but he was hungry, and what if there wasn't food left when he went out later? Before he could decide what to answer, the doorknob twisted, and Mr. McKenzie came in. Landon fought the urge to scoot back in his chair, away from the man.

Mr. McKenzie knelt in front of Landon's big reading chair. "Did I scare you, small one?"

"No," Landon insisted. It wasn't fear. Landon wasn't some scared little boy. He could defend himself. He could make people hurt—even people bigger than him. He didn't need to be afraid.

"I didn't think so. Fear doesn't come easily to those who have power, does it?"

Landon stared at the man in shock. "Power? What power?"

"Tut tut. You called me out for lying. Don't think I'll let you get away with doing the same."

Landon's heart beat faster. What did this man know about what he could do? How did he know? What did it mean? And was it a good thing or bad thing?

Mr. McKenzie stood and walked away. "Lunch is on the table. I'd like it if you joined me."

After that bomb drop, Landon couldn't really refuse.

Lunch was a type of sandwich that Mr. McKenzie called a French dip. Whenever Mom did include meat in Landon's sandwiches, she was always stingy with it. But this sandwich was almost nothing but meat. Landon liked it, even if the dip part made it way too messy.

Landon had a mouth full of sandwich and beef juice all over his face when Mr. McKenzie finally said, "You asked me what power you have. Do you truly not know?"

It's bad to talk with your mouth full, so Landon chewed carefully, using the time to think about what he'd say. The idea of talking about this seemed wrong... but it was also something he badly wanted to do. After he swallowed his food, he said, "I... I don't know."

Mr. McKenzie raised an eyebrow at him. "You're a very smart boy. Take a guess."

Landon took a sip of water. It didn't go down easy. "Is it"—the next word stuck in his throat, but he resisted the urge to drink more water—"magic?"

"There you are. Was that so hard?"

Yes, it was. It felt like Landon had said something awful. Like he'd said one of those words he sometimes heard other people say but which his mom told him he should never say because only crude idiots talked like that. She'd never said that about 'magic', and she had talked to him about it herself, but somehow this was... different. When she talked about it, it was something bad. Something that hurt people. Even if it had saved Landon's life before he was born, that didn't change that it was dangerous and trouble-causing. If that was the same thing that Landon had been doing... "How?" he asked.

Mr. McKenzie finished his sandwich and pushed his plate away. "How do you do magic?"

"How *can* I?"

"How do you think?"

Landon had a theory. He'd been wondering about it secretly inside his own mind for a long time now, though he didn't know when it had first occurred to him. But explaining his theory would mean telling this near-stranger too much. "I... don't think I should say."

Mr. McKenzie considered him but didn't push him to answer.

Landon finished the last few bites of his sandwich, then went to the sink to wash his hands. Mr. McKenzie came in with the dishes, and as he was rinsing them off, Landon asked him, "How do you know about it?"

"About magic, or about how you can use it?"

"Both."

"Let's save the first for later, but as for the second, it's easy enough to see. You don't hide it as well as you think you do. You'll need to learn to be more careful."

Landon felt his face get hot. He had thought he'd been hiding it. Or maybe he'd really thought that no one else was smart enough to notice what he was doing.

Mr. McKenzie finished with the dishes and turned to Landon, crossing his arms. "Have you used magic around anyone outside your home?"

Landon looked away, not wanting to answer.

"So that's a yes." The man's tone lightened. "I'm not rebuking you, Landon. I'm not your—well, I mean, I won't punish you. I'm only curious."

The weird hitch in Mr. McKenzie's voice for a second there made Landon look at him from the corner of his eye to find the man's face had gone slightly pink. The pink faded right away, but Landon filed what he'd seen away in his brain. "Can you use magic?" he asked the man. "Is that what you were doing this morning?"

"Yes and no."

"What does that mean?"

"Let's make a deal, shall we? If you tell me about as many of the times you've used magic as you can remember, I'll tell you what I meant by 'yes and no'."

If Mr. McKenzie already knew about what Landon could do, then he had nothing to hide. Except Landon felt like he did want to hide it. None of the things he'd done had felt like bad things at the time, but now the thought of saying them out loud, especially to a grown-up, made him feel like his stomach was full of worms. But he wanted to know what the man knew and what he'd been doing this morning that'd had him so distracted. In the end, Landon's curiosity was stronger than his fear. "Okay."

"Excellent. Why don't we go outside and enjoy the fine weather while we talk?"

Landon followed him into the back yard and they sat across from each other cross-legged on the grass. A flash of worry about grass stains on his shorts flitted through Landon's mind, but he ignored it. This was more important.

"I'm waiting," Mr. McKenzie said cheerfully.

Landon took a deep breath and let it out. *Might as well start at the beginning.* "When I was really little, I was playing outside…"

He talked for a while, and Mr. McKenzie listened. Usually, the man listened with a bland expression, nodding as if it all made sense. Sometimes he laughed at what Landon told him. Once or twice, he frowned, but he didn't say anything.

Eventually, Landon finished telling him everything—except for the most recent time, with the boys at school. Landon still didn't think he'd done anything wrong there, but he didn't like the idea of telling anyone about it. "Your turn."

Mr. McKenzie chuckled and stood up. "How about a quick break first? I need to stretch my legs. Why don't you run around and catch bugs or something?"

Landon scowled at him. "I don't do that."

"What? You're a little boy. Isn't that something little boys do?"

"Sure, when I was four. I'm not that little anymore."

"Noted," Mr. McKenzie said with a laugh. Then his expression turned really serious. His eyes locked hard on Landon's, and he said in a lower tone, "Go catch something, Landon. Something living. I don't care what it is." The next second, the seriousness was gone, and he walked off to stroll around the yard, whistling.

He's so annoying. Landon had the urge to zap the man or make him trip, but he still hadn't answered Landon's question. So Landon trudged over to the back corner where there was a tree and some rocks. A bird and a squirrel were up in the branches, but there was no way he could catch either of those. A few ants crawled up the tree's trunk, but they were too tiny to hold and they'd only end up crawling all over him. Under one of the big rocks, he found a dime-sized beetle and an earthworm. He picked up the beetle and held it in his cupped hands. *Now what?*

When both he and Mr. McKenzie had returned to their spots on the grass, Landon held out his hands, opening them to show that he'd caught something.

Mr. McKenzie quickly reached out, wrapping his much bigger

hands around Landon's to keep them closed. "No, that's fine. Hold it for now so it doesn't escape. What have you caught?"

"It's... a beetle." The feel of the man's hands on his was distracting, and the sight of it even more so. They weren't like Mom's hands at all. Something deep, deep inside Landon ached so badly he wanted to cry.

"Good." Mr. McKenzie pulled away, digging his fingers into the grass behind him as he leaned back.

"How do you know about all this?" Landon asked. "Are you... like me?" There was another word. A word that felt even more bad to say than 'magic'. Even thinking it felt bad. So Landon didn't use it.

"I suppose you could say that, yes. When I was a boy, I went through something very similar to what you're experiencing. I had to muddle through on my own. So, when I saw that you were going through it, I thought perhaps I should help."

"Show me."

"Pardon?"

"Show me you can do what I can do."

"Ah, well, I can't at the moment. Because of... circumstances I won't explain right now, I can't currently use magic myself."

That sounded suspiciously convenient. Was he lying? Was he just someone who knew that magic existed and wanted to feel special by pretending to be someone who could use it? "Then what were you doing this morning?" That was what had started this whole thing, right?

"In order to explain that, I think I shall have to teach you how to do it yourself. Do you want to learn some magic, little one?"

"Learn? Like"—a word stuck in his mouth again—"a spell?"

"Basically, yes. What you've been doing so far has been instinctive. You want something, so your will reaches into your magic and makes 'something' happen. But you can do so much more if you learn to focus those instincts in particular ways. And, eventually, to use your brain to guide your power rather than relying on your instincts. That's the only way you'll be able to do anything but the most rudimentary types of magic. Have you ever tried to do something specific with your magic?"

"Sometimes, like pick up a book, but it doesn't always work."

Mr. McKenzie nodded. "Any start is a good start. Now let's try this. Hold that beetle of yours between your fingers. Don't crush it, but make sure it can't get away."

Carefully, Landon opened his hands and grabbed the beetle between his thumb and index finger. Its little legs moved wildly, like it hoped to run through the air, but there was nothing for them to grab on.

"Good. Keep watching the beetle. Focus on it. Use your will to direct your magic into the beetle's mind. Fill the beetle with your magic. Make the beetle yours."

Landon looked at Mr. McKenzie like he'd gone crazy. "What are you talking about? None of that makes any sense."

Mr. McKenzie blinked and cringed. "It doesn't? Sorry. I've never actually tried to teach someone else any of this. Like I said, I had to figure it all out myself. I'm afraid translating that into an explanation someone else can understand is... trickier than I'd hoped."

"Maybe if you told me what I'm trying to do?"

The man sighed. "Well, it kind of ruins the drama, but I suppose we could try it that way. See, there's a fun little trick we can do. You make a connection between your mind and a creature's, and then you can see through its eyes and hear through its ears. All the senses, really. The connection won't last long on a lifeform as low as an insect, but once you learn it, you can keep practicing until you're able to make connections to birds or dogs or anything else, and that's where it really gets fun."

Landon watched the man through narrowed eyes. "And I can do that?"

He nodded. "All it takes is a bit of practice."

"Does it hurt the animal?"

"Not at all. At least, not until the strain of it overloads the thing and it dies."

Landon nearly dropped the beetle. "It dies?"

"Eventually. That beetle should last a day or two. A mouse or small lizard would last a few weeks."

"The bigger the animal, the longer it lives?"

"It's more about intelligence and level of sentience than size. A dog or cat should last several years, but you might only get one year out of a shark."

"What about a human?"

Mr. McKenzie's eyes grew sharper, but he said, "It's impossible to make a direct connection to a human. So don't go thinking of trying to do it to your mom or brother, all right?"

Impossible to make a direct connection to a human, Landon noted. It sounded like a firm answer, but there was actually a lot of wiggle room.

"I don't want to kill things," he said.

"But... it's just a beetle, Landon."

"This is a beetle. But you said if I keep doing it, then it's a bird or a dog or whatever. They'll all die eventually from this, right?"

"Yes, but... they're only animals." Mr. McKenzie sounded confused. "You use them until you can't anymore."

"We shouldn't use animals like that, though."

"You eat meat. How is this different?"

Landon frowned, thinking about it. Was it different? He never felt guilty about eating meat. Even Mom didn't say they should feel guilty about eating meat. And if using animals for food was fine even though it meant they died, then maybe using them for other things was fine, too. Where had he even gotten the idea that it wasn't? "But... it's still wrong to use people, isn't it?"

Mr. McKenzie laughed. "Ask your mother if she thinks using people is wrong. Her answer might surprise you." Under his breath, he added, "If she even gives you an answer."

Having expected a firm 'yes', Landon wasn't sure what to say next.

"You're overthinking this, small one. Squashing a bug doesn't make you an inevitable murderer." Mr. McKenzie shrugged. "It's your choice if we continue this or not, but it's only a beetle. It's hardly aware it even has an existence, so it won't mean much when it ceases to exist. And you won't really understand what I was doing this morning until you experience it yourself."

Landon studied the black beetle between his fingers, legs still moving. It *was* only a bug, after all. And he really wanted to try the thing Mr. McKenzie had described. "I want to try it."

"Good! Good! You remember what I said?"

"Yes. Let me try it by myself." Landon held the beetle up to look into its tiny black eyes. They barely even looked like eyes. No color or white or rings. Just little black dots that didn't tell him anything. Will first. Will was wanting something. *Will goes into the power. Into the… magic. And that goes into the beetle.* He stared at the beetle, trying to feel the things inside him that Mr. McKenzie had talked about. He couldn't figure it out. But those little black eyes kept staring at him, and he kept wondering what they saw. What did those tiny, waving legs feel like? The teacher had said he'd be able to see through the bug's eyes if he did this right. But how? *How?* Landon's curiosity burned hotter and hotter. How did this work? What did this all mean? And what did those weird little black eyes see?

He felt the connection latching on as a small jerk somewhere in his brain. It was like when he finally understood something he'd been studying, like that moment of *Ah-ha!* except there was some-thing almost-but-not-quite physical about it. He wondered again what the beetle saw, and then he knew.

The world looked different through the beetle's eyes, but he could recognize his own face. He couldn't feel things in the way people feel things, since the beetle didn't have skin, but he could feel the movement of the beetle's legs. It all startled him so much that he dropped the beetle, and then the beetle's-eye view of the world was tumbling flashes of shapes and movement, and then it was all sky as the beetle flew upward, and it was the most amazing thing Landon had ever felt.

He felt his own stomach lurch and his own head get dizzy, and he shut off the connection before he could even think to do so. He fell onto his side in the grass, breathing hard and trying not to throw up.

Mr. McKenzie laughed and patted him hard on the arm. "Well done, young one. Well done. How did it feel?"

Landon pushed himself back up. "I was... flying... for a second."

Mr. McKenzie beamed at him, nodding like a bobblehead. "I know. I know. Is it not delightful? Is that not a trick worth learning?"

Landon's stomach and head settled, and he looked around for the beetle. "Where did it go?"

"Can't you still feel it?"

Landon concentrated, then turned to look in the tree behind him. He couldn't see the beetle, but he could feel it back there. He could feel in his brain the exact spot where the beetle had landed. "I can."

"Once you make the connection, it won't break until either you break it or one of you dies. Try telling it to come back to you."

"I can do that?"

"You can send messages. With something as low as an insect, try sending an impulse rather than words. They can't understand words anyway, so just think of wanting it to come back to you, and will that message over to it through your connection."

That sounded like mind-reading with bugs, which sounded totally crazy, but this was all pretty crazy, so Landon did what Mr. McKenzie said, and the beetle flew over and landed in Landon's open palm.

"This is so weird," he said, watching the beetle walk around in his hand. "Do I have a pet beetle now?"

Mr. McKenzie stroked his chin. "Less a pet and more a slave. Or a servant, if you prefer," he added when he saw Landon's panicked look.

Servant. That wasn't so bad, was it? But didn't servants still have a choice? Wasn't Mr. McKenzie's first word more true?

"For the next day or two, anyway," the man added. "Play with your connection to it all you want, but I'd advise not letting your mom see. When that one dies, you can catch something else and try it again."

Landon's discomfort at the words 'slave' and 'when that one dies' were washed away by his eagerness to fly again and his ideas about what animal he should try to catch next. "That's what you were doing this morning?" he asked in wonder. "You were flying?"

"A little. But these sorts of connections have other uses, too. You'll figure that out in time."

"But you said you can't do magic."

"I can't do it right now. But forming the connection is the only time it really counts as doing magic. Once the connection's there, using it is like using your own arm. It's an extension of yourself. Does that make sense?"

"I guess. Can you do this with more than one animal at once?" Did he have to wait until he was done with the beetle before he could try it on a fish or frog?

"Yes, but it can get tricky. Think of having an extra limb, like a tail. One would be easy enough to adapt to. But think of having five extra limbs. Things could get awkward, and you'd have to learn whole new ways to make your body work in concert. Most of us make one connection at a time, with more only when there's a specific reason. And when you're learning, it's all the more important to focus on one at a time." He chuckled and patted Landon on the head. "You've got plenty of time to learn, little one. Your enthusiasm is admirable, but there's no need to get ahead of yourself."

"I have time to learn. But will you be here to teach me?" Landon asked.

The man jerked his hand away from Landon's head and held it awkwardly to his own chest. "Ah, well…"

"So I need to learn fast. If you have more to teach me, I need to learn as much as I can before you're not here anymore."

Mr. McKenzie's mouth moved; it looked like he was trying to smile but couldn't quite make it work. "Clever boy. In that case, I'll see what else I can come up with to teach you while we have the opportunity. But you know you shouldn't mention any of this to your mother, don't you? If she knew, I doubt she would allow me to babysit you again. Or see you at all, for that matter."

"I know," Landon said, offended that Mr. McKenzie felt like he even had to say it. "I won't say anything to her about this. But I do have other questions."

"Such as?"

He had to say it. He had to get it out there in the open. Landon had magic, and it wasn't all trouble like his mom always treated it as. It couldn't be, not if it made him feel this great. Which meant maybe that other word wasn't so bad either. "Are you a witch?"

The forced expression on Mr. McKenzie's face smoothed out into an easy smile. "I am. But don't go spreading it around. That's a secret between us, one to another."

"So... I'm a witch, too."

"Tell me something, young one. How long have you known? In your deepest of hearts, how long have you been keeping this secret of your own?"

Landon sighed. "I think... for almost as long as I can remember."

CHAPTER
FOURTEEN

"You want Alex to walk you home, hun?" Barb asked as she pulled out her copy of the key to lock up the store.

"No, I'm fine," Denneka said, nervously tucking her plastic bag of discount bin loot tighter under her arm. "He has to get to his next job anyway, doesn't he?"

"I have time, if you want," Alex countered, pulling on his huge backpack like it weighed nothing. He was strong and nice and handsome, and in a lot of ways he was like a second older brother. Except he wasn't her brother, so when he walked her home on nights when her parents and Jonah weren't around, it was awkward —for her, anyway. Though after this morning with Trick, she might be fine as long as Alex didn't strip naked.

As soon as she thought of it, her imagination began painting her a picture. She forced the mental image away and said, "No, really. It's barely dusk, and it's only a couple blocks. I'll be fine."

"All right," he said so easily that Denneka knew he must have nearly been running late. "Night, ladies."

It took Denneka less than two minutes to jog home. She was winded by the time she got there, but she hadn't been patient enough to walk. Not when the boy she liked was waiting there alone and her parents might be home at any time.

Luckily, there were no cars in the driveway. Denneka breathed a sigh of relief and went inside, first texting her mom to find out her parents were staying for drinks after the conference and would be home late, then her brother asking him to pick up milk on the way home and so learning that he'd be out at least another hour.

An hour, she thought, catching her breath. *Okay. Good. That should work.*

She walked down the hallway, slowing to a creep at the last few steps to her room. Trick's transformation didn't make any particular sound, but sometimes his sudden shift in size disturbed something around him. This time, though, she heard nothing at all. So she carefully knocked on her door. "Trick? It's me. I'm opening the door." She cracked the door a few inches, keeping a grip on the knob, because if Trick was the one to open it he'd probably just fling it wide.

Nothing happened for a few seconds, then Trick's human face leaned into view, only inches from the door. His shoulders and chest were bare, and she was careful not to look any lower than that.

"Here." She shoved the bag of clothes through the crack, trying not to widen it any more than necessary. "I got you some boys' clothes at the shop. Put them on, okay?"

He took the bag and looked inside. "All of them?"

"What? No. Just the pajamas is fine. And—and I brought you some underwear."

He turned away from the door, and Denneka closed it quick. After a bit, she called out, "Are you dressed?"

"Yes."

In this case, his version of 'dressed' meant pajama pants only. And possibly underwear. He was sprawled out on the bed, skin pale against her comforter even in the warm, fading light of dusk.

This is okay, she thought, staring. Except she didn't mean 'okay'. She meant… something else. Something she knew she shouldn't. *No! Not okay!* She found the pile of clothes where Trick had dumped out the bag and grabbed a t-shirt. "This too, Trick. This is meant to be part of the pajamas."

Grumpily, he sat up and pulled on the t-shirt. It took him at least twice as long as it would take anyone else.

"We should have about an hour before anyone else gets home," she told him.

"Dinner?" he asked.

He hasn't eaten all day, she realized. She'd only been feeding kitten Trick once a day, but human Trick was a teen boy and probably starving by now. "Yes, I'll get dinner soon. But you... might want to take a shower while you can."

He turned his face away as if physically rejecting the idea. "I don't like showers."

"But... you were rolling around in the grass earlier. And you're human now, at least some of the time. And... people shower." It wasn't that she didn't understand why she was having to explain this to him, but it had still caught her by surprise.

"I don't like showers," he said again.

"Um... why not?"

He shivered like the idea of showers made his skin crawl.

"Is it... the way the water hits?"

"It's like I'm being attacked by bugs."

"Didn't your mom make you shower when you were human?"

The mention of his mom earned her a quick glance of betrayal, then he admitted, "She tried, but I wouldn't. Then she made me take baths."

"Okay. Good. Take a bath, then."

His shoulders hunched, but he didn't freak out or even outright refuse like she'd expected. It was good enough.

Denneka started running a bath, then went to the kitchen to find something for dinner. They didn't have long, so it'd have to be something quick. She found a frozen pepperoni and sausage pizza and popped it in the oven, then went back to her room to try to coax a cat into a bath.

"We can have dinner after you take a bath, so hurry."

That was enough to get him on his feet, but she had to push him along toward the bathroom with a few nudges to his back. Finally, he was standing in front of the tub, watching it fill the last few inches.

"Push this down to turn off the water when it's full," Denneka instructed. "The soap and shampoo are there, and the towels are in this cupboard." She turned away for one second to point at the cupboard, and when she looked at him again, he'd already pulled the t-shirt up over his face, but his arms were still tangled in it. "Wait until I leave!" she blurted. "I'll wait right on the other side of the door, so you shouldn't change. But you have to hurry, because the pizza's only in the oven for twelve minutes, and I don't want it to burn because I can't go take it out."

"Help," he said, still struggling with the shirt.

Heat rushed into her cheeks. "I can't help you undress! I'm sure you've done it before. Figure it out." She made her escape quickly and leaned on the other side of the bathroom door.

There was a soft meow.

What?

A louder meow.

Dang it. Denneka opened the bathroom door to see a black, green-eyed kitten sitting on the small pile of Trick's clothes.

Trick pawed closer until he was a boy on all fours. "I couldn't reach the tub."

"And I forgot to measure how big the bathroom is." The tub was dangerously close to overflowing now, so she rushed past Trick to turn it off. While her back was still to him, she pulled the shower curtain closed. "You can get in now. I'll"—*What am I even doing?*—"sit on this side while you take your bath. Just keep the curtain closed, okay?"

"Okay." The side of the curtain pulled back, and Trick stepped past her into the tub. Then, just as she'd asked, the curtain closed again, and the water sloshed as he lowered down into it.

Denneka sat on the toilet lid with her face in her hands. *What even is this?* Was she really a girl with a boy? Was she a mother? A caretaker? A pet owner? As much as having Trick around was thrilling, it was also exhausting. This whole day had been exhausting. *People* were exhausting. She wanted to curl up with a book and let fictional characters be the ones dealing with all of this exhausting stuff. Real life didn't feel like it was worth the effort it took.

"Trick?" she said softly. He didn't say anything, but the splashes of movement stopped, so she knew he was listening. Even though her pulse thudded in her ears, it was easier to talk to him when she couldn't see him. "You said you like me, but... what do you like about me?" *Shoot*. That sounded like she was fishing for compliments. "I mean, why? Why would you? I... can't figure it out."

"You're familiar," he said from behind the shower curtain.

"What?"

"You're familiar," he repeated. He didn't sound flippant or casual. His tone was warm. Content, even. He meant it as a compliment.

"What—what does that even mean? We never met until your mom brought you and your brother to our shop."

"You weren't familiar *then*," he said as if she was thick in the head. "But... school was scary, and you were familiar."

Ah. That makes sense. It all made sense now. Her world was a little bit more in order now. There wasn't anything special about her at all, as she'd known. She had just happened to be the first girl he met after moving to a strange, new place. When he got more comfortable with the new place and the other new people, he would move on from her. And leave her to her books. That was the way the world made sense.

Trick peeked around the edge of the shower curtain at her. Denneka got up to pull it quickly back into place before he could see the tears about to fall from her eyes.

To change the topic, she said, "I thought cats hate baths, but you went in somewhat willingly."

"I hate having wet fur, but I don't mind water on my bare skin. It doesn't stick to me like it does when I'm a cat."

"Wet fur doesn't seem to bother dogs."

"Most dogs are too stupid to be bothered by anything."

Denneka laughed and wiped away her tears. "Spoken like a true cat."

"Well, I am."

———

Trick didn't like baths. He didn't hate them like he did whenever he was a cat and his mom insisted on giving him one, but he could never get over how weird it felt to just sit in water like that. It was so much more convenient to clean himself as a cat. He could do it anywhere, and he didn't have to get wet. But his human tongue was no good for cleaning, and he couldn't reach most of his body with it anyway. Human bodies were so stiff and awkward.

When he was done washing, he reached over and flicked the lever to let the water drain. As soon as he stood up, the girl shoved a towel at him past the curtain. *I could get one myself,* he thought at her. *You showed me where they are.* What did she think he was, some little kid who couldn't do anything for himself? When he stepped out onto the bath mat, the girl was sitting on the toilet lid with her hands over her face.

"Dry off and get dressed, then we can eat," she said.

His stomach growled. *But I want to eat now.* He was starving and something smelled delicious, but the girl didn't look like she was leaving the bathroom until he'd done as she'd told him, and he wouldn't be able to get at the food without her. Cats aren't very good at using ovens. So he shoved himself back into his new clothes. "Done. Food now?"

She looked up at him. "Sure, let's—Wait, did you not wash your hair?"

No one had said anything about washing his hair.

"Trick, you need to wash your hair too or—" A loud beeping from another room cut her off.

"You said I could eat now."

She let out a breath. "Yeah. Sorry."

He followed her into the kitchen and grabbed for the pizza as soon as she set it on the counter.

She swatted his hand away. "Wait, it's still hot, and I have to cut it."

Trick rubbed his hand and didn't bother answering. Why had she hit him? He only wanted what she'd already said he could have. She kept changing the rules on him.

Once she'd sliced it, she stepped aside and Trick slowly reached for a slice, wary of getting another smack. She moved further away, which he took as permission, and shoved the first slice into his mouth. It was really hot, but he was too hungry to care, and he didn't stop chewing until the first slice was gone.

When he reached for a second, the girl handed him a plate and said, "We've got some time still. You don't have to scarf it down like that."

He almost kept eating anyway, but something was off about the girl's mood. So he forced himself to use a plate and make it to the dining table before he continued stuffing food into his mouth.

When more than half of the small pizza was in his stomach, Trick sat back, licking his lips.

"Feel better?" the familiar girl asked.

"Mmm."

"I... I don't mean to keep harping on this, but you really should wash your hair."

Trick tried to twitch his tail in irritation at her, but he had to settle for staring at her. "Wet hair is like wet fur. I hate it."

"But it'll get gross if you don't. You don't want to feel gross, do you?"

He didn't, but he wasn't sure what she meant. His mom had never let him go more than a couple days without washing his hair during the week he'd been human. What would happen to it?

"You can wash it in the sink if you want, so you don't have to get back in the tub."

"How?"

"You've never done that?"

"No."

"Oh. Um… I guess I could wash it for you, if you want."

"You'd wash me?" he asked skeptically.

"It won't hurt, I promise. My grandma washed my hair a few times like that when I was little."

More treating him like a kid. But he was a little worried about what she meant that his hair would get gross. "Fine."

"Okay. Um, just a sec." She cleaned up the dishes, then he followed her to the bathroom, where she got a small towel and a bottle of shampoo. Back in the kitchen, she said, "Put this towel over your face like this so it doesn't get wet, then lean your head over the sink."

Trick really wasn't sure about any of this, but he followed her instructions. He heard the water running right next to his ear and the zipping sound of the hand nozzle being pulled out. He braced himself for the horrible bugs feeling of the shower spray, but when the water hit his head, the flow was soft, gentle, and warm.

The flow of water ran across the back of his head, the sides, then the top. It dripped into his ears, which made him shake his head back and forth to get it out, but the familiar girl told him that the water wouldn't hurt him and he should try to tolerate it. He was about to argue with her when he felt her hand in his hair, moving gently as the water flowed over him, and it felt so good that he would have purred like a chainsaw if he could have.

The water turned off, and disappointment hit him hard. That was it? It was so short.

"No, don't stand up yet. I'm not done. Keep the towel tight over your face so you don't get soap in your eyes."

He did as she said, and a moment later, both of her hands were in his hair, rubbing in the strong-smelling shampoo. Her fingers were gentle and firm, and his knees nearly gave out from the pleasure of it. The need to purr physically hurt, his chest aching like he'd been holding his breath too long.

Then the water was back, warm and gentle like her touch, as she washed the soap away. Then she took the small towel out of his hands and rubbed it over his head until his hair stopped dripping.

"Okay, you can stand up now."

He felt a rush as he did so, which was disorienting, and the wetness of his hair was irritating, but he felt so good and so relaxed, none of it really bothered him.

The familiar girl gave him a half-smile. "That wasn't so bad, was it?"

That was amazing. "You can wash my hair whenever you want."

She let out a weird little laugh. "Heh. Okay, well, good. Do you want me to blow-dry it so it's not wet?"

He knew about blow-dryers. They were really loud and sometimes too hot. But he was curious, so he said, "Okay."

First, they went back into the bathroom, and she gave him a fresh toothbrush and made him brush his teeth along with her. Then he had to wait just outside the door while she did some other things. When she was done, she came out with the blow-dryer in her hand, and they went to her room.

He sat on her bed while she dried his hair, making sure the heat wasn't too hot and never stayed in one place long enough to hurt. It was as loud as he remembered, but he didn't care about that once she started using her fingers to ruffle his hair all over so the hot air could dry it better. It wasn't quite as amazing as when they were rubbing his scalp harder, but it was so calming and comforting that he nearly fell asleep.

"All done," she said, turning the thing off. "Feel better?"

He looked at her with sleepy eyes that were hard to keep open. "Mmm."

The sound of a car outside startled her, and she yanked at the sleeve of his t-shirt. "That's probably Jonah. You might need to hide." But she didn't push him anywhere right away. They stayed frozen and listened to probably-her-brother come in, move around the house a little, then go into his room. Finally, she let go of Trick's sleeve. "Oh, sorry. I didn't mean to... Um, could you get in my closet for a second?"

Trick watched her, waiting for her to explain what she meant.

"I didn't get a shower today, and if I go in there now, you'll change again, so it might be more of a hassle than it's worth right now. But I do need to change clothes, so if you could go in my closet while I do that, I'd appreciate it."

"I told you I don't care if you're naked."

"But I do, Trick."

"Why do you care?" Did she think he would be mean to her about it? He didn't even know what mean thing he could say. Mock her for her lack of fur? She couldn't help that.

"I'm not getting into this again with you right now." She went to her closet and opened the door, then stared at the mess she found. Then she turned her stare on him.

"I got bored."

"So you pulled everything out of all my boxes?"

He twitched his tai—No, that didn't work. He shrugged.

"I'd make you put it all away again, but it's getting late." She shoved some stuff aside with her foot to make room on the floor. "Just stand here for a minute, please."

He did as she asked, waiting in the dark, tiny room until she opened it again. The clothes she had on weren't her usual pajamas. They were heavier and covered more of her skin. Maybe she was cold?

She locked the bedroom door and turned off the overhead light, leaving only her bedside lamp on. "My mom will think it's weird if I have my door locked, but better that than having her walk in to find you here. Anyway, I can just blame Jonah for barging in on me earlier."

Trick didn't understand any of that, but he didn't care enough to question it.

She pulled out a sleeping bag from her closet and rolled it out on the floor beside her bed. "This is for you."

"What do you mean?"

"This is where you can sleep tonight."

"But I sleep in the bed with you."

"Not as a human."

"Why not?"

"Just because!"

"But… I can't turn back into a cat while you're here."

"I know that, Trick. But you have to stay in this room or my parents will find you, and even if you're a cat, they wouldn't react well. So the only choice is for you to sleep on the floor."

Trick examined the sleeping bag. It wasn't very thick and didn't look very soft. Was this a punishment? Was the girl mad at him? This was because of messing up her closet, wasn't it? He knew at the time he shouldn't have done it. He guessed he deserved to be punished for it. So he lay down on the sleeping bag without arguing and tried to sleep.

The girl's mom did try to come into the room some time later. It was dark, with only some moonlight coming through the curtains, so Trick didn't know what time it was. He heard the doorknob jiggle and a woman's voice say, "Denneka?"

Not even getting up, the girl told her mom that it was locked because her brother had barged in earlier and she might have been changing for all he knew. Which for some reason seemed like a perfectly good answer to her mom, since she left them alone after that.

Trick lay awake for a long time after the woman left. The floor was hard, and he was starting to get chilly.

That's enough punishment, isn't it? he thought. *She can't still be mad at me. I don't think she'll mind.*

He sat up on his haunches to peer over the side of the bed at the girl. She was asleep, curled up on one side.

Good. She won't even notice.

Trick carefully pulled back the covers just enough to climb into bed beside her, where it was warm and soft, and soon fell into a peaceful sleep.

———

The police station was quiet at night. Most of the lights were off a
no one else was around. It was eerie as hell, but it did make it eas
to concentrate.

This time, Marcus had *asked* for the night shift. Unless someone
called in an emergency, he'd have plenty of time to finish typing up
his report by tomorrow. He was on the third page already.

He took a drink of coffee and checked his notepad again. Too
bad he couldn't just rip out the pages and turn those in as his report.
Organizing it all was a pain, and he sucked at writing. Though his
notepad was nothing but a random collection of names, numbers,
and facts, so it probably wouldn't mean much to anyone other than
him. Most of the information turned out to be useless and never
even made it into his official reports, but he never knew what he'd
need and what he wouldn't, so it all got scribbled onto the notepad.

They'd gotten confirmation that the body they'd found in the
grave was Haug. It would take a week or more for the final report to
come in, but the coroner's best guess was that Haug had been blud-
geoned to death. If it had happened at his home, the killer must
have cleaned the scene up, since the signs of a struggle they had
found weren't nearly enough for what Marcus would expect to see
where someone was beaten to death. Which meant that either Haug
had gone with the killer to another location or the killer knew some
things about cleaning a crime scene.

As for who the killer might be, the safe bet was on it being the
same man Marcus had seen at the graveyard. The killer had hidden
the body in a grave, then kept an eye on it to make sure it wouldn't
be found. What would he do now that it had been?

Once the sun had come up the day after they'd found the body,
Kevin had made another sweep of the spot at the edge of the trees
where Marcus had seen the man. They'd found a whole bunch of
footprints—size fourteen men's boots—and some cigarette butts
and food wrappers. The man had been staking the place out for a
while, which jibed with the theory that it was the killer keeping an
eye on the evidence of his crime.

An hour passed, and Marcus got another half-page done. He

led more coffee. He got up from his desk and went to the break
m, where he'd left the pot he'd made at the start of the shift—
lf-gone and starting to go stale, but it was all his.

On the way back to his desk, he thought he heard a footstep. He stopped and listened but didn't hear it again. Setting the coffee down, he hovered one hand over his side arm and walked toward where he thought he'd heard the sound.

"Anyone there?" He flicked the light on. It was another hallway with a couple offices. He checked the doors, and they were locked like they were supposed to be.

Eerie, he thought, shaking it off as he retrieved his coffee and went back to his desk.

As soon as he was at his computer, he opened an internet window and found some music, keeping the volume barely loud enough to drown out the silence. Then he took a few gulps of hot coffee and got back to work.

Five minutes later, he started to feel funny. He tried to look at the coffee, but suddenly his eyes had a hard time focusing. Wrapping a hand around the mug, he picked it up, trying to smell it, but it slipped out of his grip before he could get it to his nose.

I'm an idiot, he thought, reaching for his phone. But the handset wouldn't stay in his hand, and his fingers couldn't hit the buttons right.

He fell sideways out of his chair and landed painfully on the floor.

He heard a footstep again. Then another. Heavy, size fourteen sorts of footsteps. He tried to get at his gun, but his fingers were so weak he couldn't even unsnap the strap keeping it in the holster. The shape of a man approached from the hallway. Marcus's vision was blurrier than ever, but he knew it was the man he'd seen last night, out at the cemetery. The man who had almost definitely murdered Bradley Haug.

The chief's gonna kill me, Marcus thought right before he lost consciousness.

CHAPTER FIFTEEN

A sharp pain in his cheek jerked Marcus awake.

"Hey, Parkes, you alive?" David asked, then slapped him again.

"Ow, yeah, stop," Marcus groaned, opening his eyes. After a few blinks and a lot of effort, they focused enough for him to see his partner kneeling over him.

"What happened here?" David asked.

Marcus sat up. He was on the ground, his head felt funny, and there was cold, damp coffee on his pants. He rubbed his head. "Oh, man. What time is it?"

"Six."

"Is the chief here?"

"Yeah. He made sure you had a pulse and then called the rest of us in. So, what happened?"

"Pretty sure I was drugged." He found his mug—the handle now broken off—and handed it to David. "There's a few drops there. See if someone can test it. And don't drink the coffee in the break room."

"Don't worry, no one's drinking anything that was left open until we figure out what happened. You feel okay?"

"Mostly."

David reached a hand down and helped him up. "Chief wants to see you."

"Thought so." Marcus wobbled his way to the chief's office and gave his report. He didn't get quite the chewing out he'd expected, and by the end of it his head felt clearer.

"I've already got people checking the security tapes and looking for any other sign of this guy," the chief told him.

"Did he take anything?"

"Not that we've found so far. But he didn't break in here for no reason. He was after something. I want you to find out what."

"Yes, sir." Marcus turned to leave, then stopped. "He could have killed me. Do you think I got lucky?"

"No."

Marcus nodded. "Me neither." As he went back to his desk, he considered that. A normal killer might start panicking and try to take out the cops on his heels. Marcus's death might have made it a little less likely that he'd be caught. The chaos alone would buy him some time. And someone who wasn't really a killer, deep down—someone who might have killed Haug accidentally in a fit of anger or something—likely wouldn't have been meticulous enough to stake out his body and then break into the police station without being caught. "A professional," Marcus muttered to himself. Maybe it was time to double-check the bank records they'd pulled on Haug. Look for anything that could indicate a connection between a no-name schoolteacher and the kind of people who hired professional killers.

When he got back to his desk, Marcus found that someone had already come and cleaned up the spilled coffee. *What did the killer want?* His desk was always messy, so it was hard to see if anything had been disturbed. But when he looked at his computer screen, he saw it. The document he'd been working on wasn't showing the same page as it had been when he'd last seen it. The mouse was in a different place than he normally had it, too.

"Someone's been sitting in my chair," Marcus murmured. He

picked up his phone and dialed the chief's office. "He read my report."

"Which one?" asked the chief.

"The one I was writing last night. About Haug. The one that detailed everything we know about the case."

A long breath came over the line. "He was doing recon. Did he delete anything? Add anything?"

"I don't think so, but I'll read it through to find out." Maybe he'd changed the report, hoping to confuse the police on what they thought they knew, but Marcus doubted he'd have bothered trying it. If the killer was a professional, he'd have to know that they had other records besides the official report.

After telling the chief what he'd found, Marcus reached for his notepad to begin checking it against the report he'd been writing. It wasn't where he thought he'd last set it; it was on the other side of the desk. He picked it up. Something was off. What was it?

Then he noticed the tiny scraps of paper in the spiral binding at the top of the pad. A page had been torn out.

With fast, clumsy fingers, he flipped through the notepad, trying to figure out what was missing. When he realized what it was, his blood went cold.

In the official report he'd written, he'd only said that the lead about the grave had come from an anonymous source. But when he'd talked to her—that girl with a weird name he couldn't remember—he'd scribbled it down like he always did, in case he needed it later.

That was the page the killer had taken. The one with the name of the girl who'd told him where to find the body.

"What is it?" David asked from the desk across from him. "Your face just went white."

"I think we might have a problem."

———

When Denneka woke up, she was curled on her side with Trick curled up facing her. She didn't see him right away because he was lower on the mattress and completely covered by the blanket. But she could feel his head tucked against her chest, her arms wrapped around his head like a comfort pillow, soft hair under her fingers. He'd kept his hands to himself, at least, not that that made the situation much better.

I told him to sleep on the floor, she thought. The jolt of adrenaline she got on waking and seeing the situation did a lot to erase any lingering tiredness. *What is he doing here?*

Part of her was afraid of what she'd find if she threw back the covers, but most of her was instantly furious that he'd completely ignored her wishes and done exactly what she'd told him not to. She pushed away from him and sat up. "Trick!" she hissed. "What are you doing?"

He sat up languidly—at least he was still dressed—and said, "Sleeping."

Jumping out of bed, she glared down at him. "What happened to sleeping on the floor?"

"I did that for a while. I didn't like it."

"Do you even know what personal space means?"

"Not really. Why are you yelling at me?"

For a second, the hurt, confused look on his face made her waver. Then the fact that he was acting like the victim here annoyed her even more, and she said, "Never mind," then grabbed a change of clothes and stormed out.

By the time she'd taken a shower and had finished the rest of her morning bathroom routine, her head was a little clearer, but her feelings weren't. Why did he ignore her like that? Why did he act like he'd done nothing wrong? He obviously wasn't going to apologize, but she didn't think she should have to either. Wanting a little more time before she had to deal with him again, she went to the kitchen.

"Just in time," said her mom. "Breakfast is ready."

"It smells great. Thanks." Denneka got a plate and loaded it up with eggs, biscuits, and sausage. *I should let him go hungry after that stunt,* she thought, but she couldn't really put any meaning behind it even to herself. So she put as much extra food on the plate as she thought she could get away with without her mom getting suspicious.

"I got the laundry out of your room while you were in the bathroom," Mom said, and Denneka nearly dropped the plate she was holding. "If you have any more, you can leave it in the laundry room. I'll probably get to it today or tomorrow." She wasn't acting like she'd found a cat in Denneka's room. She definitely wouldn't be so casual if she had.

"You don't have to do that," Denneka said. When Mom gave her an inquiring look, she said, "I mean, I can do my own laundry now, I think. I know how to."

Mom smiled and gave her a side-hug. "You're growing up, huh? Getting mature. First you want more privacy, now taking on more of your own upkeep."

"It's not a big deal."

"Maybe. But can't a mother still notice her little girl turning into a young woman?"

Denneka blushed. This wasn't about that at all, not that she could explain that to her mom. "So you'll let me handle my own laundry and clean up my own room?"

"Absolutely. You know where to find me if you need help."

When Denneka went back to her room, she stopped just outside the door and knocked softly. She couldn't risk saying anything to him through the door in case her mom overheard. *If you want to win any points back, now's the time to do it,* she thought.

Either Trick had telepathy or he had more sense than she'd given him credit for, because when she opened the door, he was sitting calmly on the end of her bed, fully dressed in some of the new clothes she'd bought him.

I guess I underestimated him, Denneka thought guiltily as she came in.

"Your mom came in, but I hid," he said, looking at the plate of food rather than at her.

Denneka sat in her desk chair, suddenly not as hungry as before. Good. That was smart. She was getting my laundry, but I told her I'd do it from now on, so hopefully she won't come in like that anymore."

Trick's eyes were locked on the food, but he didn't try grabbing for it.

"I got enough for both of us, I think, but let me eat mine first, then you can have the rest."

His gaze moved to the floor. "You're punishing me again."

"I'm not punishing you. I just couldn't bring two plates or even two forks back without Mom getting suspicious. I have to go to school soon, so just let me eat and then you can have the rest."

He didn't answer, only kept staring at the floor.

Denneka ate a bit and drank some of the juice she'd brought in. "You shouldn't have gotten in bed with me."

"I didn't think you'd mind."

"I explicitly told you not to."

"I thought you were just angry."

"I'm angry *now*."

"Why? The floor was hard."

"I told you not to. Isn't that enough?"

"But why?"

Apparently it wasn't.

Denneka sighed and left the rest of the food on the desk. "If I leave this here while I'm gone, will that be okay? You can eat as you're hungry?"

He didn't answer. He was sulking.

"I don't know how long Mom'll be here before she goes to the shop, so you can't go use the bathroom right now. I'll leave the door cracked enough for you to get through so you can go when you need to after she's gone. But don't go wandering around, okay? Remember, my mom hates cats. I don't know what she'd do if she started finding cat hair all over."

"I remember."

It seemed like there was something else that should be said, but Denneka didn't know what it was and didn't have the time or patience to figure it out. She needed to hurry or she'd miss the bus. She left Trick in her room, alone and sulking, wondering if he'd still be there when she got home. He was only there because she was familiar, after all. He'd probably get tired of her mothering and chastising soon, and whatever affection familiarity was worth would wear away. It wouldn't be at all hard for him to find someone else to latch onto, even if he didn't want to go home yet. And then Denneka would get her usual boring, friendless life back, and everything would be normal again.

"Lisa, that police officer is here to see you again."

"Thank you, Michael. Send him in."

Marcus came into her office and closed the door behind him. He didn't look good.

She got up from her desk and came to him. "Two visits from Officer Parkes in less than a week. What's wrong now?"

"You heard about what we found?"

"My uncle already called to tell me. It's hard to believe. I have no idea why anyone would do that to Brad."

Marcus nodded distractedly. "We're still looking into it. But there's something else now, Lisa. The man who I'm pretty sure killed him broke into the station last night when I was on shift. The bastard drugged me, and by the time I came to, he was gone."

"What? Are you okay?"

"Yeah. I think he just wanted me out of the way. From what we can tell, he was trying to figure out what we knew about him and the case."

"Then why are you here?"

He stepped closer to her and lowered his voice. "I think one of your students is in danger."

Her blood raged. "Tell me."

"That girl who gave us the lead on the grave. I—I can't remember her name."

"Denneka Sparrow."

"Yeah, her. I think the killer knows she's the one who told us about it."

"How would he?"

Marcus stepped away and paced. "It's my fault. After the break-in, I saw a page from my notepad was missing. It was the notes I took when she came to give us the info."

Lisa's fists clenched, but it wouldn't do any good to hit him. Even though his bad memory was annoying, there wasn't actually anything wrong with taking notes. "You think he's after her?"

"I think he might be. Why else would he take that page?"

"Why hasn't my uncle called to warn me about this yet?"

"He doesn't think it's a serious concern. He... he thinks I just misplaced that page of my notes. I'm not the most organized guy in the world. He doesn't want to spend the money and manpower on keeping a watch on the girl based on nothing but my missing note page."

Lisa pinched the bridge of her nose and let out a tight breath. She knew the sort of pressure that her uncle was under, having to account for the minutest use of public resources. And everyone knew Marcus was sloppy enough to lose something like that and forget he lost it. But Lisa had known him since they were teens. If he was this sure about something, she had to believe him. "What can we do?"

"I volunteered to be the one to keep an eye on the girl, but the chief put me on tracking down Haug's financials instead. I think the killer might be a professional, which means Haug might have had ties to organized crime or something like it."

"You think a *hitman* killed him?"

"He doesn't have to be a hitman to be a professional."

"You think Brad was involved with the mob?"

"Maybe not anything that serious, but there are a lot of minor players in that arena."

"I have a hard time believing Brad would get involved in something like that."

"How well did you know him?"

She thought about it and had to admit he had a point. "I don't typically get personal with my employees."

"So for now, I don't know what to do. That's why I'm telling you. That girl's here most of the day. Keep an eye on her. Make sure there aren't any suspicious characters skulking around. The guy we're looking for is big, but I wasn't able to see more than that."

"I run a tight campus."

"I know. So I don't think she's in the most danger here. I wanted to warn her parents, but the chief ordered me not to. He doesn't want the PR risk, especially since he doesn't believe me that it's even a problem."

"He ordered *you* not to."

Marcus nodded. "Do whatever you think's best, Lisa. And call me if you see or hear anything, okay?"

"I will. Thank you, Marcus."

———

It was significantly more difficult than usual for Kester to maintain the stern-yet-bored expression he tried to wear in class. Not with Denneka twitching every time a boy passed too close and casting surreptitious glances at them behind their backs. Not with the way she hadn't looked Kester in the eye once all day.

That is the look of a girl who has seen the male body and is wondering if they all look the same, he thought with deep amusement.

With the sun having been down, Julia hadn't been able to watch them last night, but she'd arrived at the girl's house early enough to get a peek at their cozy sleeping arrangements—and Denneka's surprised reaction to said arrangements. Kester didn't think the kitten boy was actually trying to put moves on her, and it hadn't really looked like the girl believed that either. Which was part of what made the whole thing so entertaining. A male with obvious salacious intent is easy enough for a female to rebuff without guilt, but when his intentions are pure, the softhearted female finds herself stymied. Kester wished he could devise a way to observe them more closely, but short of turning himself into a fly on the wall, he didn't yet know how he could manage it.

The students were all focused with heads bent over a history worksheet he'd gotten off the internet. Teaching isn't all that hard when you don't care if the students actually learn anything, though he did wonder when Lisa would notice he wasn't giving them any tasks difficult enough to be challenging. Well, challenging to most of them. There were a few morons who managed to nearly fail even the very easy assignments he bothered to give them, but he supposed the world does need its manual laborers.

The bell rang, and the kids quickly packed up to head to third period. "Denneka," Kester called before she could get away. "A moment of your time, please."

She hung back as her peers rushed out, then hesitantly approached his desk. Her hands were tight on the straps of her bag, and her gaze moved no higher than the surface of his desk.

"I would appreciate being looked in the eye when I'm speaking to you," he said, careful to keep the smirk off his face.

Her wide, brown eyes darted up to his chest, then back to his desk, before finally doing as he'd instructed. They wavered, liable to run away again at any moment, but he held them with a look that promised punishment if she disobeyed him. A blush gradually but inexorably began to spread across her cheeks.

"Are my classes boring you, Denneka?"

She flinched. "What?"

"You failed to answer twice when I called on you, and you've been in a distracted daze all morning. Is this about Patrick?"

"What? I—um—I mean…" She shook her head. Most likely trying to remember what the state of Trick was as far as everyone else knew. "They still haven't found him, right? And there's no news. And no one else seems to even remember that he's missing. Or that he was ever here."

"Rest assured, that's not true. Your fellow students, perhaps, but there are quite a few adults who have far from forgotten him. I myself am still quite interested in his case. So do try not to sulk about it, if you wouldn't mind."

"Sorry, Mr. McKenzie."

"It's not for my sake. Patrick will need your help to catch up once he comes back, won't he? How can you help him if you don't pay attention in class?"

She blinked as his words sank in, then her back straightened. "You're right. Thank you."

Look at me, a proper mentor and all, Kester thought as she scurried away. But he wondered why he'd bothered to say anything to make the girl feel better. The words had fallen out of his mouth unplanned. If Trick really had been missing, they'd likely have been just the right thing to say. Not that he could be sure about that, since offering comfort was nothing he was an expert in. But knowing that Trick was at home waiting for her, he wondered why they made her feel better now. If Julia had been able to hear more of their conversation this morning, maybe he would know.

I think I'm beginning to like that girl, he realized to his own surprise. It wasn't just watching her and Trick together. He was beginning to enjoy her for herself, as well. Her awkwardness was highly amusing, and she'd figured out Julia with remarkable speed. If not for the disguise he wore whenever he was around her, perhaps she would even suspect him of being the witch he was.

With his classroom empty, Kester momentarily checked in with Julia, then pulled out a book to enjoy his free period. Before he'd even opened it, Lisa came in, shutting the door behind her. She looked as stiff and buttoned-up as ever. *I'd love to see her students' reaction to the sight of her with her hair down,* he thought. Then again, she'd probably worked in the school system for a good while. Long enough for some of her students to graduate and become bar patrons themselves. Was she the type to have a fling with a former student? It was a small town, after all.

"Good morning, Lisa. How can I help you?"

The scowl he only just noticed deepened as she approached his desk. "There's a problem, John. Some of what I'm about to tell you will likely be widely known by tomorrow, if not sooner, but some won't. I need you to keep as much as you can quiet for as long as you can."

Kester got out of his chair to move closer to her, crossing his arms and leaning a hip against his desk. "All right."

"The police found Brad Haug. He's dead."

Jacqueline had told him as much, but he tried to look surprised. "I'm sorry," he said because it's what one says.

"Apparently Denneka was the one who gave them the lead on where to find the body. I don't know the details, but they're not important. The important thing is that the man the police believe to be Brad's murderer broke into the police station last night and found out she was the one who gave them that information."

Kester's eyebrows came together in genuine concern. "I see."

"Don't tell her about it—we don't want to scare her unnecessarily—but keep an eye out for anyone suspicious."

"May I ask how you know about this?"

"I have a contact in the department. He's the one who found out the killer knows about Denneka. His boss doesn't believe him, so officially the police aren't doing anything about it. So he came to me."

"Can you tell me his name? In case I do see something and need to report it."

She hesitated before saying, "Officer Marcus Parkes." She got a sticky note from his desk and wrote a phone number down in neat, bold lines. "This is his cell number. If it's an emergency, call 9-1-1. But if it's not, call him here. And call me as well if you see anything, even if it's not something you're sure is worth reporting to the police. Our students' safety is top priority, understand?"

"Yes, ma'am."

"Good," she said and strode out.

Frowning, Kester took his seat. This interesting situation had now become a problematic one. He fingered the sticky note with the officer's number, then pocketed it. If the girl was in danger, he wouldn't be able to sit on this much longer.

No one gets to break my toys until I'm finished playing with them.

———

Trick had made a mess again, and he knew he was going to get in trouble for it. He hadn't meant to make things worse. Even though he was small now, he'd thought he could put some of the things in the closet back where they were supposed to be, but all he'd managed to do was toss them around more and accidentally unravel part of a sweater.

If I tell her right away and apologize, maybe she won't get as mad. He had really fuzzy memories of being a little kid and his mom yelling at him when she found out about bad things he'd done and then tried to hide. And when his brother did something wrong (which wasn't very often), he always admitted to it and apologized right away, and their mom went easier on him.

When afternoon came, he heard someone come into the house and then footsteps come down the hall. The twisty-pully thing happened to his body, and then he was a boy again. He jumped up and pulled on the clothes the girl had laid out for him—for some reason, his being dressed always put her in a better mood—and then shut the closet door so she wouldn't see the mess right away. When she opened the bedroom door, he was sitting as innocently as he could on the bed.

"Hi, Trick," she said softly, closing the door and leaning back against it.

"I'm sorry about the mess in the closet," he told her. "I tried to fix it, but I made it worse. Now that I have hands, I'll clean it up." *There. That should do it.*

"Okay. Thanks." She moved to the desk and started pulling books out of her backpack.

"You're not mad?"

"No. I'm... I'm sorry about getting upset this morning. I know you didn't mean any harm. But I'd just woken up, and you surprised me, and…" She shook her head. "I'm sorry the floor was hard. I'll try to figure out something else for tonight."

The hurt Trick had felt this morning clouded his head. It had taken a very long nap to clear his mind of her rejection, but now it was back. He'd half-expected her to toss him out. He'd half-considered leaving on his own. But she'd said sorry, so he had to forgive her.

He went over to where she was sitting in her desk chair and knelt on the floor, resting his chin on her leg. After a second, she took the hint and began petting his head. He closed his eyes, enjoying the feel of her fingers in his hair rubbing against his scalp. Now he felt better. If only he had his real ears so she could rub those sensitive spots just behind them.

She petted him for a while, and he sensed her body relaxing. Then all of a sudden she stopped and said, "Homework time."

"Dinner first?" he asked. He was hungry now, and it could take hours for her to finish with all those books.

"If I feed you now, how will you stay motivated to do your homework?" she said.

He stared at her. What did she mean by that?

"You can't stay hidden here forever, Trick. You'll have to go back to school sometime, and you don't want to be so far behind that they hold you back a grade."

"But… I'll be a cat all the time again. Once I find a way. Then I won't have to go to school."

The familiar girl let out a big breath. "Even if that's what you want, don't you think it's better to prepare for going back to school, in case it doesn't happen?"

Not really.

"Your mom's gonna find you eventually. Don't you think she'll be less angry about you hiding if you can tell her you kept up with your schoolwork?"

He thought about that. "Maybe."

"So will you help with the homework and let me catch you up?"

He got up and sprawled across the bed on his belly. "Okay," he muttered.

Homework was boring and pointless, but he let the familiar girl read her notes to him. When they had to answer questions, she didn't let him stay quiet but kept asking him until he gave her what he thought the right answers were. On one long question, they argued over the right answer until someone knocked on the door.

"Denneka?" It was her mom's voice. "Are you talking to someone?"

The girl stiffened and said, "No! Just talking to myself!"

"Oh," said her mom. "I thought you might be on the phone with someone."

The girl ducked her head and said quietly, "Yeah, that would have been a better answer."

"Anyway, dinner's ready whenever you want it," said her mom.

"I'm doing my homework," the girl called back. "So I'll get it later when I'm done. It might be late, so don't bother leaving it out for me."

"Okay. Try not to stay up too late. You need your rest."

By the time the girl decided they were done with homework, the clock said it was past eleven. "Dinner now?" Trick pleaded.

"Hang on." The girl peeked out of her door. "I don't see any other lights on. I think everyone else has gone to bed, but be really quiet anyway, okay?"

Trick nodded and followed her out. He kept as sharp an ear out as he could with his weak human ears as they went to the kitchen. The familiar girl got them both some food, and they ate as quickly and quietly as they could, still listening for any sound of her family being awake. Trick felt much better when his stomach was full, and he was ready to curl up for sleep, but when he tried to crawl into the bed, the girl pulled him away from it.

"Don't go to sleep yet. You need a shower," she said.

"Again?"

"It's usually a daily thing."

"Will you wash my hair again?"

"You don't really need to do that every day. Besides, we can't risk doing that in the kitchen right now."

"I don't like baths. But I like when you wash my hair. I won't take a bath unless you wash my hair."

The girl gave him a strange look, then rubbed her face with her hands. "You are so weird. Fine. Wait here first, though, while I take my shower and brush my teeth and stuff."

When she left the room, he transformed into a cat, wriggled out of the pile of his clothes, and curled up on the bed. He got a good ten-minute nap in before the uncomfortable transformation woke him. The door cracked open, and the familiar girl's hand poked through the crack, holding a towel.

"Wrap this around your waist," she said from the other side of the door.

At least she wasn't making him put all his clothes on again. He did as she asked and happily followed her to the bathroom.

"The tub's already full," she said. "I just plugged the drain while I took my shower, so... sorry about making you use my dirty shower water, but if anyone heard the bath running again, it might sound weird."

Trick didn't think the shower water could have really gotten dirty just from her using it, and he wanted to hurry and get the bath out of the way so she'd wash his hair. He dropped the towel and pulled the shower curtain aside without remembering to let her cover her eyes first. She flinched away from him so hard that she fell against the toilet and knocked the trash over.

"What's that?" he asked, caught off guard by the layer of white foam on top of the bathwater.

"It's bubble-bath," she said as she put the trash back in the plastic bin. Her face was going pink again.

"Why?"

"Just because. Hurry and get in."

He got in, and she closed the curtain between them. Once surrounded by the bubbles, Trick remembered baths like this when he was really little. Mom had prepared Brother's baths once, too, but not for a while. Another kid thing.

Trick swatted in annoyance at a clump of bubbles. It got stuck his hand, and he shook it away. The fluffy lump was suddenly sistible, and he swatted at it again. He grabbed for it several tim before trapping it against the curtain with a loud smack.

"What are you doing?" the girl asked.

Trick shoved both of his hands into the water. "Nothing." Definitely not playing in the bubbles like a little kid.

They sure were fluffy, though. And they moved funny.

He washed himself with the soap for a while. Then he tossed a big clump of bubbles high and smacked it down, slamming it into the water with a loud splash.

"Are you done?" the girl asked.

"Yes," he admitted. "Hair now?"

She hummed in a way that sounded unhappy. "Trick, gather as much of the bubbles in close to you as you can, okay?"

"Why?"

"It's a game. Just gather them up and try not to let them get away."

It didn't sound like a very fun game, but he did what she said. He hadn't noticed until now, but there were fewer bubbles than when he'd gotten in. He pulled as much of the fluffy mass to him as he could get.

When she pulled the curtain back, her eyes were closed, and she carefully cracked one open and peered down at him. Then she let out a puff and opened her eyes the rest of the way.

Trick wasn't stupid. "I figured out the game," he told her. "The game is keeping the bubbles over my boy parts so you don't have to see them, right?"

Her face turned red. "Yes."

"I still don't get why you hate them so much. I've said I won't hurt you with them."

"I--uh--" She covered her face with her hands for a second

 looking at him again. "I know that, Trick. If I thought there
chance that—that you would, you wouldn't still be here."

"then what's wrong?" It was annoying to have to keep covering
and putting on clothes and stuff.

I've tried to explain it already, but... but you didn't get it. So I
n't think I *can* explain."

She was right about that. Trick hadn't understood her explanation at all. "Maybe sometime you'll find a way to explain it," he said
optimistically. *Or maybe sometime you'll decide it doesn't matter,* he
thought even more optimistically. "Will you wash my hair now?"

The shower head could come off like the sprayer in the kitchen
sink. The familiar girl took it and pointed it at the water by his feet,
then turned it on and adjusted the flow and temperature until she
was happy with it.

"Lean your head back," she told him.

It was uncomfortable on his neck, but he did as she said, and she
soaked his hair with the shower head. He stared into her eyes as she
worked. They were so focused. As soon as she caught him watching
her, her cheeks went red again and the water stopped.

"Hold this," she said, handing him the shower head. He took it,
and she poured shampoo into her hand. "Close your eyes."

He was so relaxed, he wouldn't have been able to keep them
open much longer anyway. His eyes slid closed as her fingers
worked through his hair, rubbing at his head, making his chest ache
with his need to purr. The flowery smell of the shampoo was too
strong, but it would always remind him of her hands in his hair, so
he couldn't dislike it.

"More," he said softly, without meaning to.

"More what?" she asked.

"Rub harder."

Her hands froze, clinging to the sides of his head. "Trick? You're
not... um..."

He didn't feel any soap or water on his eyes, so he opened them
carefully to see her gaping at him as if she was afraid. "Why did you
stop?"

Her eyes darted down, to where his hands—and the shower head—had fallen into his lap. He hadn't even noticed when he couldn't hold them up anymore. "Nothing. It's nothing," she said uncertainly.

"Then keep going." He closed his eyes again to protect them from the soap.

Her hands rubbed him for only a little while more, then she said, "Can you hand me the shower head, please?"

He held it up for her, and she took it, her fingers quick and light as she rinsed the soap out. When she was done, she replaced the shower head and pulled the curtain closed. "Drain the water, and here's your towel." She set it on the edge of the tub near his head. "Dry yourself off, then wrap the towel around your waist again. You don't need to get dressed right now."

She sure made things more complicated than they needed to be. But Trick was in a very good mood, so he did everything she asked without arguing. She was twitchy on the way back to her bedroom, dragging him behind her quickly while constantly shooting looks toward the other doors. But they made it back to her room without anyone catching them.

He relaxed even more as she blow-dried his hair, enough that she had to keep poking his shoulder to stop him from melting into a puddle on her bed. When she finished and got up to put the blow-dryer away, Trick fell sideways onto the bed, seconds away from falling asleep.

"For tonight, I was thinking..." She stopped talking just as Trick heard the sound of the closet door opening and stuff falling over.

Trick sat up. He'd told her he'd clean the mess in the closet, and he'd meant to. He just hadn't yet. Making sure the towel was fixed around his waist, he went to the closet and nudged her out of the way. "I'll clean it." He dropped to his knees and worked on getting things back into boxes. They probably weren't the right boxes, but he did his best.

"Um, okay," she said from behind him. "So, the back of the closet is eleven feet from everything but the left foot or so of my bed. So I was thinking, if I stay on the right side of my bed and you get in the closet, you can sleep as a cat tonight, and we can make a sort of bed for you in the back there."

That sounded a lot like she was punishing him, but she didn't sound angry, so Trick wasn't sure what she meant by it. But he didn't want to make her angry, so as he cleaned up the closet, he used the sweater he'd ruined to make a soft spot to lie on at the back of the closet, on top of a box.

"Do you think that'll work?" the girl asked.

Her voice was weak and higher than normal, which made him a little concerned, so he said, "Okay."

He got up and stood in the space he'd cleared on the closet floor. The familiar girl closed the door—not all the way, but leaving a crack open where a sliver of light came through—and he heard her soft footsteps walking away. As soon as he changed back into a cat, he hopped up onto the makeshift sweater bed. It wasn't very warm or soft, but it was better than the floor, and the closet was cozy. He curled up and went to sleep.

CHAPTER
SIXTEEN

Denneka woke up with a heavy weight on her chest. When she opened her eyes, she was flat on her back with Trick's chin resting on her sternum, right above the top button in the v-neck of her flannel pajamas. The naked skin of his shoulders and back were visible, then the rest of his body disappeared under the blankets. Only his upper body was actually on top of her, the rest of him from the waist down lying next to her on the mattress. His arms were tucked in against her sides but not holding her, and as he slept peacefully, soft breaths of air from his nose tickled the skin of her upper chest.

Don't freak out. Don't freak out. Don't freak out. Don't freak out.

He definitely didn't mean anything by it, and she didn't want to make him sulky again. She'd woken up before to him lying on her chest when he was a cat. And she knew that, in his mind, nothing was different now from then. So she worked so hard to keep from freaking out that when she was able to speak, her voice came out unnaturally calm and sweet.

"Trick?"

His eyelids opened halfway until he was peering sleepily at her with those bright green eyes, not moving at all. The sight made her heart pound so hard it felt like it would burst out of her chest.

"Why are you lying on me?" she squeaked.

His eyes drifted closed, and without moving his jaw to speak, he said, "Comfy."

His complete nonchalance about their situation filled her with a rush of irritation that allowed her to get some sort of grip on herself. She sat up, pushing him off, and with a small, annoyed grumble, he shifted as if to curl up on the bed.

"No, don't go back to sleep," she ordered. "Tell me why you're in my bed. I thought you were sleeping in the closet last night."

Succumbing to the inevitability of the conversation, Trick pushed himself up into a sitting position on the side of the bed. Which made the blanket fall off of him. He was facing mostly away from her, but the lean, smooth lines of his shoulders, back, and legs distracted her until she rubbed her eyes and forced herself to look at his cute face and rumpled hair instead. That sight wasn't much less distracting.

"I *was* in the closet," he said in a rough voice with just enough whine to make sure she knew he wanted to go back to sleep. "Then you must have rolled too far over in the bed or something, because I turned human and couldn't get far enough away to turn back. And it's all lumpy boxes and hard floor in there, so I had nowhere else to go but here."

Denneka took a deep breath and tried to calm herself down. If he was telling the truth—and she chose to give him the benefit of the doubt on that—then it really wasn't his fault. If anything, it was hers for coming up with an unrealistic plan. She wouldn't have shoved him in the closet as a human and expected him to sleep, so from his perspective, the bed really was the only option.

"You couldn't have at least put some clothes on?"

"I didn't think of it." And he still wasn't thinking of it.

She got out of bed on the opposite side from where he was sitting. "Okay. Okay. You can go back to sleep now. I'll try not to come and go too many times before I go to school, and I'll leave some food out for you."

Trick curled up on the bed, pulled the blanket fully over himself, and became a silent lump on the mattress.

Denneka didn't think to read the paper, but as
the bus, she heard the news.

Mr. Haug was dead. They'd found his body.

And it was right where Trick had said it was.

With everything that had been going on with Trick at
whole thing with Mr. Haug had completely gone out of h
This was the first time she'd even thought of it since Tric
turned human again.

Trick had told her he'd seen Mr. Haug in a grave. Trick—as a
—had tried to show her the grave. That must have been it. Wha
had she done to make him think she wanted to see it, though? She
tried to remember. She'd been crying about Trick, about losing him.
Her face flushed at the memory. She'd cried about Trick *to* Trick. It
was humiliating. But she'd been thinking about how Trick was
missing after Mr. Haug had gone missing, so she must have said
something about Mr. Haug, and Trick had thought it meant she'd
wanted to see where he'd seen him. Not that any of it mattered now.
She hadn't needed to know the exact grave to give the police the tip
that led them to it.

"The article said they only found him because of an anonymous
tip," the girl in the seat in front of her whispered to her friend. "I
wonder who it was."

Just as Denneka started to feel a little swell of pride, the other
girl said, "Probably the killer trying to brag about it. That's how
they are, right?"

Denneka listened to the two girls argue about that all the way to
school, and it was enough to convince her that nothing good would
be likely to come of Denneka revealing herself as the anonymous
tipster. Not that she had any real desire to. Even if she believed it
was a way to gain popularity, Denneka didn't need or want
popularity.

While she was glad the police were able to make progress on
finding out what happened to Mr. Haug, she was sad to find out
that Trick had been right that the teacher was dead. He hadn't been

. or anything, but he hadn't been a bad teacher.

~e someone who deserved to get killed.

₃ot a lot worse once she got to class.

ll find that new kid next," said Peter Noncer. He sat a
of Denneka, but he was talking loudly enough for
~o hear.

₃ and her friends picked up this train of thought with gusto.

₃otally," she said even louder than Peter. "I bet that weirdo is
₃ in another hole somewhere, rotting away like the worthless
₃sh he is."

Denneka's jaw and fists clenched, but she refused to acknowledge the challenging sneer that Amy sent her way.

Trick wasn't dead. Trick was fine. She knew that and they didn't.
But they would know it sooner or later, when Trick came back. If
Denneka rose to their bait now, they'd just find some way to throw
it back in her face when Trick came back. Probably tease her about
how she was so in love with him that she had to defend his honor or
something.

And how would Trick respond if they said something like that?
Would he be confused? Disgusted? Would he try to keep his
distance from her so he didn't encourage her?

Was she in love with him?

Of course not. Don't be stupid, she told herself. She liked him, yes.
She had to admit that—to herself, even if she didn't want to confess
it to anyone else. But she was only thirteen. She didn't know
anything about that kind of love.

When she was older, though, maybe she would—

*No. Stop it. There is no 'when we're older'. He only likes me now
because I'm convenient. Because I'm familiar. That isn't going to last once
he gets over his shyness or whatever this is and returns to society. He's nice
and really cute. Even if they think he's weird, that won't last. He'll make
friends. He'll… get a girlfriend. He won't need me. Once he gets more used
to being human, he'll probably be embarrassed about how he's acting
around me now. I'd be surprised if he's even still speaking to me when
we're older.*

"Would you guys stop?" said a voice that sounded like it belonged to a fourth-grader.

Denneka glanced up to see Brook giving her a look of pity.

"You don't have to say that stuff where Denneka can hear," Brook told Amy and the others.

"Duh, of course we do," Amy said. There was a little less venom in the tone she aimed at Brook than the one she always used for Denneka. "That's the whole point."

"To make her sad?" asked Brook.

Amy rolled her eyes and was clearly working on another horrible thing to say when the bell rang.

"Quiet down," said Mr. McKenzie. He'd been sitting up front the whole time and could have shut Amy and the others up, but he'd only been reading the paper like he didn't care. For a second there, yesterday, she'd thought maybe there was something nice under all that nastiness, but maybe she'd been wrong. And now that Mr. Haug was definitely never coming back, they might be stuck with Mr. McKenzie for the rest of the year.

At lunchtime, Denneka carried her tray between the tables, steering well clear of Amy's group and looking for a quiet place to sit alone, per usual. But she got distracted by the conversation of a group of girls she passed. One was showing around a photo of a kitten on her phone.

"He's so cute!" Maddie cooed.

"I just got him last weekend," Jennifer said proudly. "His name's Chester."

"Be sure to get him used to things like trimming his nails and baths while he's young," said Wanda. "It'll make it so much easier when you have to do those things once he's grown."

"Do you have cats?" Jennifer asked.

"Oh yeah, we've always had cats," Wanda said. "We have four now."

Denneka listened until she realized she'd been standing beside their table long enough that it was getting weird. "Um, can I join you?" she asked.

The girls looked up at her in surprise, and Brook said, "Sure."

The other girls couldn't argue with her then, so Denneka took the seat beside Brook.

"Thanks for telling off Amy this morning," she told Brook quietly.

Brook shrugged. "Sorry it didn't help."

"That's just how she is," Denneka agreed.

An awkward silence fell over the table, and the other girls watched her with dread, clearly expecting that she'd bring a really uncomfortable subject into their otherwise peaceful lives.

"I'm not worried about Trick," she told them. "Just because Mr. Haug died doesn't mean that's what happened to Trick. I think he'll be back. Anyway, I don't want to talk about that. I stopped because I heard you talking about cats, and I kinda had some questions."

The relief that washed over them was palpable. "Did you want to see the picture?" Jennifer asked, turning her phone to show Denneka.

"He's really cute," Denneka said with appropriate enthusiasm.

"Do you have a cat?" Maddie asked.

"Well... sort of." How was the best way to say this? "I'm taking care of a kitten temporarily. I found a stray, but I think I know who his owner is, so I probably won't have him much longer. But, Wanda, it sounds like you know some stuff about cats, so I was... hoping to get some advice?" She hadn't thought to get advice until she'd heard the girls talking about it, but now it seemed obvious.

Still thrilled not to be talking about their missing-and-maybe-dead classmate, Wanda said, "Sure!"

"How do you... get them to behave? Like, if they keep doing something you don't want them to do."

Wanda laughed. "Well, cats aren't dogs, so you can't really train them much. Mostly, if they're doing something you don't want them to do, you have two options."

"Okay..." Denneka leaned closer, not wanting to miss anything under the noise of the cafeteria.

Wanda put up one finger. "If they're getting into stuff, see if you can just keep that stuff away from them and out of their reach."

The 'stuff' Trick was getting into was her bed, so that probably wasn't an option.

Wanda put up a second finger. "And if you can't do that, you just have to compromise."

"Compromise?" Denneka asked. She might be able to compromise with Trick, but how did one compromise with a regular cat?

"If it keeps doing something you don't want, figure out the maximum amount of that thing that you can tolerate, and then let the cat do it that much and only try to correct it if it goes past that amount. Like, if it scratches the furniture, give it plenty of stuff to scratch on. If it still scratches the furniture, see if there's one piece of furniture you can let it scratch. Then it won't feel so deprived if you don't let it scratch on the others."

Trick didn't scratch on anything... that Denneka knew of. "So... let the cat get away with as much as I can tolerate, so it doesn't feel deprived?"

"Basically, yeah," said Wanda. "If the cat feels like you won't let it get away with anything, it'll just lash out and do whatever it wants when it can get away with it. If you let it get away with some stuff, then it feels like it's getting something out of obeying you when you tell it to not do other stuff."

Denneka had always had the idea that pets were supposed to obey their owners, period. Apparently that wasn't always the case.

"Does that help?" Wanda asked.

"I... think so. Thanks." Denneka picked up her tray and got up. "Sorry to bother you."

"You can stay," Brook said.

Denneka looked cautiously at the other girls, but they were smiling. Wanda nodded. Maddie said, "Yeah, you're already here."

Denneka had never been invited to eat at lunch before. Not for years, anyway. She sat back down. "Thanks." She didn't talk much for the rest of lunch, but the other girls didn't seem to mind that she was there. It felt... strange. Good strange.

That night, once their homework was done and she'd gotten Trick fed and bathed (he'd insisted on having his hair washed again, but at least he didn't say anything weird this time), she made sure he put on his pajamas and sat him down. "I've decided to let you sleep in the bed with me," she told him. "On two conditions. You have to agree, or I'll get mad at you. Okay?"

"What?" Trick asked.

"You have to always wear your pajamas, or you're not allowed in the bed."

"But what if I transform into a cat and back and get cold?"

"*If* that happens, then you put your pajamas back on before getting in bed."

"What if I can't find them?"

"Then put other clothes on or wake me up."

Trick didn't look happy, but he didn't continue to argue. "What else?"

She turned back the top blanket. "You sleep under the top blanket only." She turned back the second blanket and sheet. "And I sleep under all of them. So the second blanket and sheet stay between us. Okay?"

Trick cocked his head. "Why?"

"Because that's the compromise, Trick. Will you agree?"

The look Trick gave her said that he thought she was being very unreasonable and may have slightly lost it. But he said, "Okay."

He waited.

She waited.

Resigning herself, she turned off the lights and got in bed, tossing back the top blanket for him. Her body felt hot, like she was blushing with her whole body, and wired, but she wasn't actually trembling. She felt like she was doing something dirty.

When Trick followed her into the bed, he didn't lie down next to her like a human would. He crawled completely under the top blanket and curled up at the foot of the bed, draping his body across her lower legs.

Gradually, and long after Trick fell into a peaceful sleep,

scratch at the
heard footsteps
be working all
asn't sure who it

was getting rest-
really wanted to
k that he knew
to be human, it
wanted to play

being
harde
Trick wa
ll these nice
up in or on, a
same size as her
t valley that her legs
erfect for stretching ou
uman, it was too small f

Softly at first.
it was, if they
utside. As long
why would she
er to leave her
m had done in

with her, but she was still
to let him sleep in the bed
had been with a couple silly

t the door. As
ver it was and

up from the foot of the bed
ly, pressing his side as much
his arms under him. She'd
to her chest, so he figured
nd tucked his nose into the
a little hard to breathe, but it
curled around him a little,

got there. The
e pawed at it,
as human, he
ldn't think of
steps came up

he felt her stir. Her body jolted
laughter. "Um, Trick? Is that

e looked a lot
alike—but he
played sports.
held him. "I
ght run away,

eck felt a little stiff. Why were
up on his heels and looked

away, but he
e him for not

turning pink. "I'd better go get

as having a goo
her closet when h
hat her parents woul
high school, so Trick w
me home to visit him?

stay quiet to be safe, but he
let him outside in days, and he
sunshine and try to catch that ha
ing him. Maybe, if the hawk used
with him. Not that he was at all sure he
d, but he was starting to get desperate.

pawed at the door, careful not to scratch
when no one answered, harder. Whoever
uld just open the door, he could escape and get
as he came back inside before the girl got home,
care? Maybe when he was human he could ask h
window open or even install a cat door like his mo
their last house.

The footsteps approached, and he kept pawing
soon as it opened, Trick darted past the legs of who
ran for the sliding glass door that led to the back yard

He hadn't really thought of what to do when he
door was closed, which he should have expected. H
too, but of course it didn't open on its own. If he w
could have opened it, but he wasn't. Since he cou
anything else, he just kept pawing at it until the foot
behind him and big hands scooped him up.

"You're still here, huh?" said the girl's brother. H
like her—brown hair and eyes, and their faces looked
was a lot bigger than her. He looked like a guy who
Trick squirmed, trying to get down, but the older bo
don't think so, little guy. If I let you outside, you mi
and Denneka will get mad at me."

Trick stopped squirming. He knew he wouldn't run
couldn't explain that to this boy. And he couldn't blam

wanting the girl mad at him. Trick didn't like it when she was mad at him either.

The older boy held him with one hand that nearly entirely circled Trick's body and stroked his head gently with the other. Trick hadn't had his head stroked as a cat in days. He started to purr, tilting his head to try to get the boy's hands behind his ears.

"Not that I'm afraid of her," the girl's brother said. "She couldn't even tell Mom and Dad on me, since she's not actually allowed to have you. But if she still has you, then maybe it's because she needs you, and as long as you don't cause problems, I'm okay with that."

Needs me how? Trick wondered. He was the one who'd asked to stay with her.

The older boy sat down on a leather chair and set Trick in his lap, continuing to pet him. "I have to admit, you're kinda cute. Makes me wish we were allowed to have pets."

Trick purred and raised his chin for the boy to scratch under it. The girl's brother was good at petting him and appreciated how cute Trick was. And he smelled kind of like the familiar girl. Maybe this human wasn't so bad.

The boy didn't pet him for anywhere near long enough. He didn't play with him, either. He started coughing and looked down at Trick with watery eyes. "Sorry, little guy. I need to take some meds and go to bed."

Oh, so you came home because you're sick. I bet if you keep petting me, it'll help you feel better.

"Kinda wish I could borrow you," the boy said, almost as if he could hear Trick, "but I don't want you to get caught, so you'd better go back to Denneka's room." He picked Trick up in one big hand and took him to the bathroom first. "You need to go while we're here?"

Trick did.

"You sure are a smart cat," the brother said when he picked him up again. "It'd be nice if she can convince Mom to let her keep you."

When he put Trick back in the girl's room and closed the door before Trick could escape again, Trick realized he had a problem.

He'd never considered that he wouldn't be able to get outside if he really wanted to. His mom had never kept him cooped up inside. But the girl's bedroom felt smaller and smaller each day that Trick was trapped in it. He needed to convince the familiar girl to let him outside more, or else he might have to go back home to avoid going completely stir crazy.

———

At lunch on Wednesday, Landon was invited to sit with a group of girls. They were all really nice, and one had offered to give him the cupcake her mom had packed, so he said yes. Mom hadn't been making very good lunches lately, still so distracted by Trick being gone, so the cupcake sounded pretty good.

He'd just gotten his lunch bag out of his cubby when Miss Cutler tapped him on the shoulder.

"There's someone here to see you, Landon." Her eyebrows were slightly pinched. He thought it meant she was worried, but he wasn't sure.

"My mom?" he asked, not sure who else it could be.

"No. It's a man. His name's Mr. McKenzie. Do you know him?"

A thrill of excitement went through Landon, but he kept it down. "Yes. He's been watching me while Mom's looking for my brother. He's teaching me how to cook."

For some reason, it had seemed like that extra bit of info would help, and from Miss Cutler's expression, it did. Landon would have to put that aside to figure out why later.

Miss Cutler smiled. "He's waiting in the school office to talk to you. I'll take you there."

Landon put his lunch back in his cubby—he'd have to say sorry to the girls later or they might be mad at him—and followed Miss Cutler to the office.

Mr. McKenzie was waiting in the office, like she'd said. He was in a button-up shirt and tie, looking more professional and teachery than he did when he was at their house.

"The two of you match," Miss Cutler said with a little laugh. "Did you plan that?"

Landon hadn't noticed at first, but he was wearing the same shirt and tie colors as Mr. McKenzie.

"Pure coincidence," the man said easily. "We must have a similar fashion sense."

Miss Cutler laughed again, then stood by the wall near the door.

Landon walked over to where Mr. McKenzie was in one corner of the office waiting area. The man squatted down to his level and talked in a voice soft enough that they wouldn't be heard by Miss Cutler or the secretary. "I've got a project I'd like your help with. I could do it myself, but I thought it might be a good learning opportunity for you."

Excitement zipped through Landon's body. "Magic?" he whispered.

Mr. McKenzie nodded. "But there's a small obstacle to overcome first. In order to do this task, you'll need to come with me. However, your mother is the only person the school is authorized to release you to."

Landon knew about that. It was never a problem, since his mom was the one to pick him up every day. Except now it *was* a problem.

"I can't currently do magic," Mr. McKenzie said softly. "If you want to come with me, you'll need to convince these nice people to let me take you."

"How?"

He winked. "Magic, naturally."

"How?" Landon asked again. His mouth felt dry.

"You'll need to get past both your teacher and the school secretary, and we'll need to act quickly before anyone else comes in who might cause a problem. Speak to them one at a time. Tell them whatever lie you think might convince them to let you go with me."

"They'll believe me?"

"Do you remember how you reached into the beetle? This is similar. Except you're not trying to bond with their mind, only nudge it. Pour your will into your words, will them to believe you, nudge their mind into believing what you say. If you come up with a plausible enough lie, it shouldn't take much. Do you want to give it a try?"

"Yeah." So much it was hard to stand still.

Mr. McKenzie stood and nodded him toward the school secretary, then went over and began chatting with Miss Cutler. When Landon saw that the man had her distracted, he went up to the counter where the school secretary sat and pulled himself up on his elbows so he could see over it.

"Ms. Olger," he said.

She looked up from her computer and smiled at him. "Yes, dear?"

Landon looked into the lady's eyes, remembering the beetle, remembering what it felt like to focus his will. Not trying to pour himself in this time, but only nudge. "My dad wants to take me to lunch. Is that okay?"

Ms. Olger frowned. "Your dad?" She gave Mr. McKenzie a second look.

"Yeah. He's my dad," Landon said. It was the most believable lie he could think of. Landon didn't have a dad, so there wouldn't be one on file, but parents were always allowed to take their kids out of school. Mr. McKenzie was still new to town, which meant that not many people probably knew who he was—or who he wasn't. Even though they didn't look alike, it shouldn't be that hard for someone to believe he was his dad, since there was no one else. Not if Landon himself said so. "He wants to take me to lunch. Is that okay?"

Ms. Olger started clicking things on her computer. "You're Landon St. Andrew, right? I didn't think we had your dad in our records."

"He's there," Landon said, his chest tightening with fear. What if he screwed this up? How could he make her see something that wasn't there? Hearing him, she met his eyes, and he focused hard on her, nudging with all his might, willing her to believe him. "He's in the system. He's allowed to pick me up." He could feel something

going out of him toward her—a thin, wispy so
had no idea if it was connecting.

Then Ms. Olger's expression went blank for a
Sure thing, dear. I'll just make a note of it here." She
the room to Mr. McKenzie and called, "Mr. St. Andrew,
him back by the end of lunch if you can."

Mr. McKenzie blinked in surprise.

"It's okay, Dad, she already checked us out," Landon
hurrying toward him.

If anything, Mr. McKenzie looked even more stunned tha
before, then he smiled over at Ms. Olger. "Ah, thank you."

"Mr. St. Andrew?" Miss Cutler asked.

"No need to correct her," Mr. McKenzie told her quietly enough
that Ms. Olger didn't hear. "But Landon's mother and I aren't
married."

"Ah," Miss Cutler said. Her frown had appeared just then, and
then went away, but now it came back. "But wouldn't Ms. Olger
have seen your name in our system?"

Mr. McKenzie laid a hand on Landon's shoulder and used it to
nudge him toward his teacher.

What now? Landon tried to think fast. He wasn't used to lying. It
didn't come easily to him. Mr. McKenzie would have already given
his name to Ms. Olger when he came in. Why had she assumed his
name was different now that she believed he was Landon's dad?
Unless Landon messed up and nudged her too hard or something.

"She did," Landon insisted, panic making him push his will toward
Miss Cutler as hard as he could. If he got caught in his lie now, it
could be really bad.

"Then why did she call him Mr. St. Andrew?" Miss Cutler asked.

"She didn't." Things were spinning out of control so much,
Landon actually felt dizzy. But he focused hard on Miss Cutler, his
eyes locked with hers, willing her to believe him even though what
he was telling her made no sense.

Miss Cutler blinked a few times. "She didn't?"

harder. "No. She called him Mr. McKenzie.
me. That's what she saw in the system."

skin got really pale, and her face went blank long
ndon was afraid she'd faint or something. But then
to normal. "Right. Have fun, Landon." She wandered
fice, not quite steady on her feet.

n's hands were shaking. "Did I hurt her?" he whispered
tely.

No," Mr. McKenzie said in a low, flat voice. "Come on." He
d his hand on Landon's shoulder to guide him out of the office
nd into the parking lot, not stopping until they reached his car. He
opened the door for Landon and strapped him in before getting in
on the driver's side. He parked the car two blocks away from the
school in a grocery store parking lot.

Landon's hands finally stopped shaking. "You're sure I didn't
hurt her?"

"She'll be fine," Mr. McKenzie said, his voice gentle now. "You
backed yourself into a corner and had to push too hard to get out.
But you're very young, and your magic is very young. She's probably already recovered."

"Will she remember? Will they know what happened when I go
back?"

"I doubt it. They experienced a sort of cognitive dissonance.
Most likely, their brains will discard the information that makes the
least sense and blur over the rest." He stroked his chin. "Your dad,
huh?"

"It was the lie that made the most sense, since people don't
usually argue about parents taking their kids out of school."

"You're right. It is obvious. I... should have considered you'd
think of that."

"You didn't?"

"You caught me by surprise is all. I've never had anyone call me
'Dad' before."

Landon looked at his hands. He hadn't really realized it in the
moment, but... "I've never called anyone 'Dad' before."

Mr. McKenzie rubbed the sides of the steering wheel like he didn't know what to do with his hands. "You can keep doing it. If you want. While we're out, I mean. To keep up appearances."

Landon shook his head. "Not unless I have to. It... hurts too much. Knowing it's not true."

They were quiet so long it started getting uncomfortable. Then Mr. McKenzie started the car and got back on the road.

"That was good practice," he said, upbeat again. "What I need you to do next is similar."

"What are we doing?"

"We're going to meet someone. Have you heard the news about that missing teacher?"

"I heard they found him dead." The kids at school had been talking about it, but the teachers were quick to tell off anyone who started getting into the gory details.

"Yes, and the killer's still at large. I've taken an interest in the case. The dead man was a fellow teacher, after all, the one I was brought in to replace. But the police aren't giving away everything they know. It's possible that the police don't even *know* everything they know."

"What does that mean?"

"I'll explain it when we get to that point. I've asked for an interview with one of the officers working the case. I want to see if we can find out anything the rest of the public doesn't know and see if it will give me a lead on finding this killer."

Landon smiled at that. He always liked a good mystery story.

———

This Officer Parkes was too trusting, or he'd never have agreed to Kester's request to meet in such a secluded place. Kester had not met many cops, but it wouldn't surprise him if they tended to have an 'us vs. them' mindset about their work. He guessed that was true for Officer Parkes, at least. Kester had introduced himself as Denneka's teacher and told him that Lisa had given him his number.

at, apparently, had put Kester in the column of 'us' in Parkes's ~ind. So he hadn't questioned it when Kester had asked to meet in a park on the far outskirts of town—one which, when they arrived, was utterly empty except for the squad car in the parking lot and a lone man sitting on a bench.

Kester parked the car a few spaces away, told Landon to wait until he called for him, and went to meet Lisa's contact.

Parkes stood to meet him, and Kester couldn't help sizing the other man up as he approached. He was tall and broad-shouldered with short, blond hair. Mid-forties, but very fit and not just for his age. Not to mention handsome in a rugged, working-class sort of way.

"John McKenzie," Parkes said, offering a handshake that was firm but not overcompensating. "I've seen you a couple times, but it's good to actually meet you."

Kester remembered him vaguely as one of the officers who'd responded to his call on the evening Trick 'went missing'. He hadn't had cause to pay much attention to him at the time, and Parkes had not been one of the officers who'd spoken to him. They'd seen each other from a distance at Jacqueline's house while Kester had been making breakfast the next morning, but they'd spared each other barely a glance. "Likewise. Thank you for meeting me." Then, because sometimes he really couldn't help himself, he asked, "Out of curiosity, how long have you known Lisa?"

"Since high school."

"Friends that long, huh?"

Parkes laughed. "On a good day."

Kester's eyebrow drew up. "She might be my boss, but I hope it's not out of line to notice that she's a beautiful woman. I'm surprised a man could know her that long and not try to marry her."

"Well, heh." Parkes scratched at his hair. "We dated in high school for a while. Didn't really work out. Why are you so interested anyway? Don't tell me you called me under false pretenses and you just want tips on how to ask her out."

Kester laughed, waving the idea away. "No, no. It's only that she referred to you as 'a contact' and I was curious what sort of contact you had with her. Now that I see you, I think I have some idea."

Parkes frowned. "Then I guess it's none of your business, is it?"

Kester held up his hands. "Easy, Officer. I'm no threat to you or her or whatever kind of relationship you two enjoy." *Because I've already had the pleasure.* Oh, how he wished he could say that aloud. He was dying to see the man's reaction. "It was only a bit of friendly banter to get to know each other. I did come, as I said, about the case involving the killer who you think may be targeting one of my students."

A mask of professional, wary interest slid over Parkes's face. "Have you seen anything at the school? Any suspicious men hanging around?"

"I was wondering if you could tell me more specifically what I'm looking for."

Parkes shook his head and shrugged in frustration. "Tall, big build. I wish I could tell you more. I've caught a glimpse of him twice now, so I should be able to say more, but I can't."

"I see." Kester turned and waved to Landon.

Parkes's face screwed up in confusion as the boy approached. "Who's this? He looks kinda familiar. Have I see him before?"

It might not be ideal for him to remember that Landon is at all connected to Trick, Kester thought. He caught the boy's eye and shook his head slightly.

"No," Landon told Parkes.

It was a simple, easy lie—if Landon even remembered enough to know it was a lie. The two of them hadn't spoken, merely been in the same vicinity. Perhaps it wasn't even necessary to do this. But better safe than sorry.

Parkes seemed to accept that answer easily. "So who is he?" he asked Kester.

"My assistant, currently." Kester took a seat on the bench. "Why don't we sit down?"

Parkes remained standing and looked from Landon to Kester. "Assistant for what?"

Let's try something. "Landon, please tell Officer Parkes to sit."

Suspicion flared in Parkes's brown eyes, but he only looked between the two of them, possibly fighting his discomfort at their strange behavior versus the knowledge that they were only a small boy and a schoolteacher. "What's going on?"

Landon approached the tall man with small steps, but when he caught Parkes's eyes, he said, "Sit."

And Parkes did.

Either Landon was catching on to this aspect of magic with remarkable speed or Parkes was unusually susceptible to it.

Now sitting on the bench beside Kester, Parkes stayed silent, the focus of his eyes slipping in and out as he fought the control that Landon had placed over his mind. Did the boy even know he was still pushing his will onto Parkes?

Kester reached out to take Landon's shoulder, guiding him to stand directly in front of Parkes so that he could keep as much focus and connection as possible. "Good. Not too forcefully, though. Remember your teacher."

Landon flinched, his intensity slacking enough for Parkes to focus alternately on Landon and Kester, but not to speak or act.

"Tell him to describe Haug's killer to you," Kester instructed.

The twitch of his eyebrows was the only sign of confusion or hesitation that Landon betrayed. "Describe Haug's killer," he repeated to Parkes.

"Big," Parkes said. "Tall."

"He knows more," Kester told Landon. "He doesn't know he does, but he does. You need to pull it out of him by forcing him to answer questions."

"What else?" Landon asked Parkes.

"Wears size fourteen boots," Parkes said.

"What kind of hair?" Landon asked.

Parkes's face strained with the effort to say he didn't know, and

stil
an to
himself,
n to push t
es forgetting
l done for the

shoulder. "Let

k himself back
car and drove

'y
the
k, may
Landon

yes. Wide mou

e was there. His
t up and went to
ne painkiller, and
ut an image kept
a man he thought

istered a whole lot m
d in on. More's the pity
d a much better idea of
He'd relay the informa-
'd have eyes combing
ty need to pull her off of

g in his head. The
ry after he'd been
n blurrier, not his
hat he'd seen then
l, not a clear image.

" Kester instructed.
ry specific on what
ame.
s.
.

If he didn't believe
awake telling him
ldn't trust Marcus's
econds from passing

iosity about what

ncentration. "It
rave'."
nough," Kester

...e o...
...by wa...
...ng the m...
...dn't see to i...
...he told Lando...
...didn't want Par...
...se or everything he'...
...ould get noticed.

...ntle hand on Landon's...

...stantly. Before Parkes could bli...
...ess, Kester hurried Landon to the...

...arcus sat on the park bench, wondering why h...
head pounded. *When did I get this headache?* He g...
his squad car, dug around in the glove box for so...
swallowed it. It was hard to think past the pain, ...
swimming up in front of his eyes. An ugly face of...
he should know.

A burst of clarity came along with a throbbin...
killer! He'd thought his vision had been blur...
drugged, but it was his mind that had gotte...
eyesight. Somehow, his brain had dragged up ...
and let him make enough sense of it to get—we...
But good enough to go on.

Not that he could tell the chief about it. ...
Marcus when he was stone sober and wide...
about the notebook page he'd lost, he wou...
memory from a time he was drugged and s...
out.

But Lisa would. He dug out his phone and opened it. He could call her and—

Lisa.

Someone had talked to him about Lisa. Someone... He'd agreed to listen to someone because of Lisa.

He pulled up the call history on his phone. His memory for names and numbers was not good, so whenever someone called who he thought there was even the smallest chance he'd want to speak to again, he added the number to his contacts list.

John McKenzie had called him two hours ago.

He racked his brain for the name. It sounded familiar.

The school. He's one of the teachers.

Why had one of the teachers wanted to meet with him?

No, wait. One of the teachers *had* met with him. Right here, at this park.

With a boy.

Marcus rubbed his head. This didn't make sense. Had he met them? It seemed like he had, but if it had just happened, why couldn't he remember anything about it?

He pulled out his notepad and wrote down everything he could remember about the meeting he couldn't remember. On a separate page, he wrote as detailed a description of the killer as he could, pulling up the face in his mind's eye easily now.

The teacher and the boy—whatever that situation had been— could wait. He had a killer to catch. For some reason, he could now remember what the suspect looked like. And catching the killer was the only lead he had on finding the missing boy. Marcus wasn't one to look a gift horse in the mouth, not even a gift horse that gave him a splitting headache.

———

Mr. McKenzie didn't stop the car until they reached the school parking lot, which gave Landon time to calm down.

He hadn't just nudged. He'd pushed, pulled, and twisted that man's mind until he'd told them everything Mr. McKenzie had wanted to know. A grown man, a police officer, and Landon had commanded him to sit like a dog and he'd done it.

The power Landon felt was a rush even better than flying.

"How did that feel?" Mr. McKenzie asked him, turning in his seat to smile at Landon.

"Good," he said because he couldn't think of enough bigger words. *Good times a hundred. Good times a million.* "Great. Amazing. Fantastic."

Landon was so busy digging up more words for 'good' that he barely heard Mr. McKenzie say, "You did very well. You have a real talent."

He needed to try it again. He turned to look at Mr. McKenzie. The teacher had said he was a witch with power like Landon, but he'd also said he couldn't use that power now. Maybe that meant he couldn't stop Landon from using his.

———

Kester wasn't sure what the right words to say here were. 'I'm proud of you' sounded far too intimate. As far as Landon knew, Kester wasn't anyone with any right to claim pride in him. Kester *didn't* have any right to claim pride in him. Even as the boy's teacher, he was doing very little. Merely giving him a few pointers in the right direction. Landon had picked up most of the magic he'd learned on his own. He'd felt it out for himself. He was becoming self-sufficient, just as Kester had said he should be. He would likely grow up to be a man who didn't need anyone, and he'd do so without any help from the man who'd sired him.

"Mr. McKenzie," Landon said, turning clear, blue eyes up to him.

"Yes, Landon?"

"Turn on the car."

It was an odd request, but Kester complied. Perhaps the boy wanted to go somewhere else before returning to school.

"Now turn it off."

I guess he changed his mind, Kester thought, turning off the engine. The corner of Landon's mouth turned up. "Tell me your full name."

"Kester John McKenzie," Kester said automatically. *Wait, why did I say that? If he tells Jacqueline—*

"Tell me where you're from."

"The backwoods of nowhere," he said. The boy's eyes narrowed slightly, and Kester felt a pressure like a weight on his tongue, and he added, "But I was born in New Orleans." *Stop it. Stop talking. What's happening?* But he knew. With a chill down his spine, he knew. He'd never spent much time around other witches, and when he did, he'd always had his guard up. But it hadn't occurred to him that a child could be a threat, so he hadn't thought twice about being around him while his magic was bound up.

"Tell me... why you want to know me."

His son's will was clumsy and unrefined, but without magic to give Kester's will substance, the boy's still pushed right through Kester's mental defense as if he had none at all. Officer Parkes hadn't been particularly susceptible to it. Landon was simply that good. "You intrigue me."

"Because I'm a witch?"

"Yes." It was the truth, of a sort, and Landon didn't push for more. But with each question, the boy was getting closer and closer to secrets Kester wanted to keep well hidden. Panic began to build in Kester's chest. He needed to stop this. He tried to break eye contact, but his eyelids wouldn't close and his head wouldn't turn. But he had some control of his arm. With a great deal of effort, he lifted it.

"Tell me—"

Kester laid his hand on Landon's head and physically turned it away from him. As soon as eye contact was broken, Kester gained full control over his body and looked away. "That wasn't very nice," he said gently, then stopped to calm his breathing and racing pulse.

"Sorry," said the boy.

"No, you're not." When the boy remained silent, Kester risked a peek out of the corner of his eye.

Landon was looking at the dashboard with a small grin on his face. "It felt good."

"Controlling me?"

"Yes."

Another chill ran down Kester's spine. "You need to promise never to do that to me again. Or I won't teach you anymore."

Landon's eyes went wide with fear, and he nodded. "I won't. I promise. Are you mad at me?"

Kester tried to give him a reassuring smile. "No. Go on, though. You're already late for class."

Landon left obediently, and Kester watched him run to the school building in his tiny, clumsy body.

Six years old, and already he had so much power. Kester had never been so proud and terrified of another person.

But why should it scare him? Landon had done nothing other than what Kester had taught him to do, only one of the many things Kester had done on a regular basis for decades.

It was because this time, Kester was on the receiving end of it. He never had been before. He didn't like it.

Is this what it's like? he wondered. He thought of all the women he'd coerced over the years with small—or not so small—nudges of his will on their mind, justifying himself that they never complained afterward. Of the men and women and sometimes children that he manipulated in myriad ways when it suited him, thinking such small things harmless. And they were, by some measures of 'harm'. Most likely, they hadn't even been aware of his manipulations. But he was.

Magic could do many, many things, though it did have its limitations. Manipulation, control, temptation, persuasion… He couldn't count the ways and types of magic he'd used to get what he wanted in life, regardless of the cost to others.

For the first time in his life, Kester asked himself, *Am I a bad person?*

———

After knocking on every business and residential door in town, Jacqueline was at her wit's end. No one recognized her picture of Trick as a cat or knew anything about a lost black kitten, and the police still hadn't found him as a human. She'd circled back to nearly all the doors that had gone unanswered on her first time around, which had led to nothing. So after picking Landon up from school and bringing him home, she consulted her notes one more time, in case there was anything she'd missed.

She found her reminder about the suspicious-acting girl from the shop who lived in the blue house. It wasn't much at all, but she had nothing else to go on right now. It was worth at least driving by to see if she could get anyone else to answer the door.

It was late in the afternoon when she drove up to the house, parking on the side street. She grabbed the photo of Trick as a cat and made her way toward the front door, hoping that one of the girl's parents was home this time. She'd gone by the girl's family's shop and asked around, but the owners were unavailable, and she'd only been able to get the young salesman to look at the photo. Maybe if she'd waited until evening, she'd have had better odds that one of the girl's parents would be home to ask, but she hadn't been patient enough. If they weren't here now, she could stake the place out and catch them when they came home.

The sidewalk paralleled a tall, wooden fence outlining the house's back yard. As she strode past, a voice froze her steps as instantly as if she'd walked into wet cement.

"Trick, come down from there!" It was a girl's voice, whisper-shouting. If there had been any traffic on the street, Jacqueline might not have caught it. "You don't want to get stuck up there!"

Rather than a boy's voice, the response was a loud meow.

Maybe the girl had been lying, after all. The girl's description matched that of the person the vet had told Jacqueline had brought in a black cat. It isn't so strange for a kid to find a stray animal and want to keep it as a pet, even if they know someone else is searching for it.

Jacqueline went to the side gate of the wooden fence, reached over the top, and hoisted herself high enough to see over it.

The girl was in the back yard, shouting at something in a tree. Jacqueline could see movement and shaking branches, then nothing else at first. Suddenly, a hawk flew out of the branches and landed on the edge of the roof. Hot on its heels, a small blur of black leapt out after it.

In midair, the black kitten transformed into a teen boy. Jacqueline lost her grip on the fence and fell to the ground. Relief flooded her body and made her weak. Trick was here. Her son was safe.

"Trick!" the girl yelped. "Stop it!"

Jacqueline's relief was soon replaced by anger, annoyance, and worry. She pulled herself back up to look over the fence. Her son—buck naked, of course—was jumping up and down by the side of the house, trying to grab at the hawk which remained well out of his reach.

"I can get it!" he insisted to the girl.

The hawk preened itself, unconcerned.

"If you're going to be human, put your clothes on!" the girl hissed at him, her face turning read. Even odds on it being from anger or embarrassment.

That's enough of this. Jacqueline put on her *you're in so much trouble, young man* face and loudly cleared her throat.

Trick stopped jumping and spun toward her, a guilty look of fear frozen on his face. The girl just gaped at Jacqueline, her mouth opening and closing, unable to land on something to say.

"Shall we take this inside?" Jacqueline suggested.

CHAPTER
SEVENTEEN

After witnessing that scene outside, Jacqueline wasn't surprised to learn that none of the girl's family members were home.

"Mom's still at the shop, and Dad took Jonah to the doctor," the girl said. She was sitting on a love seat with her hands folded in her lap and her eyes locked on her fiddling fingers. Trick sat beside her, dressed in clothes Jacqueline didn't recognize.

"Do any of them know about this?" Jacqueline asked, bracing herself for the worst.

The girl shook her head. "Jonah knows I've been hiding a kitten in my room, but that's it. Neither of my parents know anything."

Jacqueline let out a breath. At least the girl had contained the situation reasonably well. "Denneka, isn't it?" The girl nodded. "Thank you for looking after my son. I'm sorry for the trouble I'm sure he's caused you."

Denneka looked at her with surprise. "Oh! Um... it's okay."

"Mom!" Trick protested. "I didn't cause any trouble."

"You're my son. I know you well enough to know that you've caused her trouble." The girl's pointed lack of coming to Trick's defense said all Jacqueline needed to know. "Do you have any idea how worried I was?"

"How worried?"

"Very worried! Although"—she had to be fair—"I had a feeling you were in a situation like this. So I wasn't as worried as I might have been. And no, that does not get you off the hook!"

"What do you mean?" Denneka asked.

"As soon as Trick went missing, I called around at vets and shelters. One of them said a girl had brought in a black kitten. It was nothing conclusive, but I hoped that it meant someone had found him and was taking care of him."

"You're not mad at me for keeping him here?"

Jacqueline sighed. "I'm mad at you for lying to me when I came around earlier. Has he been changing from cat to human the whole time?"

Denneka shook her head. "He was a cat for about a week straight. I didn't know he was Trick at all."

"Where did you find him?"

"I didn't find him. He came here."

Jacqueline raised her eyebrows at her son. "You came here? Instead of coming home?"

"Home was too far!" Trick said. "The hawk was chasing me!"

"It wasn't chasing you," Denneka said reasonably. "It was only following you."

"I know that *now*!"

"Hang on," Jacqueline told them. "What hawk? That one you were playing with outside?"

"Yes!"

The girl was more informative. "It's not really a hawk. It's a familiar, like Trick was."

Dread rumbled through Jacqueline's stomach. *I try to get us out, but we keep getting dragged back in.* "What do you mean? How do you know? Whose familiar?"

"The witch who changed me again," Trick said.

"Witch?" Jacqueline repeated in horror.

"I figured it out when Trick explained what had happened to him when he was a kid, then when we saw the hawk," Denneka said.

"What witch?" Jacqueline's voice was hoarse.

"Trick says there's a male witch who changed him into a cat at school that day. He doesn't know who he is, though."

She'd been afraid it was something like this, but she'd really hoped it was the original spell acting up or something. She'd brought them to a new town to get *away* from all this magic crap. How had more of it found them so quickly? "A witch is messing with Trick again, and that hawk is his familiar?" she asked in a dark tone.

Maybe a little too dark, because Denneka edged away from her slightly and Trick went stiff. "Yeah," said the girl.

Jacqueline bolted out of her seat and stormed into the back yard. She made a bee-line for the perch where she'd last seen the hawk, but it wasn't there. It wasn't in the tree, either, at least not that she could see. "Hawk!" she shouted at the sky. "Come back here! I want to talk to you!"

The hawk didn't show itself. Maybe it had flown back to its master.

She waited a few more minutes, then returned to the room where her son and his friend were still waiting patiently. "It's gone."

"It's not always here," Denneka offered quietly. "But it's here a lot. I think it's been watching Trick."

Which means it'll be back later, Jacqueline thought. *Then I can catch it, or maybe follow it back to its master.*

"Is it dinnertime yet?" Trick asked.

"We're in the middle of something, Trick," Denneka told him.

"But I'm hungry."

Denneka sighed. "I can probably grab something quick. If that's okay, Mrs.—um, Jacqueline."

Watching the exchange between them curiously, Jacqueline nodded. When the girl got up to go the kitchen, Trick trailed after her like a puppy. He wasn't right on her tail but stayed just far enough away for her to work without bumping into him. She pulled something out of the freezer, microwaved it, then wrapped it in a paper towel and handed it to him.

"Let it cool," she suggested.

Trick immediately bit into the sandwich, made a pained sound, then held it out and glared at it. Denneka shook her head indulgently and led him back to the love seat. When Trick sat down next to her, he sat closely enough that their shoulders were touching.

"So Trick was a cat for a week," Jacqueline said. "How did he turn human again?"

Trick was busy taking bites of the sandwich and trying to cool them off in his mouth, so Denneka answered. "I don't know. I just, um, woke up one day and he was human." A healthy blush spread across her face and down her neck.

"The witch didn't bother making a spell that allowed him to transform back already wearing clothes, I gather." She'd seen that much outside.

"Nooo," the girl said awkwardly.

When Trick had first become human again, he'd shown no sense of modesty whatsoever. Jacqueline doubted he'd learned any since then. A chuckle escaped her at the poor girl's plight. "I'm so sorry about him."

"He's getting better about it," she murmured.

"On his own?" Jacqueline asked with a surge of hope. If he was developing a sense of modesty, maybe—

"No. But he'll usually listen to me when I tell him to get dressed, and he knows to do it before I come in the room."

So much for that. "Why didn't you contact me as soon as he started turning human? You must have known I'd have come to get him."

"I told him to go home," she said. "I told him you'd want him to. But..."

"But?"

"But he asked me to let him stay. He said he liked it here."

Jacqueline considered the two of them, not sure what to say about that or how angry to be. Trick finished his sandwich, dropped the paper towel on the coffee table, and bent his head to nudge Denneka's shoulder with it. As if it was automatic, the girl moved her hand to pet his head. As she did so, Trick's eyes drifted closed in pleasure.

Denneka caught Jacqueline watching and realized what she was doing. She jerked her hand down and pushed Trick away.

"Well, thank you again for taking care of him," Jacqueline told her. "And thank you for keeping his secret. It means a lot. I'll take him off your hands now."

Trick shot her a glare. "No."

"Trick," Jacqueline said firmly, "it's time to go home."

"I don't want to."

Jacqueline sighed at her petulant son, but before she could order him into the car, Denneka spoke up.

"Um, I don't know that he *can* go home."

"What do you mean?"

"Well, um, you saw him transform out in the yard, right?"

"Yes."

"That's not random. He changes back into a cat when he gets more than ten feet away from me, and into a human when he gets closer than that."

Jacqueline stared in bewilderment at the girl, processing what she'd said. "Why?"

Denneka shrugged. "I guess that's how the witch made the spell work this time."

"Why?" Jacqueline asked again.

"I... I don't know."

"You're sure about this?"

"I tested it, yeah. Whenever I go to school, he stays in my room as a cat. Then he turns human again when I get home. I have to be careful how far away from him I get, though."

Jacqueline rubbed at the sudden tension in her forehead. "So if I take him home, he'll be a cat all the time." *At least until I can track down the witch and make him remove the spell.*

For seven years, Jacqueline had waited to get her human son back. He'd lost seven years of his life to that old woman. No, Jacqueline had used those seven years of Trick's life to pay for all of Landon's. That was on her. And while she couldn't bring herself to regret that decision, she had so badly wanted to put it behind them. Her rambunctious, brave boy who'd been forever digging in the dirt, splashing in puddles, and climbing up trees had become someone who didn't even want to be human anymore. Even if it meant keeping him close and safe at home, letting him continue to be a cat was the last thing Jacqueline wanted.

But it was exactly what Trick wanted.

So why is he refusing to come home?

Trick pulled his legs up and hugged his knees, leaning casually against Denneka.

"If Trick is a human whenever you're around," Jacqueline asked her, "then where does he sleep?"

The girl blushed deep red, and Jacqueline had her answer.

"She made me sleep on the floor," Trick said, "then in the closet. But those were uncomfortable, so she lets me sleep in the bed again now."

Somehow, Denneka's blush managed to deepen. "I didn't know what else to do. He kept crawling in during the night anyway."

"He isn't misbehaving, is he?" Jacqueline addressed her question to the girl, not sure her son would understand what she was asking.

"No, not—not like that! He's fine! He, uh, kinda crowds me, but he doesn't mean anything by it."

When is a boy not a boy? Jacqueline asked herself. Thirteen was a confusing enough age for anyone, but for a boy who believed himself to be a cat? Something about this girl made him willing to be human to stay near her. Even if he didn't know why, even if he didn't see her the way a boy sees a girl, could that be enough to draw him closer to choosing to be human?

The girl evidently wanted to hurry on from the topic of Trick's sleeping arrangements, because she didn't wait for Jacqueline's response before saying, "I'm helping him keep up on homework and stuff."

"Oh?"

"He'll need to go back to school eventually, right? So I'm making him help with homework."

"You're an extremely responsible girl, aren't you?"

"What? No. Not really. I don't think so."

Responsible enough to take care of Trick like a good pet owner and keep up his studies like a good guardian. Strong-willed enough to discipline Trick and draw boundaries for him. Kind enough to make him want to stay by her side.

This might help, Jacqueline decided. *Though her parents will kill me if they ever find out.*

"It sounds like there's no choice but to let Trick stay here for the time being," Jacqueline said.

Trick perked up. "Really?"

"For now, yes. Under certain conditions."

He frowned. "More conditions."

Jacqueline ignored that comment. Learning to live by rules was an important part of being human, so she wouldn't relent on that count. "First, Denneka's family must not find out you're here, especially in your human form. If they find out, all of us are going to be in very serious trouble. Do you understand? This is absolutely critical."

"I know," he groused. "I'm not stupid."

Denneka nodded fervently. "Believe me, I know. I've been very careful to keep him hidden."

"Second, tutoring at home isn't enough. I want Trick to go to school."

Trick leaned closer to Denneka like he was trying to hide behind her.

"How?" Denneka asked. "My parents are home in the morning sometimes, and it's not like we can get on the bus here. Everyone would figure out we're living together pretty quickly."

"We'll work out the timing. Let him out the window if you have to. The two of you can walk somewhere, and I can pick you up and drive you to school. As long as none of your classmates actually stake out your house, they shouldn't know that he's living here."

"But we have one class period where our classes are different," she said.

"Let me know which, and I'll see if I can change his schedule. Otherwise, you might need to try to change yours. Are they required classes?"

"No. Electives."

"Then we might be able to work it out."

"But we'll have to stay within ten feet of each other all day!" The girl looked positively panicked at the idea. "What if something happens and he turns into a cat in front of everyone?"

"It's certainly a challenge, but I think you're up to it." It was a risk, but Trick needed to experience being human for more than a few hours a day and more than around a single person. "Do you agree, Trick?"

He refused to look at her, staring outside as if utterly bored, but after a few seconds, he gave a single, terse nod.

Jacqueline had to work to hide her shock. He was not only willing to be human, but willing to go to *school* to stay near Denneka? Did either of them have any idea how big a deal that was?

"Third," Jacqueline counted off, "we'll need to tell the police a story for why you're back. I'll work something out, but I'll need you —and possibly you, too, Denneka—to play along. If Trick's going back to school, obviously everyone won't keep thinking he's been kidnapped, and they'll all want to know what happened. Even if he weren't going back to school, I couldn't in good conscience keep taking up people's time looking for him or helping me out under false pretenses." She'd need to tell John soon. Was there any chance he'd be willing to babysit for her sometimes under normal conditions? She didn't have much to pay for childcare, but it would be a shame to lose someone Landon was familiar with and was beginning to adapt to. But that was a question for later.

Both kids agreed to playing along with her story without argument.

"One last condition, but this one's only for Denneka."

The girl looked surprised and slightly panicked. Jacqueline cocked a finger to beckon her closer, and she crept around the coffee table and bent close so Jacqueline could whisper.

"I'll trust your judgment on this, Denneka. When you get the impression that Trick is starting to treat you as a boy treats a girl rather than as a cat treats its master, tell me right away. I may not be the most old-fashioned mom in the world, but I do have some sense of propriety."

Denneka's face pinked. "I don't think he—"

"Promise me."

She nodded.

"Okay, then." Jacqueline sat back. "I've probably been here too long already, if we're going to maintain secrecy about all this. Trick, be good." She made sure Denneka had her number in her phone, then left her son in the girl's hands.

The weight of Trick's disappearance was lifted from her shoulders, but there was a fire inside her that didn't let up. She'd achieved the goal of finding him, but now she had a new one: finding the witch and making him turn Trick human for good.

———

Landon was still reading in the living room when Mom came home.

"Are you okay?" she asked him as she took off her jacket and put her stuff down. "Any problems?" She worried too much. What trouble did she think he'd get into if she left him home alone for an hour or two?

"No," he said. "I'm fine."

"Good." Mom sat beside him on the couch and put an arm around his shoulders. "I've got good news. I found Trick. He's perfectly fine."

Landon was so surprised and relieved, he closed his book to look at her. "You did?"

She squeezed him and smiled. "Yes. The ornery little brat has been hiding out with a girl all this time."

"What girl?"

"That girl from the shop. Do you remember meeting her? She's in his class, and it looks like he's gotten attached to her."

Landon vaguely remembered meeting a girl at the shop. Why on earth would Trick go to her house and stay there? "Does he not like us anymore?"

She laughed. "No, it's not that. It's a bit complicated to explain, but it all happened because what I suspected was right. He'd been turned into a cat again. Only now, he's changing back and forth, and he has to stay near the girl, so I told him he could as long as he didn't get caught."

That didn't sound like something Mom would agree to at all. But Landon knew there was a lot of stuff she didn't explain to him, so she must have had her reasons. "He's changing into a cat?"

She pulled away from him and frowned. "Yes. Apparently there's another witch out there, and for some reason he reactivated the spell on Trick. Or put a new one on. Or something. Who knows?"

"He?" Landon repeated.

"Trick says it's a man."

Mr. McKenzie. Landon was certain. It *could* have been someone else, but the odds of that were very low.

"What... are you going to do?" he asked.

"I'm going to find that witch and make him put Trick back to normal," Mom said in a hard, threatening voice.

"How?" he asked.

"I don't know yet, but I'll find him. If he thinks he can get away with toying with my son like that, he's got another think coming."

I should tell her, Landon thought. A good boy would tell her.

But Landon knew he wouldn't. He was too eager to learn as much as he could about magic from Mr. McKenzie. If his mom knew the teacher was the witch, not only would she refuse to let Landon see him again, she might move all of them to another town to escape him. So he kept quiet.

He'd always been his mom's good boy, but he wasn't anymore.

e, then?

———

After i. inexcusable failure this afternoon, Julia kept watc
Denneka's house until the very last minute she could. Trick h
gone home with his mother, so Julia had watched to see if
would return for him later. Only when the sun had gotten so lc
that Julia began to fear she'd transform mid-flight and fall to he
death did she abandon her post to go home.

She'd barely flown through the open kitchen window when she
regained her human body. Turning the fall into a roll, she was back
on her feet in an instant and searching for her master.

Kester sat in an armchair in the living room, staring into the fire
with a glass of bourbon in one hand.

Julia went to him and fell to her knees, bowing her head to him.

"What is this?" he said in a distracted way.

"I failed, Master," she told him, keeping her head bowed. "I'm
ready to accept my punishment." Whatever it was, she knew it
wouldn't be horrible. Kester was never cruel.

"Failed how?"

He didn't usually force her to admit her failings, not when they
both already knew what they were. He usually gave her that mercy.
Maybe she'd angered him more than usual. "I got distracted playing
with the kitten boy. I failed to see his mother approach. Because of
this, she discovered him."

Kester let out a long sigh. It sounded... sad. Worse than sad.
Anguished. That wasn't like him at all. A stab of worry pierced her
heart, but she kept her submissive pose.

His finger reached out to lift her chin. The face she loved was
somehow both sad and expressionless. "Julia. Dearest one. You did
nothing wrong. You couldn't have stopped Jacqueline if you'd
tried."

"But—"

"Get up. Get dressed."

303

and took a shower before putting on her pajamas and
while worrying. What was wrong with him? Was it
she could fix?

she returned to the living room, she found he hadn't
at all. She sat in her usual seat across from him. She wanted
what was wrong, but she knew he felt her worry for him. She
t need to ask.

"Julia," he said, staring into the glass of bourbon which had
ardly been touched, "am I a bad person?"

"No. Why would you say that?"

"Let me rephrase. Has my use of magic made me a worse person
than I might otherwise be?"

That was an entirely different question, and one Julia couldn't
immediately answer. "Why are you asking?"

"I taught the boy how to manipulate a man's mind today," he
said. "It went well. He's very good at it. A natural. He liked using
his power. So much that he turned it against me."

Julia's mouth fell open in shock. Not that the boy could do such
a thing—she knew how Kester's magic was locked away when he
wore his disguise—but that he would. Kester was her master, and
the thought of anyone attacking him made her want to fight them,
child or not.

Kester answered her emotional response. "Don't think so badly
of him. He's only six. He didn't mean it as an attack. I'd taught him
a trick, and he wanted to try it out again. I happened to be the most
convenient one to try it out on. That's all."

"If you're not angry at him about it, then what's troubling you?"
she asked.

Instead of answering her, he took a sip of his bourbon and said,
"Tell me about how we met."

Her confusion was immediate and intense. Had the boy's manipulation of his mind caused Kester to lose some of his memory?

Kester smiled wryly. He hadn't looked at her once since she'd re-
entered the room, and he still didn't. "I remember it. I want to hear
your version."

It was a bittersweet memory, and not one she wanted to dwell on, but her master had given her a command, so she had to comply. "I was eleven. My mother had died years before, and my father had just found out he had terminal cancer. He'd tried all the doctors and medical treatments he could, but it was only getting worse. He'd been told he had only months to live. Somehow, he heard a rumor about a witch living in a motor home in the woods. He dragged me out of my bed one night and threw me in the car. It was a long drive. So long I fell asleep. I woke to him grabbing me by the arm and dragging me to your door. We were both surprised to see the witch was a teenager. I think my father nearly gave up right then. But he was desperate. You let us inside and talked to him. I don't remember much about what the two of you said. I was scared. The motor home was cramped and filled with strange things and an unpleasant smell. Neither of you looked at me while you talked, except once. You looked at me once. I was a scared kid, and you were strange, so you creeped me out." She didn't like telling him that, but he'd asked for her version of events, so she had to tell it as truthfully as she could. "When you went into the back, I was glad to see you go, but I didn't know why we were waiting. It seemed like a long time, but maybe it was only minutes. Then you came back and handed my father a glass jar. He didn't give you any money, only looked at me with guilt in his eyes. I'd never seen my father express guilt about anything before. That was when I understood that I was being sold. I cried and asked him why, but he didn't look at me again. You didn't look at me either. You both ignored me as you kept talking, and I kept crying. My father left without even saying goodbye or giving me another glance. Then you looked at me again, and I was terrified. I was too young to even know what to be afraid of, but I was so scared I thought I'd die from it. But you spoke to me kindly and gave me food and a soft place on the floor to sleep.

"Near morning, you woke me up, gave me breakfast, and told me about the spell you'd put on me in my sleep. That I would turn into an animal. It sounded like something out of a movie. Amazing but ridiculous. Then the sun rose, and I turned into a bird. I was so cared and confused that when you tried to take me in your hands, I scratched you with my talons. But you were patient and didn't punish me. You did another spell, the one to make me your familiar, and explained what that meant. I didn't understand that, either, but I could feel the connection to you and could hear your voice in my head. You helped me learn how to fly, then set me free. I didn't know you could find me if you wanted to. I just soared through the sky. It was exhilarating. I felt freer than I ever had before. All my fear of you vanished because you'd made it so I could fly.

"I did try to fly home. Not because I missed it but... out of instinct, I guess. I flew for miles and miles, following the road that I could tell led to my home. Then I saw the accident scene and my father's car smashed on the side of the road. There were people around, and I perched in a tree to listen to them talk. My father's body had already been taken away. I didn't feel sad. I felt... happy. Awfully, terribly happy.

"When I came back to you, you were happy to see me, and that made me even more happy because my father had never been happy to see me. I wanted to tell you about what I'd seen, but you already knew, and you explained that it was because of our bond. That's when it really sank in that I could never get away from you, but also that I'd never really be alone. It was scary, but it felt good, too. You told me that most witches don't let their familiars be human at all, that they change them into an animal and leave them that way their whole lives, but you didn't have any need for an animal familiar when you're sleeping, so you let me go back to being human at night. When dusk came, you set out my clothes, which you'd washed and dried, and gave me privacy to change, then gave me dinner.

"You were kind and gentle, and you gave me everything I ever needed. Pretty soon I couldn't even remember why I'd been afraid of you at first." When Julia finished, she felt a little embarrassed. She'd probably made that whole thing more flowery than it needed to be. Maybe she'd talked about her feelings too much. She waited in silence for him to tell her why he'd wanted to hear all that.

After a long, long moment, he said, "You were right to fear me." He took a sip of bourbon, considered the glass, then had another before continuing. "I was eighteen, Julia. I was well acquainted with women by that point, but I was also impatient. I thought it might be handy to have one I didn't have to hunt down whenever I wanted to have some fun. That was why I crafted the spell so you'd be human at night. Not out of kindness or mercy or consideration. I planned to enslave you in my bed at night just as I enslave you for everything else during the day."

His words and the harshness in his tone bit at her heart and made her wince. When he didn't go on right away, she said, "I know."

He met her gaze sharply. "What?"

"I figured that out a long time ago, Kester."

"Why did you never say anything?"

"Because by the time I figured it out, I was in my late teens, and you would have started doing it by then if that had still been your plan."

He let out a long breath. "I see. And you don't hate me for it, knowing that all my supposed kindness when we first met was nothing but a predator grooming his prey." It hadn't been a question because he knew full well she didn't hate him. The implied question he didn't speak seemed to be, 'Why?'

"I could never hate you, Kester. The kindness then may have been fake—though I don't believe it entirely was—but how do you explain the kindness since then? Why did you change your plan?"

"I could say that it's because I realized that if I hurt you, I would feel it. If you hated me, I wouldn't be able to ignore it. And if you resented me, you'd be a bad servant."

"But none of those are the reason."

He set the glass on the table beside his chair and gazed at her, his face beautiful and woeful in the firelight. "I never knew what it felt like to love anything before I met you. It happened before I knew it, and when I finally realized you'd grown into a woman's body, you were far too dear to me to use that way. I would kill myself before destroying our friendship and companionship for a quick bout of pleasure. They're too precious to me. *You* are too precious to me."

Her heart was full to bursting with happiness and love for this man. But also sadness. "And what about the others?"

"What others?"

"All of them. All the other women in the world. Are they not precious? Are they not worthy of more than 'a quick bout of pleasure'?"

He closed his eyes in pain, his face pinching as if she'd just stuck a long needle in him. "Therein lies the problem." He reached for his glass and raised it but didn't drink. "I've had something of an epiphany. My son has given me a taste of what it's like to be on the receiving end of another's selfish, thoughtless manipulation. And I'm afraid I've come to an unpleasant realization."

"Which is?"

"Other people are... people."

Julia could hardly believe her ears. Had he really just said...

A laugh burst out of her, and she crossed the space between them in a moment, took his head between her hands, and kissed him on the forehead, the cheeks, every spot on his face she could find—except his mouth; that would have been too far—and didn't stop until he grabbed her forearms to forcibly stop her.

"Julia! Julia! What on earth's gotten into you?"

She pulled out of his grip enough to squeeze his hands in hers. "Kester, you have no idea how long I've been wanting to hear you say that."

He looked away in embarrassment. It was an extremely rare and extremely adorable look on him. "Have I really set that low a bar?"

"Please don't belittle my master. I have a lot of respect for him."

He dropped her hands. "I can't imagine why."

Because he's the man I love, she thought. She didn't want to make things awkward or push things too far by saying it, but her desire to do so and the love she felt was something that she knew would travel across their bond back to him. She never needed to tell him she loved him because she knew he felt it coming from her.

But, as always, he chose to pretend he didn't. He shooed her back into her seat, and she complied. But she couldn't help the pang of hurt she felt at his rejection.

Is it because I'm too precious to you? she thought. *Or is it because you don't even want me?* As a hawk, she was fierce and beautiful, but as a woman...

She forced herself to stop that train of thought. Kester was feeling enough sadness and uncertainty of his own right now. He didn't need her thrusting hers on him as well.

"I know you have opinions on how I live my life," he told her. "And I know I haven't exactly invited criticism. But I want to know your thoughts, dearest one. What is wrong with me? Where have I erred?"

"Other than with women?"

"Other than with women."

Julia took a deep, bracing breath. It was not her place to criticize her master. But he'd asked, so... "The children."

"Which children?"

Julia rolled her eyes. She knew he wasn't that dense. "The ones you've sired."

"Oh. Them." He looked ashamed. That was probably a good thing.

"How many are there?"

"Only seven. That I'm sure of."

"And how many have you bothered showing any interest in?"

"Three."

"Because?"

"Because those were the ones who showed signs of being witches."

"And how many of those have you bothered to actually meet?"

He was quiet, almost pouting.

"How many?"

"One."

"Why?"

He mumbled something.

"What was that?"

"Because the others weren't good enough."

"And because the others didn't have another family member to keep you entertained long enough for you to watch them develop their magic."

Kester examined his fingernails. "You're saying I'm a terrible father. I don't disagree."

"I'm saying you're irresponsible and you haven't even been trying."

"No," he countered. "I really am a terrible father. I've barely entered Landon's life, and already I fear I've led him down the wrong path."

"Why do you think that?"

He switched to tapping his fingers on the armrest and staring into the fire. "You didn't answer me earlier. When I asked if you thought my use of magic made me a worse person. I'd like to know your answer."

Julia considered it. "I think… it's possible."

A line formed between his eyebrows. Maybe he hadn't expected that answer.

"Magic came to you early, and I think it made getting what you wanted too easy."

"That's exactly what magic is for."

"Then… maybe magic isn't such a great thing."

He looked at her as if she'd just said maybe breathing was overrated. "Explain."

"I'm not a witch, so I can't really say. But if you think you've erred by treating people badly, and the thing that made it so easy for you to treat people badly was magic, then maybe magic hasn't been such a great thing for you."

Kester bit the end of his thumb and stared into the fire without moving or speaking for so long that eventually Julia quietly slipped away to go to bed. He didn't seem to notice her leave.

CHAPTER
EIGHTEEN

Marcus closed the book of mugshots and set it on the stack with the rest of them. He'd gone through all his department had and had begun requesting nearby districts to send him copies of theirs, but it was taking a while. Since he was sure the chief wouldn't believe he could remember enough with certainty to make a positive ID, he had to squeeze it in around everything else he was doing.

He wasn't even sure he *could* make a positive ID, since there'd been some distance and shadows, and he'd been on the floor. But he had to try.

An e-mail popped up on his computer screen. Finally, he had access to the date range he'd requested for Haug's financial records. Sometimes he couldn't believe the amount of red tape and paperwork involved in being a cop. He printed out the records—it was always easier for him to scan and cross-check stuff like this in hard copy—and laid them out on his desk.

After half an hour of studying them along with the more recent records they already had, Marcus had a pretty good idea why Haug had been killed.

Gathering the records and his notes, he went to the chief's office.

"What have you got?" the chief asked.

Marcus handed him the papers. "Haug's financials. There wasn't enough there to see at first, but if you go back further, it's pretty obvious." The chief flipped through the papers, but Marcus explained it anyway. "Haug had a gambling problem. A year ago, he was deep in debt. Eight months ago, all the debt got paid off, and he started making payments to an unspecified recipient. He started digging himself back into debt right away, and the mystery payment amount gradually decreased until four months ago, when the payments stopped completely."

The chief nodded as he verified Marcus's description for himself. "That simple, huh?"

"Looks like. He borrowed money from the wrong people, stopped paying them back, and they killed him."

The chief handed the papers back to him. "Good work. See what you can find about who he borrowed from."

Marcus turned to go, already dreading the report he'd have to write now while everything was fresh. He should call Lisa before he got bogged down in that, though. She'd want to know as soon—

The chief's voice stopped him with his hand on the doorknob. "Tell Lisa hello for me."

Marcus turned slowly to face his boss.

The chief waved a dismissive hand. "I'm well aware of your... let's say *friendship* with my niece. And I don't care. Even if she's getting information out of you that she couldn't get from the rest of us, she's not a reporter or gossip. This case does involve her, at least peripherally. I trust her judgment and discretion. If I didn't, I'd have done something to stop you talking to her."

The sudden tightness in Marcus's chest gave way, and he let out a breath. "Roger that." As he left, Marcus had to smirk at the old man's reminder that his people couldn't get away with anything he didn't allow.

Once at his desk, he called Lisa, not bothering to try to hide it from his partner across their desks. "I have news," Marcus told her. "And your uncle says hello."

There was the sound of an amused puff of breath through her nose. "Of course he does. What is it?"

Marcus updated her and asked if she knew anything about Haug's gambling problem.

"No, I didn't." There was a long pause before she said in a voice so uncertain that it didn't sound anything like her, "Maybe I should start getting a little more personal with my employees. If I'd known he had a problem like that, maybe I could have gotten him help."

"He was a grown man, Lisa. He made his own choices." Addiction was a serious issue, but it was no good letting her sink into survivor's guilt about it, or whatever it was called when things like this happened. "Have you seen any sign of the suspect around the school?"

"No. John hasn't mentioned seeing anything either."

John. John McKenzie. The man he'd... met? At the park. "How well do you know him? McKenzie, I mean."

"Not well, since he just started and he's brand new to town. He's too harsh with the students sometimes, but he seems normal enough and expressed concern when I told him about the possible threat to Denneka. Though to be honest, now isn't the best time to ask me my opinion about anyone's character. I'm starting to doubt I can tell anything about people at all."

He wished he knew what to say to get her mind off Haug, but no matter how long they'd known each other or how intimate they got physically, she would always keep him at arm's length in other ways. That was just how she was. "Do you think I was overreacting about the danger to the girl?"

"No. But even if you were, when it comes to my students, I'd always rather overreact than underreact."

"Yeah. Me, too. Did you tell her parents?"

"Almost. But no. With her family running that shop and all the people that come and go through there, it wouldn't take much for something to accidentally slip, and then... well, what with Trick missing already, a lot of parents could make a lot of fuss. Between that and whatever my uncle would do to punish you for letting it get out, it would only take focus and manpower away from actually catching the bad guy, which would only put Denneka in more danger."

Marcus was surprised by her decision, but after hearing what the chief had said about her, he shouldn't have been. *He knows her better than I do*, he thought ruefully.

"Thanks for updating me," she said, "but if that's all, I have work to do."

"Okay. Talk to you later, Lisa."

The next day and a half went by quickly. With more solid leads than ever, Marcus and the rest of the squad worked a lot of hours to try to track down Haug's killer and the boy who was still missing. He got home so late on Friday night that all he could do was take off his shoes and collapse, then it was right back at it Saturday morning. Luckily, Saturday saw him catch another break.

He was still on his first cup of coffee since getting to the station when his phone rang. "This is Parkes."

"Officer Parkes. Hi. I had your business card from when you and your partner were at my house the other day."

Marcus wasn't great with names, but he could remember voices pretty well, especially ones that sounded like music and belonged to beautiful redheads. "Right. You're Trick's mother. How can I help you?"

"Well, it's about Trick." She didn't sound nearly as worried as she'd been when he and David had gone to her house after her son went missing. "He's home."

Marcus almost spilled his coffee. "He is?"

"Yeah. He came in last night. Apparently he wasn't kidnapped at all." She said that with an annoyed intensity that meant she was probably glaring at Trick as she spoke. "He'd just gotten sick of school and ran off to a different town. I guess a couple weeks on the streets made him rethink how unbearable it was to live under my rules."

"That's great! I mean—not that he ran off, but—it's great that he's back." Marcus felt almost lightheaded with relief. He'd had actual nightmares about finding that boy's corpse. "Do you mind if I come over and talk to him?"

Her voice went up an octave. "Come over?"

"Yeah. I'd like to get the details squared away so I can close his case, but I'd also like to ask him some things about the murder case we're working on. That girl told us he's the one who found the body, but I'd really like to hear it from him."

There was a pause, then the woman—(What was her name? He'd have to check his notes.)—said in a measured tone, "Okay. But can you give me an hour to get the house cleaned up for company? If it's not urgent."

Fifty minutes later, Marcus knocked on her front door. While he waited, he checked his notes again. Jacqueline. She'd asked them to call her Jacqueline.

He heard a stern shout, not loud enough for him to make out the words, and then the door opened and Jacqueline gave him a tired smile.

Marcus swallowed hard, remembering how he'd been so afraid of saying something unprofessional last time that he'd let David do most of the talking. Except David had the day off now, so it was only him. There was something about this woman's looks that reached inside him and shook all the sense loose. "Good morning, Mrs.—uh, I mean—"

"Jacqueline," she said. "Not a missus. Come in, Officer Parkes."

He'd already known she wasn't married; the 'Mrs.' thing had been a slip of the tongue. Funny she thought it worth correcting, though. *No, stop. Focus.* "Call me Marcus." It always felt weird having a conversation that was only one-way formal.

"Okay. Marcus." She glanced past him. "Is your partner not here?"

"Day off."

"Ah." She moved back to let him through.

The house was clean but still littered with unpacked boxes. Jacqueline waved him to a chair in the living room. Trick was already sitting silently on the couch. Marcus had the crazy impulse to go over and touch him to make sure he was real.

For some reason, the girl Marcus had talked to at the station was sitting next to the boy. "It's you," Marcus blurted.

Her eyes darted around like she was afraid she'd been caught somewhere she shouldn't be. "Um, yes. Hi again. Um, sir. Officer."

She's adorable. He remembered how he'd wanted to root for her with that boy and smiled. "Nice to see you again. Denneka, wasn't it?" What with the recent concern over her safety, he was pretty sure he remembered it right.

"Yes. Is it okay I'm here? Trick, uh, asked me to come."

The boy leaned closer to her.

Seems he does like her. Marcus winked at the girl. "I don't mind." He sat and clicked his pen. "Good to meet you, Trick. I'm Officer Parkes."

Jacqueline sat on the boy's other side so that he was sandwiched between the two females. There was something weird about their postures. Casual but stiff, like they were trying to shield him. But then, people did sometimes get weird around cops even when they had no good reason to. Something about the uniform. Made Marcus feel like a hall monitor sometimes. He sat back in his chair and physically relaxed as much as he could to show he wasn't here to come after them for anything.

Trick's bright green eyes stared at him unblinkingly. Not challenging or lifeless. Just… waiting.

Jacqueline nudged him. "Say hello, Trick."

"Hello."

"I'm glad to see you're back, Trick," Marcus said. "We're all really glad you're back. Would you tell me what happened?"

"I ran away."

"What for?"

There was a beat, then Trick's eyes tightened in irritation for half a second, then another beat, then he shrugged stiffly. "The teacher man made me read."

"That's it?"

"The humans were mean. I mean the other humans. They're... scary. So I left."

"O... kay." *Teacher man? Other humans?* Marcus raised an eyebrow at Jacqueline, but she gave him a *what can you do?* sort of half-shrug. "Where did you go?"

"Turnerville," Trick said.

"That's fifty miles away. How did you get there?"

"Hitchhiked."

"What'd you do when you got there?"

"Not much. Sat around. Got hungry. Came back."

"And there wasn't anyone with you? No one hurting you or forcing you to do anything?"

"No."

There was something noticeably rehearsed about the way Trick answered. And the whole 'Greetings, fellow humans' way of speaking was a little creepy. But none of that mattered to Marcus at the moment. The case was that a boy was missing, and now he was back, so the case could be closed. Marcus didn't really care if Trick was an alien or robot or whatever. As long as his mom was sure it was him and didn't want anything followed up on, that was good enough.

"Okay, then." Marcus flipped a page in his notepad. "I was hoping you could help with another case we're working on. Your friend Denneka gave us some information that she said she got from you, and it was really helpful to us. She told us that you'd seen a man named Bradley Haug in a grave. We dug up the grave and found his body. That was a big help to us, and we're working now on finding his killer. But would you mind telling me about what you saw in your own words? Maybe you saw the person who was burying the body?"

When Marcus said 'in your own words', the females bracketing Trick visibly tensed.

Trick himself grew tense as well, his facial muscles tightening, and he seemed to have to work to get the words out. He sounded like he was thinking very hard about each one. "I saw... the big man.... Yes."

"In the graveyard?"

Trick nodded.

"When?"

"I don't know."

Jacqueline put a hand on Trick's knee. "He's not very good with remembering dates or things like that."

Marcus offered a reassuring smile. "Neither am I. That's what this is for." He flashed the notepad.

She looked surprised at his casual response and turned to her son. "Best guess, Trick? It was after we got here but before you started school, right? So... maybe around a month ago?"

Trick gave another jerky shrug. Jacqueline nudged him with her knee. He changed it to a nod.

"Can you describe the man you saw burying Haug's body?" Marcus asked.

"Big."

"Is that it?"

"Really big."

Doesn't have much of an eye for details, does he? Then again, it was a month ago. Marcus considered what to say next. Normally, he shouldn't do what he was considering. If his partner were here, David would probably stop him. Even though they weren't lawyers, 'leading the witness' was usually not a great way to get accurate testimony. But this was an exception. Marcus knew what he'd seen, and if he could get corroboration from Trick on what the suspect looked like, the chief might actually take him seriously. So he described to Trick what he remembered from his own recently-recovered memory of the man who'd broken into the police station. When he finished, he asked Trick, "Does that sound like the man you saw?"

Trick nodded.

"You're sure?"

Another nod.

The kid's face was so blank, Marcus wasn't all that sure he'd actually understood. "I'd appreciate if you could verbally confirm that what I said is an accurate description of the man you saw."

The boy didn't say anything. His mother nudged him. "That is the big man I saw at the grave."

"Thanks. Can you tell me what you were doing there? Did the man see you?"

"Yes," Trick said.

Jacqueline shot the boy a look.

"No," Trick said.

"Trick," Jacqueline hissed under her breath.

What is going on here? Marcus asked himself.

"I can... tell," Trick said, his face tightening again. "I was only... exploring. It was dark. He didn't see... me."

"You're sure he couldn't recognize you if he were to see you again?"

"Yes." No hesitation that time. Did that mean that he wasn't lying when he chose his words carefully?

Maybe he has a speech impediment.

Marcus asked some more questions, but Trick didn't have much else to offer. Everything he told Marcus was information they already had. "I guess that's it," Marcus said when it was clear he wasn't getting anything useful. But as he stood up to go, he caught a glimpse of something around the corner, then heard a shift of movement. He leaned forward to see what it was.

"It's all right," Jacqueline said. "It's only my other son." Then she turned toward where Marcus was looking and said, "Landon, come out already. You shouldn't lurk at police officers."

A small boy with pale blond hair and light blue eyes carefully edged around the corner, watching Marcus like a hawk.

"Sorry to scare you," the boy said.

Marcus laughed and held up his hands. "It's all right, kid. You didn't scare—" A chill of fear crawled down Marcus's spine as something inside his brain recognized the boy. Not in any specific way. There was no name or event or anything. Only the fear.

He lowered his hands, hardly noticing that he'd stopped talking mid-sentence. As he worked to try to place the boy, he remembered seeing him from a distance when they'd investigated the scene of Trick's supposed disappearance.

That's probably it, he thought.

But that wasn't it, and his spiking pulse didn't slow down.

The little boy's expression was starting to turn guilty.

"Landon?" Jacqueline sounded worried. "Marcus? What's going on?" She went to stand behind her younger son, her hands on his shoulders.

Marcus stepped closer to them and asked the boy, "Did I see you with a—"

"Trick!" the boy said. "Wanna play tag outside?"

"Yes!" Trick leapt up from the couch and ran toward the back of the house, Denneka hurrying along after him. The little boy tore away from his mother and followed them out.

Suddenly, Marcus found himself standing alone in the room with Jacqueline. All the confusion and unexplained fear of a little boy faded in embarrassment as he raised his eyes to meet her concerned look. She watched him, wary and calculating.

Marcus laughed awkwardly. "Sorry. Didn't mean that to get weird. I just recognized him and was trying to remember from where."

Her expression softened. "He shouldn't have startled you. He's quiet and stays out of the way, but he doesn't always know when it's better not to do that."

Now that the boy was out of the room, Marcus's brain was working better. He remembered those light blue eyes. The little cherub face. And a splitting headache. For a second, he thought of pressing Jacqueline for anything she knew about it, but his body was coming down from an unexpected rush of fear, and her eyes were smoldering with a languid, mother wolf intensity that was turning him on in ways that could get him in real trouble if he let it continue.

He checked his watch. "Shoot. I need to see the chief before he takes off for a meeting. I appreciate you letting me come and talk to Trick."

She relaxed a little more. "And I appreciate you and all the other police officers doing all you did to try to find him. I'm sorry it was just him being a stupid kid."

Marcus shook his head. "It's nothing. I wish all cases involving kids ended up with it being harmless stupidity."

The intensity in her eyes bored into him like she was trying to crack him open and see what was inside.

He backed toward the door, caught his heel on the carpet and stumbled, then righted himself and kept going. "Anyway, thank you, ma'am."

"Jacqueline," she corrected, opening the door for him.

He dared to make eye contact again. There was a little smile on her face. He returned it before he knew what he was doing. "Jacqueline. Have a nice day."

"You too, Marcus."

———

Been a while since I've met a man like that, Jacqueline thought, watching Marcus go out to his car. She'd noticed his good looks when they'd met before—(How could she not notice a man who looked like one of the heroes from her books?)—but what really caught her was the look he'd been wearing when he talked about cases involving kids. Like he cared. A lot.

She shut the door before he reached his car and pushed thoughts of the hot cop out of her mind. Now that the issue with Trick's non-kidnapping was settled, she had a witch to find.

———

As Kester parked and walked up to Jacqueline's door, he could feel Julia's presence in a tree fifty feet behind and above him. When Jacqueline had appeared at Denneka's house and picked both her nd Trick up, Julia had followed, but Kester didn't want to risk her getting close enough for any of them to spot her. The kids had more or less gotten used to Julia's presence, but he wasn't sure what Jacqueline would do.

"Thanks for coming," Jacqueline greeted him as she let him in. "Sorry for calling on Saturday again."

"I already told you I'm happy to help, and I wasn't busy with anything. But you said you had something to tell me?"

"Yes. This is pretty embarrassing, but—"

A girl's squeal interrupted her, followed by pounding footsteps, then Denneka barreled in from somewhere past the hallway with Trick right behind her. "Trick, no biting!"

Trick didn't listen, chasing her around some furniture, reaching out with one hand to grab her arm and in the same motion pulling it toward his open mouth. He repeated this several times, and she managed to get away from him each time before his teeth more than grazed her. Kester had to put his hand over his own mouth to keep from laughing at them.

Jacqueline grabbed Trick by the collar as he went by, and Denneka stumbled to a halt as soon as she realized he'd been caught. "Trick!" the girl shouted, her eyes blazing. "It's touch tag, not bite tag!"

"That's less fun," Trick muttered, most of his attention now on trying to pull away from his mother.

"Enough!" Jacqueline gave her son a light shake. "Game's over! We have company."

Denneka gave a surprised squeal when she spotted Kester. "Mr. McKenzie?"

Trick glared at him and made a sound approximating a growl until Jacqueline shook him again. When he stopped moving for what she deemed an acceptable length of time, she released him.

In an exasperated tone, she told Kester, "As you can see, Trick's back."

"Indeed. Well…" He'd had his surprised reaction all planned

out, but Trick had thrown him off his game by his entrance. "That's a relief."

"He wasn't kidnapped at all. He'd just run away," Jacqueline continued. "I'm sorry he made you worry and do all those things for me. Turns out you never had anything to feel guilty about. I know it's asking a lot, but I hope you won't hold it against him."

Trick moved to stand beside—and slightly behind—Denneka. "Why're you here?" he asked Kester.

Jacqueline answered. "Because I called him. John's been very kind in offering his time and assistance in helping me while I was *worried that you were lying dead somewhere.*"

"He has?" Denneka blurted in disbelief.

Kester spread his hands genially. "I am an exceptionally kind and helpful person."

"No, you're not!" Denneka blurted again, then slapped her hands over her mouth.

Kester couldn't stop the laugh that came out of him even as Jacqueline gaped at the girl.

"Sorry!" Denneka's face was turning red. "I mean—it's just—you're..." Her gaze dropped to the floor, and her voice dropped to a murmur. "You're not very nice."

Jacqueline was still staring at Trick and Denneka in shocked embarrassment.

Kester chuckled. "Don't worry, Jacqueline. I'm not offended. It's normal for kids to think of their teachers as mean, especially ones who've given them detention."

Briefly, Denneka's face screwed up like she was going to protest that the detention wasn't the only reason she felt that way, but she held her tongue.

Jacqueline got her keys out of her purse and tossed them to Denneka. "Get him out to the car and settled down, will you? I'll be out in a minute."

The girl picked up her bag and started for the door, but Trick didn't follow. She had to push him to get him going, and he still glared at Kester the whole way until they were outside.

Once they were gone, Jacqueline sighed. "Sorry about that. I love Trick to death, but he's a bit of a handful."

"Well, I'm glad he's returned to you. You'll be able to relax now."

"Yes and no," she said, not quite loudly enough for him to be sure he'd been meant to hear it.

He tilted his head inquiringly.

"I've got a new project I'm working on. Something that'll probably take up a lot of my time until I get it settled."

"A book?" he asked.

"Sadly, no. I… can't really get into what it is. Not right now, anyway. But now that Trick's back, I wanted to make sure you knew right away. So you don't feel obligated to keep helping me."

"I haven't been doing much helping lately except watching Landon," he said. "And I don't mind doing that at all."

She frowned like she wasn't sure she'd heard him right. "Do you mean you're willing to keep babysitting him for me?"

"Certainly."

"Really? That would be amazing. I still don't know many people here, and he's gotten used to you. I'd hate for both of us to have to break someone new in right now. I'll pay you, of course—"

He held up a hand, her words cutting into him unexpectedly deeply. "No need. I enjoy it, and I don't have anything better to do on my days off."

"Of course you do. Everyone has better things to do than babysit someone else's kid. Julia is probably already getting annoyed with me for taking up your time as much as I have been."

"Julia works every weekend, so we couldn't go out even if I were free."

"Really? Every weekend? Her boss must be a real dick."

Kester smiled wanly. "Yes, I suppose he is."

"But I have to pay you anyway. I'm not a worried mother with a missing child anymore, so you can't do it out of pity. And you don't have any responsibility for my situation, so you can't do it out of guilt. And we're not such good friends that it would make sense for you to—"

"We're not friends?"

That stopped her short. "We—well, not *good* friends."

"How good of friends must we be before you'll allow me to babysit for free?"

Her eyes narrowed. "Why are you pushing this so hard?"

Because he's not 'someone else's kid'; he's mine. Because I am responsible for your situation. "Because, if I can be perfectly frank, you need the money more than I do, and I'd feel like I was taking advantage if I let you pay me for spending an enjoyable time with a person I like on what would otherwise be a dull and lonely day."

Jacqueline looked between Kester and Landon, who had come in after the other kids and been sitting quietly on the couch this whole time.

Kester took a step backward toward the door, bowing slightly as he did so. "I see. You suspect me of being a deviant. You're afraid I might corrupt him." His heart ached with the knowledge that she was absolutely right, if not in the way she feared. "Not friends, then. I'm sorry." He opened the door to leave. This was for the best. He suspected he was a bad influence on his son, but he couldn't manage to break off contact with him on his own. But if the boy's mother drove him away, he was too much a coward to fight her.

"Wait, John, hang on! I didn't say that!"

He stopped. "Why would you trust someone you pay—or someone who acts out of pity or guilt—but not someone who acts out of friendship?"

She reeled back as if he'd pushed her. "I... I..."

He stepped back inside and closed the door. "You what?" he asked gently.

"I understand pity and guilt and payment. But I've been so focused on my kids and my work, I haven't had a good friend since college. I haven't had a good male friend since I was a child."

"You don't understand friendship, so you don't trust it."

"Maybe. Yeah."

Kester had the irrational urge to reach out and hug her. He, at least, had Julia, even if he'd never had any other friend. Not that he had let Julia even attempt to make any friends of her own. He smiled. "Good news, then. Your lack of friends has made me pity you. I think I'll have to babysit your child so you can get out and make friends."

Jacqueline looked at him in shock, then laughed. "You know, John, you're a weird guy, but I think I like you. As a friend."

Such a simple statement, but it made Kester want something he didn't think he'd ever wanted before. Not that it mattered. Truly being Jacqueline's friend was impossible. He had no intention of maintaining his 'John' disguise for the long term, and if Jacqueline ever found out how he'd been deceiving her, she'd loathe him. "By the way, how's the search for Charcoal going?" he asked because it seemed like something 'John' might say at this juncture.

"Charcoal?"

"Your cat. Or Trick's cat, wasn't it? Have you told him the cat is missing?"

"Oh! No, I haven't told him. It's probably best not to bring it up. I'm hoping I'll be able to find him before Trick notices."

"Ah. Speaking of Trick, you told the kids you'd be outside soon, didn't you? I assume you have somewhere to go?"

"Right! I hate to—"

"I'll be happy to watch Landon while you're out. I assumed that was why you called me over here, so I was already planning on it."

"Thank you. I do appreciate it." She got her purse and jacket, then kissed Landon on the head. "Be good. Call if you need anything."

After she left, Kester and Landon remained where they were, not speaking until they heard the car leave the driveway.

Then Landon said in a very calm voice, "You're the witch. The one who made Trick a cat again."

Kester sat next to him on the couch. "Yes."

"Mom's really angry at you. That's what she's doing now, after she drops them off. She's looking for you."

"Why haven't you told her about me?"

Landon looked at his hands in his lap. "I know I should. But I don't want to."

There it was. Proof of what Kester had suspected. His bad influence. Landon had done something he knew was wrong. "Why not?"

"I don't think she'd let you come over if she knew."

"I'm certain you're correct."

"And I want you to keep coming over."

"I want that, as well." Though it was selfish of him. And not good for anyone else. And getting more and more dangerous for him the closer Jacqueline came to finding out the truth. By rights, he should have already abandoned this game and left town.

"Did you use magic on her just now?"

"What?" Kester asked sharply.

"She was close to making you leave, wasn't she? Then you talked to her and she changed her mind."

Kester felt a heavy weight in his gut. He'd been honest and genuine with someone other than Julia for once—even if not *totally* honest—and hadn't intentionally manipulated Jacqueline into getting what he'd wanted. But Landon was right. Kester had turned the conversation so it was about his hurt feelings, making her feel guilty, making her question her own instincts. *God help me. It's such a habit, I do it even when I don't mean to.* "No. That wasn't magic. And it wasn't very nice, either."

Landon squinted at him like he was trying to understand some strange word he'd used. Then, sounding just a little bit disappointed, he said, "Oh." In the lull that followed, there was a sudden movement, and a small, green lizard crawled out of Landon's breast pocket and came to sit on his shoulder.

"A familiar?" Kester asked.

Landon nodded, watching him expectantly.

"A lizard. That's pretty good. Did you have any trouble?"

"No."

"Landon, would you mind terribly if we didn't do magic today? If we did something else?"

"Like what?"

"Maybe I could teach you some more cooking?"

Landon considered this suggestion. "Okay."

By checking in periodically with Julia, Kester knew exactly how Jacqueline spent the rest of the day. Mostly, watching Julia. Now that they had a description of the dangerous man who might be after Denneka, Kester had told Julia to keep an eye out for him—especially if he got anywhere near Denneka and Trick. When they got back to Denneka's house, Julia perched high in a tree where she could see the surrounding area and know if anyone entered or exited the house. It wasn't nearly as entertaining as when he had her watching the kids closely enough to see and hear what they were doing, but it was more important. And Kester was beginning to feel a bit guilty for treating them like his own personal reality show.

Jacqueline let the kids go inside and pretended to leave, then brought out a pair of binoculars and spotted Julia almost immediately. On Kester's orders, Julia stayed well away from her no matter how much Jacqueline threatened and called to her.

Jacqueline kept up her surveillance all day.

I believe she's waiting to follow you home, Kester told Julia through their bond when the sun began to set. *She expects you to lead her to your master. I don't think you'll be able to wait her out. Go on home. If she's able to follow you, she deserves to find out.*

Julia did as he instructed, flying home as the dusk light shone sideways across the sky. She lost Jacqueline's car easily.

When Jacqueline walked into her house just after the sun had set, she appeared tired, hungry, and irritated.

Kester looked up from the book he was reading on the couch. "Welcome home. You were out late. How did it go?"

She tossed her bag and coat on a chair. "How did what go?"

"Whatever you were doing." He didn't ask where Trick was. There was no point in forcing her to make up a lie.

"Not so great," she said. "But I'm not giving up yet. What smells good?"

"Eggplant Parmesan." He pointed to the dining table. "Landon has already eaten and is studying in his room."

"You didn't have to make dinner."

"I ate some, too, and you already had all the ingredients in your fridge, if that makes you feel any better."

She sat down to eat, and he went over to join her.

He wasn't entirely sure why.

"Have you been able to get any writing done?" he asked her.

"Not much," she said with her mouth full.

"Have you been getting enough sleep?"

"I'm used to not sleeping much."

He pulled a slice of garlic bread from the loaf on the table and slowly ate half of it. "Now that Trick's back, what is it that's troubling you enough to put your health and finances at risk?" he asked because he was curious what she'd tell him. But as soon as he saw her start fumbling for a lie, he regretted his words. "Never mind. I see it's personal. Forget I asked."

She flushed slightly in embarrassment, obviously realizing he'd known she was about to lie. "It is, but…"

She was going to say something she didn't really want to, he could tell. Because he'd asked an awkward question and then retracted it in a way that drew attention to it. He wondered if it was possible for him *not* to manipulate people anymore.

Jacqueline stopped eating but poked at the remains of food on her plate with her fork. "Do you believe in magic, John?"

That wasn't something he'd expected her to say, and the surprise delighted him. "Me? I'm not sure. I suppose it depends on what you mean."

"Let's say… fortune-telling. Bad luck. Superstitions. That kind of thing."

He thought about it. "I would say… I believe in making my own luck."

She nodded, the corner of her mouth curled in a hint of a smile. "I'm more like that now, too. But when I was young, I was a lot more naïve. Every superstitious fad that was ever popular with American teens—tarot cards, horoscopes, Ouija boards—I was into all of it. Anything that could help me find my Prince Charming, I think was why I started with it."

"Really?" He'd known all of this. It had been one of the topics they'd hit on when they'd met at that nightclub seven and a half years ago. "But you don't believe in that now?"

"Not the superstitions. But…" She tapped lightly at the edge of her plate. "I've seen and experienced enough weird stuff… I don't know *what* magic is, but I know *that* it is. If you get what I mean."

"You mean that you do believe in magic."

"You probably think I'm still a superstitious idiot."

"Your belief is based on your experiences. I can't discount your experiences, especially without even knowing what they are."

Her eyes searched his for a while, and he thought she was trying to decide how much more to tell him.

"There's someone out there," she said. "Someone who's messing with my family. It has something to do with… well, with magic. So I doubt the police would take me seriously or be able to help even if they did. No one would. So it's up to me to find this guy."

"And what will you do with 'this guy' once you find him?"

Her daintily-arched brows lowered into a scowl. "Whatever I have to until he leaves my family alone."

If Kester hadn't known that the power gap between those who could use magic and those who couldn't was less a gap and more a canyon, he might have been frightened.

Then again… *If she catches me while I've got my disguise on and I'm not able to remove it to unlock my power, I might actually be in danger.*

Jacqueline was worn down, tired, and determined. The ferocity in her eyes was so hot that for a moment, he actually considered coming clean.

The reason he didn't wasn't because he was afraid that if he did so right now, she might actually murder him before he could get the watch off and restore his power. No, his reason was much more altruistic. Right now, Jacqueline's search for the witch meant that she was staying close to Denneka—because she was looking for Julia, and Julia was staying close to Denneka. Which meant that if the probable killer who might have nefarious intentions toward Denneka approached the girl, there would be another set of wary eyes nearby to spot him.

It was concern for the girl that stopped him from coming clean to Jacqueline. That was all. It definitely wasn't because he still wasn't ready to end his game, even if a growing part of him felt worse the longer he kept playing it.

"You're clearly a woman on a mission," he told her. "Far be it from me to hinder you in any way. I'm happy to watch Landon whenever you need while you hunt down your prey."

"Really? You don't think I'm delusional or stupid?"

"You've never struck me as either. I don't see why what you've just told me should change my mind."

"Thank you, John. I... That means a lot."

———

Having gotten absolutely nowhere by trying to follow the hawk familiar back to its master, Jacqueline decided to try another tack. So on Sunday, after calling John over to watch Landon, she headed to the town library.

It was a small building that looked like it had been built in the eighties and not updated since. The paint was faded, but the windows were clean and the lawn was lush and trimmed.

When she went in, a tall man with glasses greeted her. "Can I help you find anything?"

"Do you have a local history section?"

He guided her to a single floor-to-ceiling bookshelf in the back. After perusing the titles, she grabbed an armful and went to a table to spread out.

Her thinking was this: Maybe she'd unwittingly brought her family into a witch's territory and, perhaps sensing the magic of Trick's spell, the witch had been drawn to them. If this was the case, the witch might be warning them off—or possibly playing with them. He might even have a darker plan for them and messing around with Trick's transformation was only a predator toying with its prey before striking the killing blow.

If there was a witch local to Agreste, he might have been there for a while. And she really had no idea how long witches lived. A lot of stories about them made it sound like they were supernatural creatures that could live for hundreds of years. She knew they could die of more-or-less natural causes, as the witch who had made Trick her familiar had done, but Jacqueline had never learned how old that old woman had actually been. She'd looked around eighty, but she'd claimed to be much older, which could have meant ninety or five hundred. So if the male witch was local to the area and if he had been there for very long, there might be stories in the local histories that could lead to him.

For the rest of the morning, Jacqueline pored over the books, searching for any stories of spooky or haunted places, any unexplained mysteries or local legends involving the supernatural.

Near lunch time, a pair of young women sat at the end of the table she was working at. They slammed a couple of heavy hardcovers down and proceeded to natter on too loudly to be ignored.

"So then when we took down the third boss and it dropped some legendary plate leggings, this rogue tries to ninja loot it, saying he super duper needs it for his alt and he got the last hit in so technically the kill was his anyway."

"No way. You didn't let him, did you?"

"What do you take me for, a noob? I told him to give the leggings to the tank or he'd be kicked out of the guild. TBH, I might kick him anyway after that stunt."

The page that Jacqueline had been trying to focus on blurred as the woman's words rang in her head. 'What do you take me for?'

'What kind of witch do you take me for?'

John had asked her that when they'd first met. Jacqueline had found it strange and startling, but something had happened and it had gone out of her mind. But now that she knew there was a witch in town...

A male witch.

Her head swam, and she almost bolted from the libr. desperate rush to get home. But she forced herself to stop and If John were the witch and meant harm to Landon, he'd already plenty of opportunity to cause it.

Besides, she had no reason to think he was the witch, other tha a single odd comment he made when he was trying to make a joke. It would be stupid to judge anyone based on a bad or poorly-worded joke. It would be an idiotic thing to actually accuse someone based on. His support even in the face of her illogical (to anyone who hadn't experienced it) belief in magic was surprising and not something she took for granted. If she accused him of being a witch based on nothing but an offhand comment he probably didn't even remember making, he really would think she was a lunatic and break off contact.

And Landon really seemed to like him. He didn't say much about John, but Landon wasn't a very affectionate boy on the whole, so he wouldn't. The fact that he had stopped acting suspicious of John and the way he calmly accepted being put in John's care spoke volumes. Trick had never seemed to lack anything from not having a father, and Jacqueline hadn't thought Landon had either, but when she saw the small but powerful changes in her younger son, she felt immensely guilty for not providing him any kind of male role model before now.

Maybe one day she'd meet a man she wanted to marry and give Landon a father, but until then, John seemed to be filling that void which Jacqueline hadn't even been aware Landon had. For her son's sake, even if not for her own, she wouldn't risk that without hard evidence.

She continued to search the local history, and when she got home that afternoon, she found John and Landon playing a board game at the dining table.

"A teacher playing a six-year-old at Scrabble?" she noted, going over to them. "Isn't that a little unfair?"

John looked over his shoulder at her. "You'd think so, but he d me to let him use a dictionary, and now he's trouncing

queline watched them finish the game, examining John for signs of being a witch. Problem was, he was the most plain, assuming person she'd ever met. He had an interesting person-ity under the nondescript appearance, but it was nothing she would call witchy. The old woman who'd taken Trick in exchange for a potion had seemed fairly normal on the surface too, though. If real witches were all hiding in plain sight, maybe there were no reli-able ways of spotting them.

Landon won the game, and Jacqueline saw John out. When he was gone, she sat at the table with Landon and said, "You seem to get along well with him. Do you like him?"

Landon was focused on putting the game pieces back in the box. "Yeah."

"Do you think there's anything weird about him?"

He looked at her. "Weird how?"

"Just anything he says or does that... seems weird."

He went back to the game pieces. "No."

"What'd you guys do today?"

"Cooking. Games. I told him what books I like."

He was engaged. Doing things with another person. Not just reading in his room all day. "Sounds fun."

"Yeah."

Jacqueline didn't like suspecting John. She didn't want to. But she couldn't erase the suspicion from her mind until she knew more. Maybe if she did some digging on him, she'd find evidence that he wasn't hiding something and she'd be able to stop worrying.

CHAPTER
NINETEEN

Denneka still wasn't sure how she felt about Trick's mom. In some ways, Jacqueline was kind of like her own mom. But in other ways, she definitely was not. Denneka would never in a million years have expected any mom to let Trick continue to stay at Denneka's house, even considering the whole he's-not-human-when-he's-not-near-her thing. More than that, to not only allow them to continue keeping it secret from her parents but to insist on it. If Trick were the girl and Denneka were the boy, would Jacqueline still have done that? Denneka wanted to ask but couldn't summon up the nerve.

Especially not after Jacqueline had made her promise to tell her if Trick started treating her like a boy treats a girl. What did that even mean? No boy had ever treated Denneka that way—she'd been a nerdy loser for a long time—so she wasn't sure she'd even know what to look for.

She tried to put it out of her head. There was no point trying to imagine what that would look like because he didn't see her that way. She was only convenient for him. Familiar. Right now, she was the only one he found easy to be around, and that was the only reason he'd ever given for being around her. Okay, he had said he liked her, but when she'd asked why he liked her, all he'd said was that she was familiar. And now that his mom was forcing him to go back to school, that wouldn't stay true much longer. Soon, there would be a lot more girls who were familiar to him. Ones who were also pretty and charming and athletic and lots of other things Denneka wasn't.

"You're awfully quiet over there," Jacqueline said, glancing aside at her as she drove.

"Sorry," Denneka mumbled.

Jacqueline laughed. "Don't be. After Trick and Landon, I don't think I'd know what to do with a talkative kid. Although... Trick was talkative, before he was transformed. I wonder if he ever will be again."

They'd already dropped Landon off at his school and were on their way to the junior high. Denneka had only met Trick's brother briefly a few times, but he seemed normal enough. And one of the few things she'd heard about him was that he liked to read, which made Denneka both like him and worry for his social future.

"If you're worrying about Trick turning into a cat during school, don't," Jacqueline said. "I know both of you will work hard to stay on top of it. And I'm going in right away to get his schedule changed so it's the same as yours."

"But what about if one of us has to go to the bathroom? Or—oh, no! What about PE?" She hadn't even thought about PE. There was no way to stay near him then. Their plan was ruined!

Jacqueline's brow furrowed. "I'll write him a note to excuse him from it. He was supposedly living on the streets for a couple weeks, so it's not unreasonable that he wouldn't be feeling well."

"But what about me? I can't... Well, I guess I could say I'm on my period and don't feel well."

She heard sniffs from right beside her ear and turned to see Trick leaning forward. "You don't smell like you're in heat," he said in a questioning tone.

Jacqueline's arm whipped around so fast that Denneka barely saw it, smacking Trick in the chest and shoving him back in his seat. "First of all, Trick," Jacqueline lectured, "don't sniff people. It's rude. Second, never talk to a girl about her period. Third, humans don't go into heat, and if you can't remember that, then you'd better ask your health teacher for a refresher lesson on human reproduction."

Since he was sitting behind her in the car, Denneka had kind of forgotten about his presence when she'd made the suggestion. But now she was blushing again and whispered to his mom, "Can he really smell... ?"

Jacqueline sighed. "As a human, I doubt it. As a cat, I wouldn't be surprised. Cats' noses might not be as good as dogs', but they're a lot better than humans'. I don't think he cares one way or the other about it, though. I wish he did; any sign of being a normal teen boy would be welcome at this point."

Denneka peeked around the back of her seat to see Trick slouching with his shoulder pressed against the door. "The teacher man would make fun of me if I asked," he grumbled in his mom's general direction. "The familiar girl can explain it to me."

"Which teacher man?" Jacqueline asked. "Do you mean John? Is Mr. McKenzie your health teacher?"

"Yeah," Denneka answered. "He teaches most of our classes. PE too. Wait a minute. What did Trick just say?"

Jacqueline chuckled. "You mean 'the familiar girl'? I think that's you."

Denneka's heart sank. "Trick! Do you not know my name?!"

He looked at her with a face free of any expression. "Your name's... Denneka."

"DID YOU HAVE TO THINK ABOUT IT!?"

He jerked at her outburst, pressing himself into the seat back and holding himself very still, his eyes quite round all of a sudden. "Just for a second," he said in a tiny voice, moving his mouth as little as possible.

She turned around and slumped into her seat. He'd been living with her for like two weeks now and still had to work to remember her name. This was so much worse than she'd known.

"Trick," Jacqueline said calmly. "Who am I?"

"Mom."

"Who was in the car with us earlier?"

"Brother."

"Who else did you see at home on Saturday?"

"The teacher man and the police man."

"Can you remember anyone else you met at school?"

He thought about it. "The aggressive boy and the mean girl."

"Try not to take it personally, Denneka," Jacqueline said. "I think it's just the way his mind works. He hasn't been around all that many people in his life, so he can still get away with classifying them with descriptors. I think he'll have to grow out of it once he knows too many people for that to work anymore. That kind of thing is exactly why I want him to go to school. Do you get it?"

She nodded. "Yeah. I think I do." Didn't really make it hurt any less that Trick couldn't call her by her name. Whenever he got to know other girls and they became familiar to him too, she really would become nothing to him.

They pulled into the school parking lot, and Denneka's sense of dread grew.

"Pulling the 'female problems' card is always a good call with male teachers," Jacqueline said. "As long as you don't play it too often, it usually stops them asking questions. But I'll talk to him, too. I know you guys think he's mean because he's your teacher and he gave you detention, but he really has been going out of his way to help. I think I can come up with a reason to explain Trick needing to stay near you after his running away episode. I really doubt John'll give you trouble about it."

Denneka was a little offended that Jacqueline thought all she had against Mr. McKenzie was being a teacher—and the detention *had* been unjustified—but she didn't have enough spare energy to argue about it. Any that hadn't gotten sucked out of her by Trick's barely knowing her name needed to be focused on keeping his secret.

As if school wasn't draining enough already.

———

338

Everyone was looking at Trick. They had lots of expression. faces, but he couldn't be sure what any of them meant. Wr came close, he met most of their eyes—not challenging b showing weakness. The familiar girl was in front of him, mc through the pack of humans like a fish through water. Staying r on her heels, he was able to get through, too.

On their way to their classroom, they passed through a space where there weren't as many humans, and the familiar girl said, "The paper already reported you were back, so most of them should already know the story your mom told. Most of them are just curious, I think. There was a lot of talk about you the first day or two after you went missing."

They made it to their seats in class, but as soon as they did, a boy yelled, "Whoa!" and leapt over some seats toward them. Trick froze, but the boy stopped right in front of him. "Dude! You're back, new kid!" His teeth were bared and his mouth was open, but Trick was pretty sure it was a smile. The loud boy was... happy to see him?

Trick waited for the boy to move away or say something else, but he watched Trick like he was waiting for something.

"Yeah, he's back," the familiar girl told the boy. "But he's kinda nervous around a lot of people, so could you maybe back away a little, Ian?"

The loud boy only looked between the two of them. "Nervous? Why? Did ya get hassled by gang members while you were on the streets or something?"

"Nothing like that," the familiar girl said. "He's just stressed out from all of it and being around people stresses him out more."

The loud boy gave her a funny look. "Hey, are you guys going out now?"

"W-what?"

"You keep answering for him, and you seem to know a lot more than the rest of us."

A girl from a few seats away said, "Ian, can't you just say, 'We're glad you're back' and leave them alone? Look how tense Trick is."

okay," said the loud boy. "Sorry." He went back to his
Trick unclenched his muscles.

of the other kids either said nothing to Trick or greeted him
. Then those three came in—the aggressive boy, the mean girl,
their friend. They sat at desks near the windows and talked
dly enough to drown out everyone else in the room.

"Looks like the weirdo's back," said the mean girl.

The aggressive boy sneered at Trick across the room. "Hey,
weirdo. You talking yet?"

Trick stayed quiet, watching in case the boy decided to attack.

"Nothing to say for yourself?" the mean girl added. "Shouldn't
you be apologizing to everyone for wasting police time when there's
an actual murderer on the loose?"

The police man hadn't said Trick should apologize. Besides,
Trick's mom had already done that for him when the police man
was over. Trick looked to the familiar girl to see what she thought.

"He's still sticking to the other weirdo like her lap dog," said the
mean girl's friend.

Trick couldn't stop the challenging look he gave the girl. "I'm not
a dog."

The three mean humans laughed, and the familiar girl whispered at him. "Trick. Ignore them. Don't say something you
shouldn't."

The bell rang just as the teacher man came in. "Quiet down,
everyone. Yes, Patrick has returned. I expect most of you already
read the details about that in the paper. For those who haven't,
here's the short version: He wasn't kidnapped, it had nothing to do
with Mr. Haug, and there was no foul play involved. He ran away,
and now he's back. For those who did see the paper, I hope you
paid attention to the more prominent story about the police
releasing a description of the suspect in Mr. Haug's death. I urge
you not to take this lightly. If any of you sees someone who matches
that description, especially anyone acting suspiciously, I expect you
to tell the police or *some* authority figure right away. Lives could still

be at stake." That quieted the room down, and the teacher man started the lesson.

When third period came, Trick followed the familiar girl to her class instead of his usual one. She had to ask another girl to go to a different seat so Trick could sit beside her, but the girl moved without getting upset.

A lady teacher wearing an apron came up to him. She was small, her movements delicate, and she didn't make much noise. Already, he liked her better than the big, loud teacher he'd had in his drama class.

"Hi there, Trick," the apron teacher said in a soft, sweet voice. "I'm Ms. Cast. It's nice to meet you. Your mother spoke to me and explained why you wanted to transfer into this class. Even though you're a few weeks behind, I think we can make it work." Her attention shifted to the familiar girl. "Denneka, Trick's mother said you volunteered to help him catch up?"

"Yeah."

"That's wonderful. Well, Trick, I won't make you try to catch up on the practical work, so you can start from today. We're working on drawing basics. It doesn't matter how good you are; just give it your best. I'll leave it to Denneka to help you get set up with supplies."

When the apron teacher left, the familiar girl whispered, "I think your mom must have made it sound like you'd gone through some trauma or something. Ms. Cast is usually nice, but she's really handling you with kid gloves. At least that means we shouldn't have any problems from her. So that's a relief."

After art, they went back to their homeroom for science, and then it was time for PE. When the rest of the class left to head to the gym, Trick stayed back with the familiar girl to talk to the teacher man.

"Um, Mr. McKenzie," she said, creeping carefully toward his desk.

He came around it to lean against the front, and Trick could see the familiar girl fighting not to retreat. "Denneka." He sounded happy. Trick was instantly suspicious. "Do you have something to say to me?"

"Uh... um..." the girl fumbled.

"Perhaps something like, 'Wow, Mr. McKenzie, you were right. I should have listened to you. I got all worked up over nothing.'"

"What?"

The teacher man nodded toward Trick, who was standing a couple steps behind her. "Your friend. Safe and sound. Didn't I say he would be?"

What was the man getting at? Had they talked about Trick and she hadn't told him?

The familiar girl fingered the bottom hem of her shirt. "I guess. You said someone was taking care of him. But he was out on the streets, wasn't he?"

"Was he? But he looks fine to me. I still think someone must have been looking out for him, for him to have come out of that without any evident damage." His eyes shifted to Trick. "Was someone looking out for you, Patrick?"

Trick raised his hand to point at the familiar girl, but she saw and grabbed his hand. "You don't have to talk about whatever happened." She faced the teacher man, her back straighter. "He doesn't like to talk about it. It's... it's not nice to try to force him."

The teacher man smiled in a way that reminded Trick of a fox. "You've got a good friend there, Patrick. She was really worried about you. I hope you appreciate that."

Trick closed the distance between himself and the familiar girl, pressing his chest against her back and wishing he had a tail he could curl around her. Was the teacher man threatening to take her away from him? Or only toying with him? He didn't know, but he didn't like it. This man made him feel like all the fur down his spine would be standing on end if he had any.

The girl stiffened, so Trick dipped his head and pressed the side of it against hers. He wanted to purr to reassure her even more, but he couldn't, so he had to use words. "I do," he said, answering the last thing the teacher man had said.

The man laughed. "Good." The laugh died suddenly to a weak, humorless chuckle. "Good."

The familiar girl stepped away from Trick and let go of his hand. "A-anyway, Mr. McKenzie, I wanted to ask if I could be excused from PE today. I don't feel good. It's a lot of, um, cramping and—"

"That's fine. Patrick's mother already wrote a note to excuse him, so you can sit it out together. Though from the looks of you two, it would be hard to pry you apart even if I wanted to."

Yeah, it would be, Trick thought fiercely.

So while the rest of the class played soccer, Trick and the familiar girl sat on the grass at the sidelines. The weather was nice, the sun was shining, and the familiar girl was by his side. Even though the teacher man didn't let him lie down and fall asleep, he was more relaxed than he almost ever was at school. He even had fun watching the ball zip back and forth across the field, and when it zipped by very close to where he was sitting, he nearly ran out to catch it. He would have, if the familiar girl didn't grab his shirt every time he tried.

"Um, Trick," she said after a while. "I've been trying to hold it, but I really need to go to the bathroom."

He waited for her to get to the point.

"Which means you have to come with me."

Now that he thought of it, he did need to go, too.

"Mr. McKenzie," she called to the teacher man who stood a little way off, watching the game, "can we go to the bathroom?"

He checked his shiny watch. "It's almost lunch break."

"Yeah, but I really need to go now."

He waved them off. "Okay, fine."

Trick followed her off the field, back to the gym building.

"We should hurry. I should have realized this sooner, but it's better if we get there before anyone else is likely to be there. That's why I didn't want to wait for lunch break."

She headed into a room. He followed. She stopped all of a sudden and pushed him back out into the hallway. "We probably shouldn't use the girls' bathroom. You'd get in more trouble for going in there than I would for going in the boys' bathroom, if we get caught." She made an unhappy sound, then pushed him toward another door. "Go in and make sure it's empty. Don't go too far, though!"

In the time he'd been away from school, he'd forgotten what the symbols on the doors meant, but it came back to him now. When he checked, there didn't seem to be anyone inside, so he told her that.

She pushed him through the door. "Okay. I'm going in that stall. If you need to go, um, just don't get too far from there, okay?" She glanced nervously between the other stalls and the line of urinals, then darted into the stall she'd pointed at.

Since he only needed to pee, Trick used a urinal. While he was waiting outside her stall for her to finish, the bathroom door opened and the aggressive boy came in with two others. They were still in their gym clothes.

They stalked toward him. Trick tried to run, but they were too quick. They surrounded him, trapping him against the stalls. He pressed against the stall door. He couldn't even dive under it or jump over it because they were too close to let him move, and they'd grab him as soon as he tried. His heart pounded with fear, and his body froze up. If they attacked him, he had no option but to fight.

"Why so scared, weirdo?" The aggressive boy smiled, but it wasn't nice.

Trick's eyes darted between the three of them, watching for any move they might make to attack.

"Cat got your tongue?" asked the boy on his left.

Trick had never understood that phrase, so he didn't know how to answer.

"Does he ever talk?" asked the boy on his right.

"Sometimes. When the weird girl lets him," said the aggressive boy. "Seriously, weirdo, I gotta ask. What do you see in her? You *are* going out, right?"

None of these questions made any sense. What did they want

maki

"You're ki
at coming."
to ask. How is

had seemed fine
probably wasn't

ri
but

ne!" he repeated,
He started to calm
initely make Amy

es?" The
ddenly looke

essive boy enough
d up to Trick, and
t dropped Trick to
eye as the left side

t either, but it woul
her."

ggressive boy spat.
ys walk out of the

staring into Trick's
now. If he showed
nto him. "Because
r, but she can't let
now you're back
has to be a good
ll make it make
irl like Amy. So
er so much?"
get out of this
oys away from
f. "She lets me
are of me. She

r girl was kneeling
She pawed at him,
e."
d you get hit, too?"
on. Get up. We have
u need to get a cold

head into Lisa's office
spoke. "There are a

ed like they'd

...ar girl

...o hear her.

...I didn't see th...

...ling off. "I have

...ic shift. The familiar girl

...few minutes ago, though i...

...r right now. "She's... fine?"

...ive boy roared with laughter. "F...

...much he was wheezing. "She's fine!"

...thanks, man. Seriously. I think this'll de...

...etter about you turning her down."

Just when Trick thought he'd pacified the agg...

...to be left alone, the boy stopped laughing, stepp...

...punched him in the face. Pain like he'd never fe...

...the floor in an instant. He curled up, clutching hi...

...of his face throbbed.

"And that makes *me* feel better about it," the ...

From the floor, Trick watched the three bo...
bathroom.

The stall door opened, and then the famili...
beside him. "Trick! You stupid, stupid idiot!"
...pulling his hands away from his face. "Let me s...
He let her see. Her face was red and wet. "D...

"Kind of," she said in a tight voice. "Come...
...to leave before anyone sees me in here. And y...
pack or something."

The look on Michael's face when he stuck his
...made her adrenaline spike even before he...

couple kids here," said the secretary. "Looks like there was an incident."

"Send them in." When she saw Denneka's bloodshot eyes and Trick's hand over his face, she feared the murder suspect had made a move. "Sit down. What happened."

As Denneka babbled about Trevor cornering Trick in the bathroom, Lisa coaxed his hand away and saw the swelling and redness around his eye socket. She let out a breath of relief. Only a schoolboy altercation, then. Not an attempt on their lives.

Still, Trevor's father was a rich banker and held a lot of pursestrings—and therefore influence—in town. Trevor probably thought he could outright assault another student and get away with it. And he was probably right.

"Do you know why he attacked Trick?" she asked Denneka. Trick seemed to have been scared silent by the attack.

"It was about Amy. She… tried to get Trick's attention on the first day of school, but Trick ignored her."

Of course. Trevor was violently protective of both Amy and Flora. It could be an admirable trait under the right circumstances, but they were all three too young and spoiled to have any kind of discernment.

Michael came back with an ice pack. When Lisa pressed it against Trick's face, he hissed and recoiled.

"It's okay, Trick," Denneka told him. "It's good for you. You need to hold it over your eye and leave it there for a while."

Trick let out a barely audible growl under his breath, but he took the ice pack from Lisa and held it in place. Lisa told Michael to keep the kids here until she got back, then went to find Trevor.

———

Kester had a feeling something was wrong when he saw three boys in his class sneak back onto the field. He hadn't seen them leave. He'd been zoned out, checking in with Julia as she surveilled the town from the air, keeping an eye out for the killer.

It wasn't the fact that the boys had left that put the sinking feeling in his gut. It was the pleased looks on their faces and the direction they'd come from when they'd returned.

He was standing too far away to hear what they were talking about with their friends when they rejoined the group, but judging by the other students' reactions, it was something disruptive.

He strode over to them, and they stopped talking. "What's this? No need to clam up on my account. I came over because some of you are looking quite scandalized, and I love a good scandal. Please, do share."

Most of them hesitated, but Trevor grinned. "That weird—"

A boy whose name Kester didn't remember elbowed Trevor. "Dude!"

Trevor shrugged. "It's nothing. Just this weird cloud shaped like boobs. It's gone now."

"I see." It was time for lunch, so Kester dismissed the class and followed them back to the gym. He tried to stay close enough to overhear them, but although he could see they were clearly worked up about something, he couldn't make out what it was.

Ten minutes later, he went into the cafeteria and tried to be unobtrusive. A quick scan of the room showed that Trick and Denneka were missing. Not a good sign.

As he passed a table of girls, he finally heard something interesting.

"I don't think Denneka's like that," said a quiet girl. What was her name? River? Creek? Something like that.

"But Trevor said that's what the new kid said," another girl whispered. Juniper? Or maybe Juggler?

I should probably pay more attention to their names.

"I've known her since third grade," Creek said. "She's not a—"

They caught Kester listening and fell silent.

He braced his hands on the table, looming over them, and smiled. "Not a what?"

If he'd had his normal appearance, the combination of intimidation and confused attraction would have made them flustered enough to answer him. But it seemed he couldn't make even thirteen-year-old girls flustered the way he looked now. They just shoved bites of food into their mouths and stayed quiet.

This was getting frustrating.

He heard the quick clip of heels behind him and turned to see Lisa approach, concern creasing her brow.

"I need to talk to you." She walked away without waiting for a response.

———

It was the first time Denneka had seen Trick turn away food.

The school secretary, Mr. Kendrick, had brought a small bag of popcorn to them. "It's from the vending machine. Lunch is almost over and you've been here the whole time, so I thought you might be hungry."

Trick shook his head. He'd been curled up in a chair in Ms. VanBuren's office for a while now, holding the cold pack to his face and not doing much else.

"Thank you," Denneka said. She took the popcorn but didn't open it. Any appetite she'd had was long gone. Her stomach was too full of humiliation and dread.

Mr. Kendrick left, and after a bit, Ms. VanBuren came back. "Trevor claims Trick's injury was an accident. That Trick fell, and it had nothing to do with him."

Denneka shot to her feet. "That's not true!"

Ms. VanBuren held up a hand. "I know. He didn't even try to lie well. But the situation is difficult. His two friends vouched for his story—"

"Of course they did! They were—"

"Denneka. Please don't interrupt me. I know Trevor and the other two boys are lying. But I can't prove it. There are no videos or photos, and without even another witness to back up Trick's side of the story, there isn't much of a case against Trevor."

Denneka bit her lip. "What if there was another witness?"

Ms. VanBuren raised an eyebrow at her, but then shook her head. "It would still be two against three. And I'm not sure if you're aware of who Trevor's family is, but any case against him would need to be rock solid to avoid serious backlash, much less get anywhere in punishing him."

So, it hadn't been Denneka's imagination all these years that Trevor, Amy, and Flora got away with more bullying than most kids would be able to. "You're letting him get away with it?"

"The matter is being worked on, but it requires delicacy. I've called Trick's mother to come pick him up. He should see a doctor."

Filled with sudden panic, Denneka opened her mouth to ask to go with him, but Ms. VanBuren kept speaking.

"I've offered to allow you to go with him, since it's clear that for some reason he needs your support." She paused to give Trick a chance to weigh in on that statement, but he didn't even look at her. "You'll need to call one of your parents to get their approval before we can let you go with her. Do you want to do that?"

"Yes. Of course." Denneka pulled her phone from her pocket with fumbling fingers.

"There was... something else." The uncomfortable expression on Ms. VanBuren's face told Denneka exactly what the 'something else' was. "There is a rumor spreading. A rumor that Trevor confirmed he started, though he insists he didn't make it up."

Denneka felt her face heating and couldn't push any words past her clenching throat.

"The rumor is that Trick said... that you let him sleep with you. Trevor insisted that those were Trick's exact words."

Suddenly, Denneka wanted to throw up from embarrassment. "That's... technically true."

A wave of something intensely uncomfortable washed over Ms. VanBuren's face. "Denneka, it's not my place to pry into your personal life, but you two are only thirteen. You might want to wait a few more—"

"I mean it's true that he said that, not that—" It was so embarrassing, she couldn't even say it. And if the rumor was already

spreading, then everyone out there actually believe
She wanted to leave school and never come back. S.
move out of town tonight.

When Denneka pulled herself out of that sudden c
despair, Ms. VanBuren was scowling at Trick, moving in
him to make him look up at her. "So it was some juvenile lie:
you trying to impress the other boys?"

Utter confusion was Trick's only response. "I thought he w
gonna hit me, so I gave him the answers he wanted. Then he hit me
anyway!"

Ms. VanBuren processed that, and then she was all calm sympathy. She even let out a little sigh of relief. "I see. So Trevor bullied
Trick into saying that." She went to sit down at her desk. "That
makes things more complicated. The rumor is true but not true.
Trevor is being careful not to say that you two are sleeping together,
only repeating what Trick actually said. We can't prove that Trevor
forced the words out of Trick, but since Trevor's claim is technically
true, we can't rightfully accuse him of lying or slander, either.
Gossip, however damaging, is not actually illegal or even against
school rules."

Hopeless tears gathered in Denneka's eyes. "Then what do
we do?"

"Call your parents. Help Trick's mother take him to the hospital.
Get a good night's rest. We'll work on finding a solution to this
problem, but even if we can't, try to keep things in perspective.
There are more dangerous things than rumors, and more important
things than your reputation that can be threatened." There was
something too dark—too serious—in the way she said that.
Denneka didn't know what it meant, but it made her feel cold.

———

Luckily, Trick's injury wasn't serious. *If he were a normal boy,*
Jacqueline thought, *maybe he'd have learned to take a punch by now.*
She was driving them back to Denneka's home and wondering

...at was the right thing to do. The girl was upset and
more trouble at school now than she was already
it was largely Jacqueline's fault. Her fault for not
...at Trick learn more practical social skills while he was a
though he didn't think he'd need them. Her fault for
, Trick and Denneka in this unusual situation together in the
place.

But if she brought Trick home now, he'd be a cat all the time and
ould lose any motivation he had to be human. Maybe she could
get Denneka to meet them near the junior high and force him to go
to school that way, but there was too much chance of something
going wrong. The best way to keep Trick human as much as
possible was still to have him around the girl. And no matter how
much Trick moped about what had happened today, he needed to
get back in there and deal with life as a human.

It would be so easy for all of them to have Jacqueline take him
home now. He'd be happy, away from humans and living as a cat.
Denneka wouldn't have to keep hiding him and taking care of him.
And even though Jacqueline wanted her son human, he was easier
to take care of as a cat.

But that would be the coward's way out on all counts, and it
wasn't what was best for Trick.

That was a decision she could make for herself and her son, but
she had no right to make it for Denneka.

"Are you sure you want to keep going?" she asked the girl in the
passenger seat.

Denneka's brow furrowed. "Keep going?"

"With Trick. Are you sure you want to keep dealing with him?
He's made your life complicated."

The girl fidgeted with her hands. "He has. But I don't mind.
What happened today wasn't his fault. Not really. I—I like having
him around..." Her voice trailed off, but Jacqueline just barely heard
her add, "while I can."

Jacqueline took a deep breath and let it out. "Thank you. I know
this is hard on him, but I think it's better for him to face it." She

glanced at Trick in the back seat. He was staring out the window, the left side of his face swollen and purple. "Trick, you can have the rest of the day off, but you're going back to school tomorrow."

His eyes snapped to her, full of fear and surprise. "No!"

"Yes."

"But they'll kill me!"

"They won't."

"What if they do?"

"Then I'll be very sad. But they won't."

"What if they try?"

"Then either fight back or call for help."

Twitchy with fear and uncertainty, he clenched and unclenched his hand. "But I don't have claws."

"Then learn to use what you do have, if you have to."

"But what if—"

Jacqueline's phone rang. There was a lot of traffic at the moment, so she asked Denneka, "Can you see who's calling?"

Denneka picked it up from the middle console. "It says 'John'."

Maybe it was news about the boys who'd attacked Trick. "Please answer and put it on speakerphone."

Denneka did, holding it up near Jacqueline's face.

"Hello, John."

"Hello, Jacqueline." The phone almost fell when Denneka jerked in surprise. The girl apparently hadn't remembered that 'John' meant 'Mr. McKenzie'. "I'm... sorry about what happened today."

"It's not your fault."

There was a pause before he continued in a graver tone than she was used to hearing from him. "How's Trick?"

"It's only a black eye. He'll be all right."

"Good."

"Has Lisa figured out some way to punish those boys or deal with the rumor they spread?"

"No. But I wanted to let you know you needn't worry about it." An edge of menace slid into his tone. "I'll handle it."

He hung up.

That hadn't sounded much like the John she knew, but maybe the road noise and distortion from the speakerphone was to blame. "There you go," she told the kids. "He'll handle it, so don't worry so much."

"That's not very reassuring," Denneka said, putting the phone down. "He's on the bullies' side most of the time."

"I find that hard to believe," Jacqueline said.

"It's true," Trick groused. "He's mean."

Their insistence pricked at her motherly instincts. She would have asked for more details, but they arrived at Denneka's house. "Give him a chance to fix this. If you still think he's mean after school tomorrow, you can tell me all about it, okay?"

Denneka murmured, "Okay," and got out. Trick fought with his seat belt for a while before getting it off. Jacqueline reached back and pulled him in so she could kiss his cheek before letting him get away.

She watched them go into the house, considering her next move. She wanted to trust John. He hadn't really given her any reason not to. But there was something odd about him, and the last few minutes had only strengthened that impression. She decided she would go forward with her plan.

———

The familiar girl made Trick take a bath sooner than normal, since they were home a few hours early and had more time before anyone else got home. Trick couldn't work up much motivation for it, though. He sat in the water, unmoving, until it started to get cold.

"Can you wash my hair now?" he asked through the shower curtain.

"Are you done?"

"No."

She sighed. "Fine."

The warm water flowing over his body felt really good, and the girl spent longer rubbing his hair than she normally did. She was careful not to touch the hurt part of his face, but when water trickled over it, he jerked at the pain.

"Sorry," she said, and she was careful so it didn't happen again. When she was done, she said, "Did you wash yourself at all?"

"No."

She let out another sigh, this one sounding more annoyed, and reached for the loofah and soap. "I'm only doing this because I know you're not feeling good, so don't think you don't have to do it yourself anymore." She dipped the loofah into the water at his side, soaped it up, and scrubbed his back. It was too rough to feel very good, but he liked the attention, so he let her wash his back and arms and under his arms. She started to scrub at his chest, but stopped almost immediately. "You can do it from here."

He took the loofah and managed to get the rest of himself clean while she waited on the other side of the curtain.

After his bath, she fed him, and then he spent several hours curled up in a ball under the blankets on her bed. Not sleeping, just listening to the sounds she made as she moved around her room.

"Trick," she said after a while.

He didn't answer.

She pulled back the blanket. "It's after nine. Time for bed."

He pulled the blanket back over himself.

But she didn't chastise him like he expected. When he didn't hear anything from her at all for what felt like a while, he peeled the blanket back enough to poke his head out.

She was in her pajamas, sitting in her desk chair, staring right at him with an expression he didn't like.

Sad, he realized after examining it for a while. *She's sad.*

"Your poor face," she said. "I'm sorry I didn't try to stop them."

He had wondered why she hadn't, but he didn't want to make her feel bad. "Why did they attack me?" Before, he'd always been able to get away from threats without fighting. If it was a dog or something, he could always run faster and squeeze into spaces they couldn't fit in to get away. With bigger cats, he could either run or submit completely enough that they stopped seeing him as a threat and left him alone. But the boys had cornered him without warning, ganging up on him so he couldn't run, and even when he'd submitted, the aggressive boy had pretended to be satisfied and then attacked him without warning. Trick didn't understand humans at all.

"Because they're jerks, and it's fun for them."

"Fun?"

"Cats play with their prey, right?"

Trick nodded.

"It's like that."

Fear made Trick's muscles tighten. Trick never played with a mouse or lizard unless he was going to eat it soon. "They want to kill me," he whispered.

"I don't think so. Humans have laws, and that gives us some protection that animals don't have."

Laws were sorts of rules, right? Trick still didn't like rules, but if some of them would keep the aggressive boy from killing him, maybe they were okay. "Laws stop humans from killing other humans?"

"Well... no. Laws punish people for doing it, but they can't really stop them. Just look at Mr. Haug."

Trick *had* looked at him. He remembered the corpse's face clearly. "Humans kill other humans. For fun. And laws can't stop them."

"For fun or profit or revenge or a bunch of other reasons that don't make any sense if you're looking at it like an animal would. The laws do help, though. If Trevor killed you, he'd probably go to jail. He knows that. So if someone wants to kill, they know there's a risk, and the risk is from something bigger than the person they want to kill fighting back. I don't really think he wants to kill you, though. He's a bully, but that doesn't make him a killer. Humans also hurt each other for fun. And it doesn't have to be physical."

This was all scary and complicated, and Trick didn't want to think about it anymore. "Why aren't you getting in bed?"

"You—you need to get out, so you can get on your side of the blanket, like we agreed. And you need to change into your pajamas."

He didn't want to get out of the warm bed, but he did. She straightened the blankets, then got in, facing away from him while he changed. Then he pulled back the top blanket enough to crawl under it and curl up against the backs of her bent legs.

Her body stiffened, but when he shifted to rest his chin on her lower leg, she slowly relaxed, and they both fell asleep.

———

Kester swirled the hot chocolate in his mug and asked Julia, "Should I turn him into a frog or a salamander?"

"Who?"

"The boy who attacked our Trick."

Her eyebrows arched at him. "*Our* Trick?"

"Well," he said, stalling for time. When had he become so possessive of the amusing kitten boy? "He's mine until I'm finished with him."

Julia smirked, crossed her toned legs, and adjusted her robe to cover them. The robe was long, but the nightgown under it was short. "If you say so. But if you're asking my opinion, I don't think you should turn him into anything."

"Boils, then? Or perhaps blindness?"

"Don't you think that's a little much for a single punch to the face?"

"Don't forget the hateful rumor he spread."

"So the girl is yours until you're finished with her, too?"

"Yes." He internally winced at the petulance he heard in his own voice.

Julia's smirk spread into a grin. "Do you think it's possible that some of the anger you're directing at the bully, you really feel toward yourself?"

He turned his gaze to the fire and took a slow sip of hot chocolate. "Why would I feel any anger toward myself?"

"You tell me."

Blast her. How did she know him so well? He hardly knew himself these days. "It was my fault. For not watching those boys closely enough."

"And?"

He gripped his mug harder. "And for causing the whole situation to begin with."

"Can I ask you something? Not judging, only curious. If you feel bad about it, why don't you end the spell you put on Trick?"

He'd considered it more than once in the past few days. "Because... I'm afraid that if I make Trick fully human again, Jacqueline will have no reason to need me. I will become irrelevant. To her, to Landon, to all of them."

"Kester," Julia said with quiet surprise, "it sounds like you want a reason to stay in their lives."

"Maybe I do."

Julia got up, crossed the center of the living room, and stood beside his chair. With gentle fingers, she stroked his hair affectionately.

"I'm not your pet, woman," he growled with mock offense.

She kissed the top of his head. "No, Master."

He took her hand and held it. Her fingers were long and soft. She looked like the type of woman who would have callouses, but she did most of her work when she had no hands, only wings. "I don't know what's happening to me," he said softly. "I don't know who I am anymore or what I want."

"You will."

"And will you be here? Will you stay with me even if I change into a different man?"

"Do I have a choice?"

He wanted to say yes. But the thought that she might one day choose to leave him made his chest tighten and throat constrict. And, given the chance, why wouldn't someone leave the person who'd controlled their whole life from a young age?

"You know I won't leave you, Kester," she said. The sadness

and resignation that he heard in her voice and felt across their bond made his heart ache with guilt. "You know I can't. But you're not changing into a different man, so the question doesn't matter."

"But I am changing."

"Yes, but not into a different man."

"Into what, then?"

She looked as if she would answer, but then she changed her mind. "I don't want to spoil the surprise."

He frowned at her, brought the hand he was still holding to his mouth, and nipped at the tip of her finger hard enough for her to yelp and pull it away sharply. She gave him such an adorable look of irritation that he couldn't help but laugh.

It was hard to tell in the firelight, but it looked like her cheeks went slightly pink. She couldn't hide the emotions he could feel across their bond, though. Annoyance, embarrassment, and... something else he didn't dare acknowledge, even to himself.

Maybe it wouldn't be prudent to do that again.

"If you're not going to let me curse that boy, then what do you suggest?" he asked.

She resumed her seat across from him, took a sip of her drink, and frowned at what was probably by now a lukewarm mug of hot chocolate. "Find out what you can about him and his family online. Then let me follow them around tomorrow and see if I can find out anything else."

"Have it your way." He could always enact some magical vengeance later.

———

The small-town junior high building was not difficult to break into. It had no security cameras or alarm system, only locks on the doors. Why would anyone want to break into a junior high school, after all? To make matters easier, one of the windows in the main office had been left cracked open a good four inches. It took very little effort to sneak around behind the bushes, push the window open, pop off the screen, and climb inside.

The secretary's computer took five minutes to fully start up, and while it was password-locked, there was a sticky note under the keyboard with a list of passwords on it, all but the last crossed out. Sometimes systems that require people to reset their password every thirty or ninety days do more harm than good to the security of their information.

The school directory program was right there on the desktop, and it opened with the same password as the computer login. A quick search by name brought up the contact info—including home address. Then it was a simple matter of shutting off the computer, exiting through the window, and replacing the screen.

In and out. Quick and easy.

Too quick and easy, really. They ought to have been more careful, what with a killer on the loose.

CHAPTER
TWENTY

On Tuesday morning, it took Lisa a full pot of coffee to work up the willpower to go to work. She was overworked on a good week, but now there was a student to figure out how to punish, a rumor to figure out how to quash, a murdered teacher to find a permanent replacement for, and a different student to save from becoming the murderer's next victim.

Not that that last one was really her job, but she'd do her best about it anyway.

So when she arrived at the main school office and saw a trail of dirt leading from the open window to Michael's computer and back, the first thing she did was walk into her office and pull a bottle of iced coffee out of her mini-fridge. Then she called the police.

Michael got in a few minutes later. "Morning, Lisa."

"Morning, Michael. Don't go to your desk."

Michael froze like he was expecting her to tell him he was fired. Or that his desk was covered in ants. "Okay. Why not?"

She nodded toward the dirt on the floor. "Did you leave that window open yesterday?"

"Oh, crap. I opened it in the afternoon when I got hot, but I thought I'd closed it."

Two uniformed officers walked into the office: Heather Blackwell, who Lisa had known since kindergarten; and her partner, Leonard Cherry, who was relatively new to town but married to a woman who... had certain recreational acquaintanceships with some of the same men that Lisa did. Or used to have, before she'd met Leonard.

Sometimes knowing almost everyone in town felt a tad strange.

"Hi, Lisa," said Heather. "What's the problem?"

Michael looked from the officers to Lisa in confusion. "You called the police?"

Lisa ignored him and pointed to the dirt trail. It wasn't much of a trail, really. Not anything like nice, clear footprints. She might even have missed it if she weren't so caffeinated. "I think someone broke in last night."

The officers looked over the evidence, discussed amongst themselves, and came back to her. Heather said, "I gotta tell you, Lisa. I don't really see it."

Lisa had never liked Heather very much. "Are you serious? There's obviously dirt from the window to Michael's computer, but nowhere else around. And the window had been left open. That doesn't seem strange to you?"

"I'll make a note of it, but we've got bigger things to focus on right now."

"I know. That's why I'm taking this so seriously. I think it could be related."

"How?"

Lisa let out a frustrated breath. "Never mind."

"Check the computer," said Leonard. "If anything's missing or looks like it's been tampered with, give us a call."

"Sure." Once the officers left, Lisa went to Michael's computer with him. "Turn it on and see if anything looks different than normal."

Michael set his things down, turned his computer on, waited for it to start up... and then pulled out a note with his password written on it.

As he entered the password, Lisa rubbed her forehead. "I'll be ⬝ my office. Let me know if you find anything out of sorts."

"Sure thing, Lisa."

When she was back at her own desk, she used her computer to check the shared systems they used, going straight to the access logs. Sure enough, one of them had been accessed late last night: the one that they kept all the personal details for staff, students, and any other employees or volunteers in.

She called Marcus and explained the situation to him.

————

"There was only one record accessed?" Marcus asked. It was too early in the morning for bad news.

Lisa's voice was calm—which was unexpected, given the circumstances. "Yes."

Not good. "Bet I can guess which one."

"You'd lose that bet."

Marcus wondered if they'd heard each other right. "Huh?"

"The record that was accessed," Lisa explained, "was John McKenzie's."

Him again. That man kept popping up in the weirdest ways. "What does he have to do with anything? What connection does he have to the suspect?"

"Maybe none. Maybe it's unrelated."

"That sounds like an awfully big coincidence, doesn't it? Who else could be out there, breaking into places to dig up information on people?"

"I don't know. I'll ask him."

Marcus wasn't certain that was a good idea. Something about John McKenzie felt dangerous... but Marcus couldn't for the life of him say what it was or why he thought that. *Not* remembering something about someone isn't a very good reason to suspect them of anything. So even though Marcus wanted to warn Lisa to be careful about him, he didn't. "Let me know if he tells you anything

eresting. Meanwhile, I'll see if I can find out anything about him
any connection that he might have had to Haug."

"Thanks, Marcus."

"No problem, Lisa. It's what I'm here for."

———

Kester typically tried not to get to the school earlier than absolutely necessary, which meant he was usually in around ten minutes before the first class started. Today, he was surprised to find Trick and Denneka already sitting in their seats when he entered.

It wasn't a bad idea. He'd heard plenty of rumor-mongering about them as he'd worked his way through the crowded hallway. They'd probably arrived well before most of the students in order to avoid walking through that gauntlet. None of the other kids had come in yet, usually putting off getting to class until they had to, which meant their presence was likely to go unnoticed until a few minutes before class.

When Kester stepped into the classroom, Trick eyed him warily while a flash of panic lit up Denneka's face. They were afraid he'd say something that would alert the kids in the hall to their presence, and they'd have to suffer several more minutes of teasing and taunts than they might otherwise.

Kester said nothing and went to his desk, then took out a book and started reading as if they weren't even there.

Five minutes before the bell, Lisa came in. She took one look at the pair of kids, then ignored them. "John," she said when she was close enough to speak quietly, "can I speak with you for a moment?"

He glanced at the clock.

"It won't take long."

She was his boss, so he didn't have much choice. "Of course." He followed her down the hall to her office, where she explained that the office had been broken into and his records—only his—had been accessed.

"Do you have any idea why someone might do this?"

He mulled it over. "No," he said honestly. "Do you?"

"I'm afraid it has something to do with the killer on the loose."

That was an intriguing thought. He'd never been the target of a killer before. "Why?"

"You took the job of the man he murdered, and you're the home-room teacher of the girl who gave the police information that he was trying to hide. Maybe he thinks you're connected? Or that he can get to her through you?"

The idea sent a thrill through him. A normal person would probably feel fear at this point, but all he felt was anticipatory excitement. Facing off with an honest-to-god murderer? That would be quite the diversion indeed. But he tried to keep a concerned expression on his face. "This sounds serious."

"I've told Marcus about this, but the other police aren't taking it seriously. I hope I'm only overreacting. But keep an eye out—for Denneka, but also for yourself. And let me know if you can think of any reason someone might want to get at your information in such an illegal manner."

"I will certainly do that. Thank you for the warning, Lisa." As Kester wended through the hall on the way back to his classroom, a thought occurred to him. He felt a small tingle of fear and suffered a momentary hitch in his gait.

If Lisa was correct, then this murderer was after John McKenzie, the teacher—not Kester, the witch. And the only way he could find John was if Kester were wearing his disguise. Which meant his magic would be locked away as it was now. Which meant he might actually be vulnerable.

If he meant to attack me while I'm out, he wouldn't need my home address, he told himself, shaking off the fear. *And I never wear my disguise when I'm home. If he wants to break in, let him. Maybe I'll get to turn someone into a frog after all.*

———

Even though Denneka had worried for a moment when Mr. McKenzie had come in, she worried even more when he left. When the other kids started coming into class, surely his presence would have kept them from badgering her too badly.

Or so she thought.

The first several kids that came in only gave her and Trick curious glances. Or judgmental glances. Or, in the case of a boy Denneka would never have expected it from, suggestive glances. But then more people came in, and the whispers started. And the laughter. And a few rude gestures.

No one bothered to ask about Trick's black eye. Maybe Trevor had preemptively spread around his lie about that, too.

When Denneka glanced aside to Trick, she saw him watching all of the chatter with confusion obvious in his expression. Obvious to her, anyway. He didn't express as much with his face as most people did, but either he was doing it more lately or she was getting more used to reading him.

Then Trevor, Amy, and Flora came in, and all Hades broke loose.

"Well, look who came back to school!" Trevor said loudly enough to draw the attention of everyone in the room. "What were you two doing all afternoon yesterday that you couldn't even make it back to class?"

"I bet I know," cooed Flora.

"You couldn't wait to get alone, could you?" taunted Amy. "You weirdos are so shameless."

"Would you guys take it easy?" Brook said, almost too quietly to be heard.

Amy laughed. "Someone's easy and taking it, but it's not us."

The three bullies laughed the hardest at that, but a lot of other people joined in.

Denneka tried to bury her face in her hands and shrink down as small as she could, but it didn't help.

Trevor perched on the back of his chair with his feet on the seat —the better to look down on them. "Hey, weirdo, does—"

Mr. McKenzie came into the room, and silence instantly fell over the class. He looked around in a bored way, but he had to have heard at least a little of what was going on before he came in. Everyone waited for him to say something.

Please say something, Denneka thought urgently. *Please say something. You said you'd help.*

Mr. McKenzie didn't so much as give the bullies a warning look. He just sat at his desk, picked up a book, and started reading like he was trying to tune them all out.

"Do you think they went to a hotel?" Flora asked somewhat quietly, testing the waters. "Or just found an empty closet somewhere?"

Trevor and Amy laughed. Mr. McKenzie didn't even look up from his book.

More whispering started. More barely-suppressed laughter. Then Trevor said, "How much more practice you think she needs before she gets better than 'fine'?" and the trio were on a roll again.

It went on for at least a couple minutes. When the bell rang, Mr. McKenzie set his book down, walked over to close the door, and took position in the front of the room. He didn't wait for the class to settle down on its own but clapped his hands to get everyone's attention.

"So, about this rumor," he said, scratching his eyebrow distractedly. "You're all getting a lot of mileage out of it. But really, I thought most of you had more sense than this."

Denneka perked up. Other kids shifted in their seats or made whispered, annoyed remarks to each other.

Here it came. The lecture. He was going to do what teachers are supposed to do and tell them how mean and disrespectful they were being and say how he wasn't going to tolerate it.

"It seems to me," Mr. McKenzie said, "that the lot of you have greatly overestimated Patrick's intelligence."

The room fell into stunned, confused silence.

Mr. McKenzie folded his arms impatiently. "Patrick, who else besides Denneka has let you sleep with them?"

Paying no attention to the surprised sounds around them, Trick thought, then answered, "The old woman."

The classroom erupted in gasps and groans of shocked disgust.

"And sometimes my mom," Trick continued.

Disgust turned to confusion.

"And my little brother."

Confusion turned to disappointed understanding, and everyone gradually quieted down.

Mr. McKenzie waved a dismissive hand at Trick. "You see, Patrick isn't remotely as interesting as that rumor gives him credit for. He probably napped beside her on the couch once or something." He paused to see if anyone would argue with him. No one did. "Now that that's settled, would you all kindly pay attention so I can get class started?"

Mr. McKenzie had tried to take care of it like he'd said he would, in a way. Not a very nice way, but it worked better than a lecture probably would have. Trick was grumpy all day from Mr. McKenzie calling him stupid, so he didn't seem to see it, but Denneka did.

Maybe Trick's mom is right, she thought. *Maybe Mr. McKenzie isn't so bad.*

When Jacqueline picked them up at the end of the day, Denneka told her what had happened.

"Does this mean your rumor problem is solved?" Jacqueline asked.

"He called me stupid!" Trick protested from the back seat.

Denneka ignored him. "Well… it's better. Most of the people in our class have dropped it, but Amy must really have it out for him. For us. She keeps spreading it around and making jokes, even though Trevor and Flora have stopped joining in and even try to stop her when she gets going too much. I think maybe Trevor's annoyed at Trick for just being stupid instead of… you know."

"I'm not stupid!" Trick insisted.

"We know, Trick," Jacqueline said. "But this rumor was your fault, so if you have to pay the price to make it go away, that's only fair."

"What do you mean my fault?" he asked.

Denneka didn't want to explain it, so she ignored him again. "But because of Amy, a lot of the kids from the other classes still think it's true. I keep getting weird looks in the hallway. It... makes me really uncomfortable."

"It sounds like most of the steam has gone out of it, though," Jacqueline said. "Give it a few days, maybe a week, and I bet Amy will be the only one who bothers to keep talking about it, and then she'll look dumb for harping on about something no one else cares about."

Denneka wanted to believe her, but the whispers and looks from so many kids kept replaying in her mind. "I hope you're right."

———

The house Kester now lived in came with an expansive back deck which faced west. A small river ran behind it, and beyond that, green hills. It made for stunning sunsets. They were especially stunning from the comfort of the outdoor hot tub which some previous owner had thoughtfully built into the deck.

He sighed in pleasure as hot water churned around him and the sky painted itself with incandescent hues. "An honest day's work certainly is tedious. How do people do it, day in and day out, year after year?"

Julia didn't answer. Not that she could have, being a bird. She only sat perched on the deck railing to his right, watching the sunset with him.

The moment was quiet and peaceful, a slice of absolute perfection.

It went on for half an hour, and he didn't speak again. Eventually, the curve of the sun slipped behind the hills and the hawk on the railing transformed into a nude woman. She sat there, face turned toward the fading light, perfect and beautiful as a burnished sculpture.

"So, how was your day, dearest?" he asked. "Did you discover

ıything useful?" He'd been so busy, he'd rarely had time to check
ı with her.

"The bully boy's family is normal enough, I guess, for rich
bankers. I didn't see anything to make me think they're especially
evil or corrupt."

Kester nodded. He hadn't seen anything like that in his internet
research of the family either. "So you're saying we shouldn't utterly
ruin them."

She shrugged. "No reason to. I did find out one thing you might
like, though. The boy's dad has a prescription for a certain drug
popular with older men."

Ideas began to swim around in Kester's brain. "Indeed. That is
interesting." The ideas arranged themselves into a very pleasing
shape, and his mouth spread in a grin. "Good work, my darling."
He swept his hand in a stately gesture from her perch to the hot tub.
"Would you care to join me? The water's very comfortable."

She looked down at him from her vantage point, and he was
suddenly, acutely aware that he was as nude as she was. The half-
second's pulse of longing that came to him across their bond nearly
knocked the breath from his lungs.

Not a bit of it showed on Julia's face. She simply shook her head
politely and dismounted from the railing. "No, thank you, Master. I
do think I'll take a bath, though. Please excuse me." She padded into
the house, and Kester could do nothing but stare in frozen silence at
the place where she'd been sitting.

Kester had never been shy about being naked—or, in fact, about
anything he might do naked—in front of Julia. Not even when she'd
been a child. Because he'd never seen her as a child. She was always,
only, his slave. A beloved slave, yes, but still only a slave. In fact, at
first, he'd wanted her to get used to seeing his body because it
would make things easier later. By the time he'd decided he couldn't
use her as he used other women, they were both simply too
comfortable around each other to give either's nudity a second
thought.

It wasn't as if he'd never sensed any hint of desire from her. It was only that slaves were not allowed desire of any kind, so it didn't matter to him. He'd grown used to brushing it aside as he brushed aside the pain in her heart when he was with other women. As he brushed aside the romantic feelings she had for him which would make things difficult and inconvenient for him if he acknowledged them.

So why had he felt her reaction so keenly now? Why was it so difficult for him to brush aside?

He considered this question until the sky grew dark and the stars twinkled in brilliant abundance overhead.

"Because I don't wish to enslave her anymore," he murmured to himself. He wanted to give her a right to her own feelings and her own desires. Even if it meant giving her the choice to leave him and live her own life. Even if it meant risking the most precious thing he had in this world.

In that moment, with that realization, it felt as if he had already lost her. Tears began to flow down his cheeks, and he let them, knowing that she was safe inside and too far away to hear him weep.

"Why did you tell Mom the teacher man is all right?" Trick asked. He hadn't understood any of what was going on that morning or why those humans were saying such strange things to them, but he *had* understood when the teacher man had called him stupid.

They were already in bed together, the familiar girl lying on her side and Trick curled up by her feet. It was dark and warm, and he should have been sleepy, but he was too annoyed at being called stupid and at the way his mom and the familiar girl kept dismissing it when he complained.

"Because he helped us," she said from somewhere above him.

"He called me stupid," Trick complained again.

"I guess that's… true." She let out a breath. "He helped me, then. As much as he could."

"By calling me stupid?"

"Yes."

Trick wished he had his tail so he could lash it to show his annoyance. "I'm not stupid."

"I know that. You're not stupid. Everyone else will see that eventually. But for now... It's complicated."

"Explain."

"I can't. It's too embarrassing."

Trick was beginning to get annoyed at the number of things the familiar girl found embarrassing. Why couldn't she just *not care* what other humans thought? But he decided to stop pressing it. She had been sad last night, and she'd been almost as bad tonight.

He lay on her feet and tried to go to sleep.

A while later, her voice woke him from the light doze he'd fallen into. "Trick." Her voice sounded strange and tight. "Please don't tell people again that I let you sleep with me."

He had to think back to remember what she was referring to. It was something he'd said when the aggressive boy was attacking him with questions. The suit lady had brought it up, too. "Why? Is it a secret?"

"Yes. And... and they'll take it wrong."

"How?" How many ways were there to take it? It sounded like a direct statement to him.

"They'll... they'll think we're... intimate."

"Aren't we?"

"Not like that! 'Sleep with' means... it means... 'mate with'."

Trick thought about that. This was why he hated using human language. "Sleeping and mating are completely different. How can they mean the same thing?"

"They just do."

"That's stupid."

"I guess so."

"So those boys think I said you let me mate with you?"

"Y-yes. And so did everyone else, after they started talking. Mr. McKenzie helped me by making it sound like you didn't know what you were saying—which you didn't. But a lot of people at school still believe it."

So, Trick really had been stupid. "And... is that why you're sad?"

Her body hitched, and she made small sounds that troubled him. "Yeah."

"Why do you care what they think?"

The sounds were louder this time. She was crying. "I don't know, but I do."

Trick had no idea what was happening now. He crawled up so he could stick his head out of the blanket and look at her face. "Is it because they believe something untrue about you?"

Her face was wet, and her eyes were clenched shut, but he was pretty sure she knew he was there and could see her. She nodded.

This was a difficult problem. If the problem was that everyone believed something untrue about her, there were only two solutions: either correct everyone's thinking or make the thing true. If Trick understood her right, the teacher man already tried to correct everyone's thinking, and it had only partly worked. So, if that option had already been tried, did that mean... "Do you *want* me to mate with you?"

"No!" She turned and shoved him so hard, he nearly fell out of the bed. But his reflexes in this body were getting better, so he caught himself on the edge and regained his balance.

"Good," he said. "Because I'm a cat, so that wouldn't make any sense."

She stared at him, her face wet and red, and burst into laughter. Then she threw her arms around his shoulders, squeezing him tight. He struggled at the sudden confinement, but she only squeezed him harder. So he froze, more confused than ever about what was happening or what he should do.

"You're unbelievable, Trick," she said, her voice muffled because she was pressing her wet face into his shoulder. "I really like you."

"I... really like you, too."

Her body bounced, and she made a sound, but he couldn't tell whether it was crying or laughing. "I really wish you wouldn't leave me."

"I won't."

She pulled back, smiling now. He was pretty sure that was a good sign. "You will. But it's okay. I'll deal with it."

Trick felt his eyebrows lower involuntarily. He didn't like being accused of telling a lie when he hadn't. "I won't."

She wiped her eyes on her sleeve and lay down on her side, facing away from him again. "I'm tired. Let's go to sleep."

"And by 'sleep' you mean—"

"I mean sleep. 'Sleep' only means 'mate' when followed by 'with'."

That was a really overly complicated rule about what should have been a simple word, but he would try to remember it. He made sure he was on his side of the blanket, then settled down by her legs. It took him a lot of shifting before he found a position he liked, finally relaxing with his chin propped on her hip and one arm and shoulder draped over her thigh.

Why had he never noticed before how nice and soft that part of her was?

CHAPTER
TWENTY-ONE

Things always looked brighter and less hopeless in the morning. As long as Kester didn't think too much about Julia or his desire to free her or the inevitable cost of doing so, he was able to maintain his cheer and good humor.

He even brought treats in to class.

When the students came back into his classroom for fourth period, they were manifestly shocked to see the large tray of cookies he'd set out on his desk. Most of them walked right by it, suspicious of a trap. Or perhaps, since fourth period was the science class, they suspected that the cookies were to be used in some sort of laboratory experiment.

"I haven't poisoned them," Kester drawled after everyone was at their desks and only two students had taken a cookie.

"You mean those are for us?" asked a girl in the front row.

"Yes."

"But why?" asked a boy.

"I've seen other teachers bring treats to class. Do I alone need some ulterior motive?" No one seemed to want to question him further. When some of them started to get up and come forward, he pulled out a gallon of milk from behind his desk. "Ah, I brought this s well. But seeing as I don't want to spend the next half-hour mopping it up, I'll pour."

As the kids came to get their treats, Kester carefully poured milk into small paper cups and firmly secured plastic lids to them before sliding them across the desk to each student in turn.

And that was how he got the potion into Trevor.

Even though it was an easy enough potion to brew, Kester hadn't had to expend any energy doing so because it was one of the standard potions he kept in stock in his lab. Not for himself, of course, but for his customers.

Kester didn't work, as a general rule. He had many ways of acquiring funds that were far easier and more enjoyable than brewing and selling potions. But potions were a useful currency when there were items, favors, or services which could not be easily purchased with cash. And this particular potion—being more customizable and more discreet than the pharmaceutical alternative —was a popular one.

Trevor took four cookies and the spiked milk back to his desk, inhaling it all without pausing.

Teenage boys can always be relied upon to be hungry for a mid-morning snack, Kester observed with satisfaction. For a brief moment, he almost felt sorry for the boy. But then he shifted his gaze to the back of the room and saw Trick and Denneka sitting in silence, the girl working hard not to be noticed.

It might have been a mid-afternoon snack, leaving Trevor to suffer his punishment safe in his own home with only his family's reactions to deal with, were it not for the rumor. Kester had kept an ear out all morning, hoping the rumor might have died down to nothing. Sadly, there were still students in the hallway talking about it, largely egged on by Amy's insistence in continuing to spread it around and to taunt Denneka and Trick, even when her friends urged her to quiet down about it.

You should have worked harder to quiet your friend, Kester thought in Trevor's direction. *Now you'll have to pay the price.* Because the only way to get the kids to stop talking about Trick and Denneka now was to give them something more interesting to talk about.

———

Marcus leaned back in his chair and tapped all ten fingers on his desk. He'd just finished going over everything they had on Haug, and he couldn't find any mention of John McKenzie or anything that even hinted at a connection between the two. Nothing that would explain why their suspect would break into the school to look up information on the teacher. But if they could find out what the connection was between Haug and the killer, would anything there lead to McKenzie?

They wouldn't know that until they knew who the killer was and what he had to do with Haug. In the mean time, maybe looking into McKenzie's background would lead to something about Haug. Marcus had to be careful, though. McKenzie wasn't a suspect in anything. He wasn't even a victim of data theft—officially—since the officers who'd responded to Lisa's initial call hadn't thought a crime had taken place. Given the personal connection between Marcus and Lisa, it wouldn't look good to go behind their backs and open a case on it without something more concrete. And Lisa hadn't followed up with the investigating officers about the data access. Which meant that he had no good reason to go digging into McKenzie's personal information.

He picked up his desk phone and dialed the main school number.

The secretary answered. "Hello?"

"Hello. This is Officer Parkes. Principal VanBuren called me yesterday to follow up on her report about a possible break-in. She said some information had been accessed."

"Of course. She said it was something about John?"

So, she had told the secretary. That should make this easier. "It's probably nothing serious, but I'm looking into it for her."

"Right. I don't think I can help you, I'm afraid. I wasn't able to see anything strange on my computer. Do you want me to transfer your call to Lisa?"

"No, that's not necessary," Marcus said hastily. The whole reason he'd called the main number was to talk to the secretary. "I was wondering if you could fax me a copy of Mr. McKenzie's personal information that you have on file. As well as his resumé and job application, if you've got it." Marcus held his breath while he waited, wondering how much this secretary trusted the police and how that compared to what he knew about information security and private records. But he didn't have to hold his breath for long.

"Oh, sure. I think I can find that."

"That would be very helpful, thanks." Maybe Marcus should talk to Lisa about her secretary's over-helpfulness. After Marcus had gotten what he wanted.

The fax came within five minutes. Marcus hoped the secretary wouldn't say anything to Lisa about it, but it was too risky to specifically tell him not to. One of Lisa's best qualities was how protective she was of her charges. That mostly meant her students, but it also —to a lesser degree—included her employees. And if she knew Marcus was prying into John McKenzie's life as if he were a suspect rather than a potential victim, she'd tear him a new one.

Marcus sat at his desk and organized the pages of the fax containing McKenzie's records. Work history, schooling, parking information, social security number... Yes, this would give him plenty of places to start digging. For the next hour, he made notes and wrote e-mails. Hopefully, he'd soon have a better idea of who McKenzie was and if he had any connection to Haug.

Or the boy, he thought, trying to blink away the strange image of the two of them that suddenly floated in front of his eyes.

The lizard was afraid. The lizard was always afraid, except when it was asleep or curled up in Landon's shirt pocket. Right now, the lizard was afraid of the boys Landon had sent it to spy on. They were the ones who'd gone after him in the hall on that one day. They hadn't tried to bully him again, but lately he'd seen them watching him and had heard them whispering to other kids, and he knew it was about him.

Landon sat on a swing, holding the chains tightly but not moving. He was concentrated on the lizard. He could see through its eyes and feel the breath in its tiny lungs as it skittered under the see-saw and closer to the boys hanging around the monkey bars.

"Look at him over there," said the biggest boy, who Landon had learned was called Cliff. "Just staring off into space like a zombie."

"Hey, look," said another boy.

They all turned to face toward the swings. He could have pulled his attention away from the lizard, but he wanted to hear what they were saying about him. So instead, he told the lizard to climb up the ladder part of the monkey bars so he could see himself through its eyes.

In the distance, he saw a couple girls go up to the swings, but he was so connected with the lizard that he couldn't hear anything through his own ears. The lizard was too far away to see his face very well, but he knew that he looked the same as Mr. McKenzie had looked on that day he'd pretended to read all morning. One of the girls poked Landon in the shoulder. He felt it. He'd probably need to pull out of this to deal with her.

But the moment before he was going to do it, something tight wrapped around his body so hard, he gasped for breath.

No, not *his* body. The lizard's.

Any thought of the girls left his mind as his vision spun wildly. Cliff's face was suddenly there, huge and grinning. "Look what I caught."

Terror made the lizard's heart beat so fast, it physically hurt. It was too much. Landon jerked away from the lizard's mind, coming back to himself, but he could still feel its fear and pain through the familiar bond.

Ignoring the girl who'd been trying to get his attention, Landon pushed away from the swing and sprinted toward the boys. His anger was so hot that the only thing going through his head was, *Mine. Mine. Mine!*

Before he could reach the boys, the lizard's fear was joined by terrible pain as Cliff pulled off its tail.

Landon skidded to a stop ten feet away from them, grabbing at any self-control he could find. If he attacked the boys without any clear reason, it wouldn't look good for him. All the work he'd done to make people like him would be wasted. "That's mine," he said through clenched teeth. "Give it back."

It was the wrong thing to say. Landon knew it as soon as he saw the sneering grin on Cliff's face. Without a word, Cliff dropped the lizard on the blacktop, lifted his boot, and crushed it to death.

The pain the lizard felt only lasted a second, but it dropped Landon to his knees and left him panting for air. The connection was gone. Poof, like blowing out a candle.

Cliff laughed. "You shouldn't let your pets wander around like that. They could get hurt."

Landon pulled himself to his feet and glared at Cliff. He could feel the magic pooling in his body, making his hands tingle.

Cliff stepped closer to him. "You gonna do something about it?"

The boy had clearly forgotten the lesson Landon had taught him last time. He needed another one.

Even though Landon could see other kids on the edges of his vision—the other boys, the two girls who'd come up to him at the swings, and more—none of it seemed to matter. *Not here. Not in front of them*, he begged himself. But that was only a small, quiet part of his mind. Much louder was the blind rage he felt. "That was mine," he said. There was an edge to his voice, something he didn't recognize.

Cliff took a step back, his cockiness turning into uncertainty.

Let it go, said the small part of Landon's mind.

Don't let him get away, said the big, angry part.

Landon stretched out a finger, pointed to the middle of Cliff's chest, and said in what he thought was a very calm voice, "Die."

Cliff jerked and collapsed. Girls screamed. Boys screamed. A

shouted from somewhere not as far away as L.
.ked.

Cliff kept jerking on the ground, curling into a ball, g.
his chest.

"Out of the way!" shouted the teacher. It was Mr. Thom
fell on his knees beside Cliff, putting out his arm to get two
boys out of the way. "He's having a seizure?" He sounded scar
He looked at the nearest boy and asked, "What happened?"
The boy pointed to Landon, backing away. "Landon cursed him
or something!"

Mr. Thomas made an impatient sound. "Never mind. You." He
pointed at a girl who hadn't screamed and was only standing and
watching with wide eyes. "Go tell Miss Cutler to come out here."
The girl ran off.

The anger faded from Landon's mind. His chest stopped burning
with it. He looked around and saw the other kids watching him in
fear. *I ruined it,* he thought. *I ruined it all.*

Mr. Thomas grabbed Cliff and held him down while he jerked.
When Cliff stopped moving, Mr. Thomas said a bad word under his
breath, put his fingers to Cliff's neck, and then started pushing on
Cliff's chest.

Miss Cutler ran up. "What happened?" she yelled. She was
scared, too. Everyone was scared.

"I don't know," Mr. Thomas told her. "Call an ambulance. His
heart's stopped."

Miss Cutler fumbled her phone from her pocket and fumbled
more while she dialed.

I did it, Landon thought. *I killed him with magic.*

He really wasn't a good boy anymore. He wasn't even a bad boy.
He was a killer. He was... a murderer.

For a minute, nothing seemed real. He felt like he was watching
a movie, like he wasn't even in his own body anymore.

But when he thought of how his mom would react when she
heard about this, the shame and guilt were a heavy pain in his chest.
His head swam with it. He couldn't let her find out.

...s was still pushing on Cliff's chest. He wouldn't do ...were dead, would he?

...e on the way," Miss Cutler said. "They said to keep doing ...pressions until they get here."

...ly and trying not to be noticed, Landon went up to Cliff, on ...ner side of him from the teachers. Cliff's eyes were closed, and ...erked from Mr. Thomas pushing on him, but he wasn't moving ...his own at all.

"Watch out!" one of the other boys shouted at Mr. Thomas when Landon got close, but Landon shot him a look and the other boy shut up. The teachers were so focused on Cliff, they didn't act like they'd even heard the boy.

Landon crouched beside Cliff, not quite close enough to touch him, and pointed at him again. It wasn't easy this time. The magic wasn't there, bursting to come out. He had to dig for it, to gather it all together in his hand. He closed his eyes, trying to focus. When he thought he had enough magic, he opened his eyes and willed the magic into Cliff's heart. "Live."

Cliff let out a huff of breath. Mr. Thomas stopped pushing on him and felt his neck again.

"His pulse is back," said the teacher.

Cliff's eyes opened.

Mr. Thomas leaned over him. "Cliff, can you hear me? Can you speak? No, don't get up."

"Yeah," Cliff groaned.

"Good," said Mr. Thomas. "The ambulance is coming. Do you have any idea what happened to you?"

Cliff blinked like he was trying to remember.

One of the girls—the one who'd gone to get Miss Cutler—stepped forward. "Landon killed him," she told the teachers. "And then he brought him back to life."

Mr. Thomas frowned at her. "That's ridiculous. Besides, Cliff wasn't dead. His heart stopped, but that's not the same thing."

The ambulance people ran up from the school building, holding equipment. Everyone stepped aside to let them put Cliff on a stretcher and check him. Mr. Thomas talked to them about what had happened.

Mr. Thomas hadn't believed for a second that Landon could do what the other kids said he'd done. But all those kids were still watching Landon like he might attack them next. They knew what he'd done. None of them understood it, and they couldn't explain it, but they knew.

"Landon."

He looked up to see Miss Cutler's eyebrows come together. "Yes, ma'am?"

"Did you... do anything to Cliff?" she asked.

Inside, Landon was shouting in victory and crying in fear all at once, but he kept his face and voice calm. "Of course not. How could I?"

She didn't say anything after that, but he could see the doubt in her eyes.

———

It was a gray sedan from the eighties, but it looked like it was worth more than most new cars today. Not that Julia was any expert. She couldn't even tell what the make was and couldn't be sure she could name any manufacturer logos accurately, but the car had the shiny, cared-for look that a car that old usually didn't have unless it was worth something.

The car had been parked a hundred feet away from the school for the last four hours.

Julia had been doing air patrols of the area around the junior high all day, and things had looked pretty normal on the surface. But something about the placement of that car had made her pay more attention to it. It was facing the school, for one. Facing with a clear line of sight to the windows of Kester's classroom, to be precise. And when Julia had flown lower, she'd seen a man in the car. Perching where she could watch him, she did so for the next two hours. The man never got out of the car and frequently lifted a pair of binoculars to his eyes. Julia flew even closer, to a tree across the street.

She was almost completely certain that the man in the car was the same one the police were looking for: the killer—or suspected killer, anyway. He'd parked the car on a little-used side street, so no people had walked by and noticed him. If they had, they might have recognized him from the description in the paper. Had he picked that street deliberately for that reason? And if he had, did that mean he'd been lurking around town for long enough to know the best spots to not get noticed?

The interest and alarm she felt was enough to get Kester's attention. Eventually, he found a spare moment and checked in with her.

That's him, he said in her mind. *It has to be.*

She couldn't speak directly back to him, but she knew he would feel her expectation and curiosity, awaiting orders.

Be careful, Kester told her. *Keep an eye on him, but don't get into an altercation.*

Julia swiveled her head so her gaze swept from the car to his classroom and back.

I see. He's watching us. But is he watching Denneka or me? And why?

Julia couldn't answer any of that for him. But she didn't like the idea of a killer stalking her master.

As she watched, someone started to make their way down the street. It was hard to tell through all the layers of scrubby clothes, but the person was probably an older woman. She dragged a tattered duffel bag on wheels behind her.

The woman got closer to the car, approaching toward the front, walking on the sidewalk. The man in the car lowered his binoculars and pretended to read a book, but Julia didn't believe he was actually doing so.

Keep walking. Keep walking, Julia thought.

No such luck. When the woman was even with the front of the car, she looked at the man inside. Then did a double-take, leaning closer. Her mouth fell open.

Make it a little more obvious, would you?

The man got out of the car and growled something Julia couldn't make out, but the woman started backing away fearfully, hands up to ward him off. The man came around the hood, reaching for something in his pocket.

So much for that, Julia thought. Then she spread her wings and swooped toward the back of the man's neck. Just as the man reached to grab the woman with one hand and pulled a switchblade from his pocket with the other, Julia stretched her talons out as if diving for a mouse. They hit resistance and dug in deep. The man cried out and flailed, giving the old woman time to shuffle away as fast as she could.

The man swiped at Julia with his knife and tried to grab her in his meaty hands, but Julia took off into the air, circling to make sure he didn't try to go after the woman again. But all his attention was on her, cursing her out, grabbing at his bleeding neck. Her aim had been off, and she'd ended up mostly getting the collar of his jacket, but she was sure one or two talons had dug nice and deep into his flesh. She flapped higher and higher into the air. She could see from the man's red-faced fury that he wanted to strangle her, but she was well out of his reach. He wanted to shout at her, but he quickly clamped his mouth shut lest he be heard and others arrive. Julia watched from a high branch as he got back in his car and drove away. She tried to follow him back to whatever hole he was hiding in, but there were a lot of tall trees in Agreste, and somehow she lost him.

"How was school?" Jacqueline asked.

"Um…" Denneka mumbled, "school was… weird."

"Weird? What does that mean?"

"Well… um, Trevor, the boy who punched Trick… he, uh, kept getting… excited… during class."

"Excited?"

"Like he wanted to mate," Trick clarified helpfully. "I don't understand why, though. It didn't smell like any of the girls were in heat, and none of the other boys had that problem."

Annoyance lines appeared at the corners of Jacqueline's mouth. "Seriously, Trick, next time you're home, we're going to have 'the talk' again. It clearly didn't stick the first time. And—wait, you mean he—" She raised her eyebrows at Denneka.

Denneka winced and nodded. "It was… really disturbing. First it was during PE, and he tried to blame it on all the running?" She made it a question because she was still doubtful about whether that excuse was even plausible. But, not being a boy, she didn't know. "But then it happened again during lunch and then math and…" She shook her head to clear out the unpleasant images. "Thankfully, I wasn't very close whenever it happened, but a lot of people laughed at him and some of the girls got grossed out and ran away. I heard from someone else that his mom came to get him right before our computer class and didn't even wait until they got out of school before she was chewing him out about stealing one of his dad's pills and what did he plan to need it for and saying he wasn't allowed to hang out with Amy and Flora at their house anymore unless she or his dad was home."

"That does sound like quite the eventful day. So, when you say you heard it from someone else… ?"

"I don't remember who. It was all anyone was talking about by the end of school."

"Really? As in, they weren't talking about you two anymore?"

"No. It seemed like everyone forgot all about us once all that started. We sure got lucky."

"Luck? Sounds more like dramatic irony or karmic retribution. Just don't forget that it's not nice to gossip about people, okay?"

"Believe me, I didn't want to. Trevor getting 'excited' is *not* something I want to remember or think about ever again."

———

Trick's evening nap was ended by a sudden transformation into his human form and a light scratching on the bedroom door. "Hurry," he heard the familiar girl whisper from the other side.

He tried, but he had trouble with the sleeves of his sweatshirt, so he'd only gotten half-dressed by the time she slipped into the room, and he was tangled up with his arms partway in the sleeves. Her face turned pink like it always did when she saw his skin, then she set a plate of delicious-smelling food on the desk and helped him figure out the shirt.

Once she was happy with him, he dove for the food. He wasn't sure what it was called, but there was meat and sauce and noodles shaped like bows.

"Good?" she asked.

"Mmm," he answered with his mouth full of food.

"Sorry that took so long. Sometimes when everyone's home at the same time, my mom gets into a 'family dinnertime' mood and everyone has to answer questions about how their day was. And since today was so weird, it took a while to get through everything. Especially since I had to mentally edit it first to figure out what I could talk about without making them suspicious about you. The news of you being 'missing' was all over the place, so they know about you in general, and Mom already knew about us being friends. I... I also told them about the rumor, sort of. Now that it looks like it's over, I think it's safe. I didn't want them to hear about it from outdated town gossip later. I think I said it all in a way that makes it clear we're only friends. Of course, my mom will probably still tease me about you."

Trick paused for breath and asked, "Only friends? What else would we be?"

There was a small change in her expression. Trick was able to see it happen, but he couldn't tell what it meant. "Right?" she said in a quieter voice than before. "That's what I mean."

Trick didn't know what 'that' was, but it didn't seem worth stopping eating again to ask. By the time he finished, she was lying on the bed, watching a video on her phone. She was on her belly, feet kicking lazily in the air, smiling at whatever she was watching. He licked his lips, making sure his face was clean, and finished off his water.

When he climbed onto the bed and stretched out next to her in the same position, his side against hers, she didn't do anything more than look up and turn a little pink before going back to her video. He watched it with her, but even though she smiled and even chuckled, he didn't understand a lot of the jokes.

But then he noticed a piece of her hair on the side of her head sticking up weird. And once he noticed it, he couldn't not notice it. He tried to watch the video, but that lock of hair was there in the corner of his eye, nagging at him. Eventually, he couldn't take it anymore. He shifted to his hands and knees to get a better angle and licked the piece of hair into place.

The girl jerked, which made the hair even more out of place. So he held her head still with both hands and went back to trying to tame that irritating lock of hair.

"Trick!" she hissed. "What are you doing?"

He couldn't talk and groom her at the same time, so he didn't talk. He shifted his chest over her shoulders to hold her down with his body weight while he worked at getting her hair back into order. She struggled again, but he kept licking, and after another try she gave up and let him work.

Finally, he got that piece of hair into place. Then he saw more that had gotten messed up when she'd tried to get away from him, so he had to get those sorted out, too. Once he was satisfied, he sat back on his heels to examine the effect.

"Better," he declared.

She looked up at him with wide eyes, then the corners of her lips curled, then she made a sound like she was choking on a laugh. Her hand flew up to her mouth to hold back the sounds she was making. After a few seconds, she rolled onto her back and laughed.

Trick had no idea what she thought was funny now, since she'd dropped her phone on the floor, and he stared at her in confusion. *She's happy*, he realized. He didn't interrupt her laughing. He didn't think she'd been happy like that in a while, and he liked seeing her laugh a lot more than he liked seeing her cry. It was nice. It made him feel good.

Somewhere in the back of his mind, Trick noticed that his own mouth had curled into a smile, just like a real human.

CHAPTER
TWENTY-TWO

"Good morning," the middle-aged woman behind the counter greeted Jacqueline as she walked into the clothing store. There wasn't anyone else in the store at the moment other than the young salesman folding shirts near the back.

Jacqueline smiled and went to the woman. "Good morning."

The woman—her name tag said 'Barb'—set a book down and sat up. "Can I help you find anything?"

Jacqueline couldn't help glancing at the book as she stepped up to the counter. "Oh, I've read that one. What do you think of it?"

Barb perked up even more. "I'm enjoying it. I do love a good secret marriage story. Not quite as steamy as I'd like, though." She added that last part in a quiet, confidential tone.

Jacqueline chuckled. "I'll bring you one of mine some time."

The woman blinked in confusion. "One of yours?"

"Oh, I'm an author. Jacqueline St. Andrew."

Barb beamed. "No kidding? I've read one of yours. *Behind the Curtain*, I think it was. I liked it."

"I'm glad to hear that. Thank you."

"I recognized your name in the newspaper article about your son, but I didn't think it could be the same person. I mean, what are the odds?"

"We all have to live somewhere. Though my sons and I only moved to town recently."

"How is your boy doing now? That must have been quite an ordeal, living on the streets like that."

"He's doing fine, relatively speaking. School's hard for him, and he's not very comfortable with other kids. Denneka is helping him adjust, though."

"Yes, I understand they're friends." Barb winked. "I watched the two of them when you all came in a while back. I think our Denneka may have a little crush on him."

Jacqueline leaned across the counter and said softly, "Between you and me, I think he's a bit taken with her as well. Not that he realizes it. Boys can be stupid at that age."

Barb laughed. "What brings you in today? Are you looking for something specific?"

"Yes, but it's not clothes. I'm doing research for an idea for a new book. I've been trying to find out if there's any local lore regarding supernatural occurrences or legends. Any haunted places or mysterious sightings or people in local history who were thought to be witches. Anything like that. I've looked through all the books I could find at the library, and there wasn't much of anything. So I've started going around and asking locals if they knew of any legends like that. Do you happen to know of any?"

Barb considered this for a while. "I can't say that anything comes to mind." She raised her voice. "Alex, do you have a second?"

The young man came over to join them. "What's up? Oh, hello again."

Jacqueline repeated her query.

Alex said, "Well, some people in school told me that the old dance hall above the pub is haunted because some girl died there. Something about being killed by her mother, I think. Not sure I would call that a legend, though, since that story's only about ten years old and no one really believes it. Just kids trying to spook each other, I think."

Jacqueline tried to hide her disappointment, but made a mental note of the story anyway. "Is there anything else you can think of?"

He shook his head. "Sorry, no."

Jacqueline thanked them and left, making her way down the sidewalk. Usually locals were a good source for this kind of gossip, and a good place to find locals was in locally-owned businesses. But so far she wasn't getting much. A few stories like the one the young man had shared, but nothing that sounded at all like it might indicate a male witch living in the area.

She entered a small electronics store. On her way to the counter, she passed a display of strange-looking cameras which caught her eye. She took a closer look. They were nanny-cams.

She wanted to trust John; she really did. But... it couldn't hurt...

————

Marcus stared at the reports and notes laid out on his desk. He'd checked up on everything reported in McKenzie's resumé, run the info on his car and house, and even done a background check. And the one inescapable conclusion was that John McKenzie—or, at least, *this* John McKenzie—didn't exist.

No one by that name had graduated from the University of Minnesota in the year that McKenzie's resumé said he earned his degree. None of the places where he'd supposedly worked previously had any idea who he was. Oh, there had been someone to verify his supposed history when he'd called the numbers on the resumé, but when he'd looked the places up independently, he'd found different contact information, and those contacts had told a different story. Neither was there any record of him having a teaching license in this state. He didn't appear in any criminal or other governmental database Marcus had checked. His driver's license number was fake. And—this was where it got really interesting—his car was registered to someone called Kester McKenzie. That last could have been chalked up to him borrowing a family car, if not for the fact that the purc.

also signed by Kester—not John—Mck

ing was up with that guy, and Marcu.

wondering what it was. Even though he'd turned up

that there was any connection between McKenzie anc

case, the man was obviously hiding something.

Marcus called Lisa and asked without greeting, "Has M.

ever mentioned someone named Kester?"

He could hear in Lisa's voice and in the faint sound of shuff.

papers that she was busy. "He didn't have to. I've met Kester."

"You have?"

"Yes. At Bruno's." She didn't need to elaborate.

"Ah," Marcus said awkwardly. Lisa's adventuresome preference

for variety had always been weird to Marcus, who preferred to

maintain a few casual relationships with women he knew rather

than risking the wild waters of the open sea. Maybe it was all the

crazy and psychotic sides of people that he'd seen thanks to his job.

Or maybe it was just his nature.

Before he could figure out how to move past this strange curve

in the conversation, Lisa added, "He's the one that gave me John's

resumé."

"So he's local?" Marcus had never heard the name before this,

but if he was new in town too—

"No. He was only in town to help John move in. They're

cousins."

Cousins. All right. That could explain the car. But who bought an

entire house for their cousin to live in? "Are you sure they're not

roommates or something?"

"John's never mentioned him after our first meeting, and Kester

was clear that he was leaving shortly. I've never seen him around

town again, either. What's this about, Marcus?"

He considered telling her, but he knew by the impatience in her

voice that she wasn't in a great mood. And despite the fact that

McKenzie had clearly falsified the information he'd given his

employer, Marcus's interest in him was still mostly based on vague

.nfortable feelings. Those wouldn't do much to
         ...e was happy with the job McKenzie was doing,
             ...ouldn't care all that much about the mercenary
             ...ed to get the job—at least not as long as he was only a
             ...'m still looking to see if McKenzie has any connection
        ...he said instead. "I haven't found any yet, but the name
        ...icKenzie came up. If that's his cousin, then that clarifies
        ...nings. Thanks, Lisa."

"You're welcome. Is that all?"

"Yeah."

She hung up.

Marcus went back to staring at his paperwork. Why would McKenzie's cousin put his name on a house if he wasn't living there himself? Was McKenzie paying him rent? He could try to pull McKenzie's financials to find out, but he'd get in trouble if he was caught. If they'd used Kester's name to buy John's house, what were they trying to hide, since John had no criminal records that Marcus could find?

David's loud footsteps interrupted his thoughts. "Come on," said his partner. "Someone reported a break-in. We've got to check it out."

Marcus gathered his things and followed David, but his mind was still on John McKenzie and whatever he was hiding.

———

"What's that, Mom?" Landon asked. He'd been watching Jacqueline unpack a box while he did a math worksheet on the couch. It was mostly books and things which she was putting away on a bookshelf, but she'd just pulled a new thing out of a box and was hiding it in with the books and decorations.

"It's a camera," said Mom.

"Why are you hiding it?"

"It's a secret camera."

"What do you mean?"

She finished hiding it so that even though Landon knew where it was, he had to look really hard to see it, then she came to sit next to him. "I just want to see how you and Mr. McKenzie get along when I'm not here."

"It's a spy camera?"

"What? No, I'm not spying. I'm only curious."

Landon had read enough books to know what spying was.

"It's only that you don't tell me much of what you guys do when he babysits you, and neither does he, but you both seem to enjoy it so much. I just want to see what kind of fun you're having."

"Oh. Okay."

"But you can't tell him about it or it won't be as fun, okay?"

This could be a problem. They wouldn't be able to do magic now. Except Mr. McKenzie hadn't wanted to do magic lately, anyway. Not since Landon had controlled his mind. He'd said he wasn't angry, but he must have been angry because whenever Landon'd asked if he could learn more magic, Mr. McKenzie had changed the subject. Landon wanted to ask about what he'd done at school yesterday—how he'd almost killed that other boy. Except with the camera, he wouldn't be able to.

Landon had made people scared of him. He'd made *himself* scared of him. He didn't want to be scary. He wanted to be a boy people liked. He wanted to be a good boy, like he always was before.

Even though Mr. McKenzie wasn't teaching him magic like he wanted, Landon still liked being with him. He liked the attention. He liked doing stuff with him. It made him feel less lonely.

Landon still couldn't manage to tell his mom about Mr. McKenzie being the witch. But he wouldn't tell Mr. McKenzie about the camera, either. If Mr. McKenzie said or did something to out himself to Mom, then that was what would happen. The best Landon could manage to do was not get in the way.

"Okay," he agreed.

Kester's house was at the end of a very long driveway, the beginning of which was on a rural street where the nearest neighboring driveway was at least a hundred yards away. So even though his mailbox was at the street end of the driveway, he didn't think twice about checking it after changing out of his work clothes and removing his magical disguise.

His mistake.

He was halfway back to his house when he heard tires behind him and saw the police car turn the corner onto his driveway. He was too far from the house to get back—whoever was in the car had doubtless already seen him. But he was also carrying a bundle of mail (mostly junk mail and the electric bill), so he couldn't pretend to be a neighbor either. As he stood watching the visitor and considering what to do, the car steadily approached until it came to a stop right beside him and the driver's side window rolled down.

Oh, dear, Kester thought when he saw the face of the man whose mind he'd helped Landon violate. Anyone else, and he could most likely safely use magic to urge them on their way. But he wasn't at all sure how well Landon's attempt to erase Parkes's memory of their encounter had been, and if he remembered or suspected anything, he'd be much more likely to pick up on any use of magic Kester might attempt. So Kester put on his cheeriest smile and said, "Hello, Officer."

Parkes gave him an appraising, narrow-eyed look. "Any chance you might be Kester McKenzie?"

Kester tried to hide his shock and knew he failed. "I am. May I ask how you know that?"

Parkes jerked his chin toward the house. "Mind if we talk inside?"

"I'd be happy to," Kester replied automatically, mentally checking on Julia's location. She was two miles away, searching for the car she'd seen the killer in the other day, and he'd know if she approached in time to keep her out of the house until Parkes was gone.

By the time Kester reached the house, Parkes had parked his car and was waiting on the porch. Kester ushered him inside with all politeness and offered him a beverage.

"No, thanks," said Parkes. But he took a seat on the couch when Kester sat, both men maintaining neutral, non-aggressive postures. "Is your cousin John home?"

"Ah, no. He's out. Didn't say where."

"Do you know when he'll be back?"

"Late, most likely. I believe he and Julia, his girlfriend, are on a date."

"Oh. That's too bad." Parkes pulled out a notepad and tapped his pen on it absently.

"Do you know John?" Kester asked by way of making conversation.

"Mutual acquaintance," Parkes grunted. "One we share too, so I hear. Lisa VanBuren."

Kester smiled. "Ah, Lisa. Lovely woman."

"Scary woman," Parkes said, not disagreeing.

But since the other man had brought it up, Kester added, "We had quite an enjoyable evening the last time I visited town."

Instead of scowling at him as he'd done when he was 'John', Parkes only grimaced a little. "Yeah. Anyway, does that mean you're only visiting now?"

"Indeed. I'm only in town for the weekend."

"But your cousin left you to go on a date?"

"They'd had it planned already, and I invited myself over at the last minute. I can hardly hold it against him. But if you don't mind me returning to my prior question, how did you know who I am?"

"Educated guess. So, you don't live here? This isn't your residence?"

"No. Why?" As soon as he said it, he knew he'd made a miscalculation from the way the policeman's eyebrow quirked up.

"Then would you explain why your cousin's car and his house are both in your name?"

Blast it all. Kester hadn't expected to be in Agreste as long as he had been. He certainly hadn't expected anyone to do this sort of deep digging on him. Trying to gain some time, he asked, "Not to be rude or uncooperative, but could you tell me why that sort of information is of interest to the police? Is John suspected of a crime?"

"No, but he may have had some of his personal info stolen. I'm trying to determine if that has any connection to an ongoing murder investigation."

"Murder? That sounds serious."

"Murder usually is. So, in looking into it, I found your name where I was expecting to find his, and I thought, 'That's odd. I wonder what that's about.' So I'm asking."

"So, this is merely some routine data gathering."

"Yeah. That's all."

"I see. Well, it's nothing terribly interesting. We inherited some money when our mutual uncle died. John had been wanting to make a change, so he asked if I'd go in with him and buy this house. He'd live in it for a few years or until he got bored, then we'd sell it and split the money, hopefully making a profit. Real estate is usually a good investment, after all. But dual ownership can be a hassle, so we decided that I'd be the one to buy it."

"Do you have a contract between you two?"

"It was a gentlemen's agreement. No need for a contract."

"He must trust you a lot."

"Yes, we're very close. Neither of us would ever try to cheat the other."

Parkes pursed his lips but couldn't argue. While situations like Kester had described were perhaps odd, they were neither unheard-of nor illegal.

"As for the car," Kester continued, "it's mine. Cars are not good investments, you know. I already had two of my own, and he lived in a city before he moved here, so he didn't have one. I told him he could borrow my weekend car until he decided to buy one of his own or no longer needed one."

"Weekend car?" Parkes repeated.

"Yes."

Parkes muttered something about rich people.

"Does that satisfy your questions, Officer?"

Parkes huffed as he got up from the couch. "For now, yeah. Could you tell your cousin that I'd still like to talk to him? I'll be calling him later to see about setting up a meeting."

"I'll be sure to mention it to him when I see him." Kester led the officer out and watched him drive away. "Another unforeseen complication," he murmured to himself. "How much longer can this continue?"

Lisa's week had been terrible. The search for a new teacher was slow and tedious. It would have been so much easier if John had consented to come on permanently, but he'd flatly denied her. Then there was the matter of Trevor and the rumor—which seemed to finally be settled, at least, though she'd never found a good way to punish him for assaulting Trick. Plus, the break-in, the ongoing murder investigation, the potential danger to Denneka and now possibly to John...

By the time she got home Friday night, she had no energy to get dressed and go out, but she also badly needed some stress relief. She scrolled through her contacts list, finally deciding that Marcus was likely as overworked as she was lately.

He picked up on the second ring. "What's up, Lisa?"

"You off work yet?" she asked.

"Just."

"Come over."

There was a pause, then, "Yeah, okay."

Two hours later, Marcus lay in Lisa's bed, staring at the ceiling. She was on the other side, sprawled out on her stomach with one arm hanging over the side.

That had been... fun, as usual. He got some satisfaction out of seeing her go from wound tight as a spring and irritable as an angry weasel to the boneless relaxation she was in now. But his mind was still whirring with all that had been going on this week, and especially with the mystery that was John McKenzie. His cousin's answers had been reasonable, but Marcus just couldn't shake the feeling that there was something very strange about that man, and the lack of any record of him anywhere was only half of it.

"Lisa," Marcus said quietly, not wanting to wake her if she was already asleep.

"Mmm," she answered groggily.

"About McKenzie—"

"What's the rule about work talk in bed?"

"Sorry. I know. It's just, there's something weird about—"

She raised herself on her elbows to glare at him. Even in the near total darkness of her bedroom, he could see the irritation in her eyes. No matter how relaxed she got, the angry weasel was never that far under the surface.

"Sorry," he said again.

She flopped back down.

He knew better than to talk about work now. And she was probably the wrong choice to talk about it with anyway, given her connection to McKenzie. But he was desperate to talk it over with someone. The lost memories, the faces of McKenzie and the boy that kept flashing in his mind, the overwhelming feeling that something strange had been done to him but he couldn't remember what... There were moments when he felt like he was going crazy.

He didn't consciously realize he'd reached across the bed and laid his hand on her arm until he heard her growl, "Don't make me kick you out, Marcus."

He withdrew his hand and rolled to the far side of the bed, giving her plenty of space. Lisa liked her space.

———

Trick had hoped that they could go do something fun outside on Saturday. All week, he'd been mostly trapped inside, either at school or at the familiar girl's home. The one chance he might have had to run around outside was in PE, when he had to sit on the side while all the humans got to run and have fun and he couldn't do anything but watch. Though at least he'd been able to lie in the sun.

So he'd had high hopes for the weekend. But when Saturday morning came, the familiar girl's brother was sick again, so the familiar girl had to work at her family's shop all day.

"I'm sorry," she told him, setting his breakfast on the desk. "But either you stay here or you come with me to the store and follow me around. Which would be boring for you and look weird to everyone else. I tried calling your mom to see if she'd take you somewhere, but she said she had plans."

He stretched out on the bed, too disappointed to be hungry right now.

"Sorry," she said again. But he knew it wasn't her fault.

A couple hours later, Trick was woken from his doze by the sound of the door slowly opening. He raised his head to look, wondering if the familiar girl had been able to come home early— and then remembered that if it were her, he'd have already turned back into a human.

It was the familiar girl's brother. He wore baggy sweatpants and a t-shirt, and his nose and eyes were red. "Hey, little guy," said the brother.

Trick only watched him, not sure what was going on. The brother had seemed okay when he'd met him before, and he didn't look threatening now.

"Did you hope I was Denneka?" the brother said with a chuckle that turned into a cough. He covered his face with his arm and coughed a few more times. "Nah, just me. But since our parents aren't here either, I thought you might want out for a while." He opened the door fully and moved aside, leaving the path into the hallway wide open.

Out? Trick didn't need to be asked twice. He launched himself off the bed and through the open doorway, sprinting for the door to the back yard. He pawed at it, meowing to be let out so he could roll in the grass and climb the tree. But the girl's brother came up behind him and scooped him up, settling him into the crook of an arm that was much bigger and harder than the familiar girl's.

"Sorry, I can't let you out," said the brother, scratching under Trick's chin. "If you run away or get lost, Denneka'll kill me. But you can be out in the house for a while."

Disappointment made Trick limp again. But having the run of the house was better than staying in the girl's room, and she had never let him out to run around like that. There was plenty to explore.

He squirmed enough to let the girl's brother know he wanted down, and the brother set him back on the floor. Trick spent a while thoroughly exploring the brother's room and the laundry room and anywhere else in the house he could reach. There were two doors that stayed closed even after he pawed at them. "No, I don't think you should go in the garage," the brother said about one of them, and, "Mom'll have a fit if she finds cat hair on her bed," he said about the other.

While Trick was exploring the kitchen for the third time, he heard a sound that set all his nerves to attention.

Mouse, he thought, eager and ready. He hadn't had a chance to kill anything for weeks now. He carefully stalked and sniffed until he found the mouse in one of the lower cupboards. It tried to run, but he pounced on it and bit down hard. He wanted to play with it, but it was no good giving it the chance to get away from him. Like his mom had always told him, rodents didn't belong in the house.

Even though Trick's mom never wanted him to be a cat, she always praised him when he caught a mouse that had gotten inside. Maybe the familiar girl would praise him, too. It occurred to Trick that she'd done so much for him and had given him so much food, but he'd never done anything like that for her. So, eager to show it off to her, he left his prize on her pillow where she'd be sure to see it.

The hunt, short though it was, had made him tired. So he went back to the living room, where the girl's brother was sitting on the couch with his socked feet propped up on the coffee table while he watched TV. Trick hopped up to join him, picking his way around the food wrappers and used tissues, and curled up on the brother's lap.

"Finally," the brother said softly, his hand stroking Trick's fur.

Jacqueline wasn't proud of herself for calling John over to babysit that morning, considering what she was going out to do. It was somehow made worse by the fact that he didn't even bother asking her what her plans were for the day, apparently assuming that she was continuing on with her research or something equally valid.

She wasn't proud of herself—but she did it anyway. She had to. There'd been no opportunity earlier in the week. If John was the witch and the hawk was his familiar, then she had to be careful that the bird didn't spot her. Although John had been at school, so had Trick and Denneka, which meant the hawk wouldn't be watching them at Denneka's house, which meant its whereabouts were unaccounted for.

Which was still a bit of a problem, thanks to Denneka being made to work at the last minute. After Jacqueline left her house, she drove by Denneka's place. She searched as closely as she could without looking like a stalker, but she didn't see the hawk. With her fingers metaphorically crossed, she went to Sparrows'. To her relief, she spied the hawk in a tree across the street.

Why is it watching her? Jacqueline wondered, but she didn't have time to ponder it. If the hawk was here and John was at her house, she needed to get moving before either situation changed. Watching carefully to make sure the hawk didn't follow her, she drove to the address she'd pulled from the school computer.

Even though John had made references to having plenty of money, she was still surprised at how nice his house was. It was on the outskirts of town on what must have been at least a couple acres of land. Most of that land was an enormous front lawn gone slightly wild, with a few clusters of flower bushes around the edges. She parked and strode up the steps to a modest front porch. The front door was locked, and there was no key under the mat, which didn't surprise her because John was not an idiot.

As she circled the house, looking for a convenient entrance—she knew how to pick a lock if she had to, but it took her a while and made her feel even more like a criminal—she admired the lawn which wrapped unhindered around the sides of the house and spread into a smaller but still massive back yard and the small river running behind it.

If I lived in a place like this, I don't think I'd ever leave, she thought. Why on earth did John drag himself to work at a school every day when he had the money to just relax out here? Maybe she'd eventually find a non-rude way to ask him. For now, she noticed an open window on the back side of the house. *Maybe he has fallen a little into the small town sense of security, after all.*

Jacqueline pulled herself through the open window, which turned out to be over the kitchen sink. She managed to get to the floor without tumbling too badly or knocking anything over.

Now, what did one look for when one was looking for evidence of a witch?

———

Just as Kester was gently tapping an egg against the side of a bowl, he felt one of the wards on his house alert him to an intruder. His hand clenched in surprise, smashing the egg to bits, and Landon gave him a concerned look.

"Oh, dear," Kester murmured. "Butterfingers. Let me clean this up." He took the bowl to the sink, turning his back on his son, and focused on his connection to Julia's mind. She was perched in a tree, watching the front of Denneka's family store, and utterly bored.

Julia, he told her, *someone or something has set off the war* *and investigate it, would you?*

The inside of John's house was spacious, modern, and clean. Th were no leftover packing boxes like Jacqueline had. Everything w neat, orderly, elegant, and almost impersonal. She found no photos —family or otherwise—very few wall decorations, no knick-knacks... nothing that she was used to associating with a place feeling lived-in. Of course, he was a bachelor, so maybe that explained it.

A bachelor, but not exactly single, she reminded herself. She knew that John and Julia lived together, but she'd never have guessed this house had a woman's presence from the elegant but generic design of the living room and kitchen. The small bedroom she came across next looked far more lived-in than the living room, with a few pieces of clothing laid out, a bed not quite made to exacting standards, and plenty of other items which gave the undeniable impression of someone residing in the room. A female someone, if Jacqueline had to guess. It wasn't overtly feminine, but the colors and styles edged more toward feminine than masculine. And one of the pieces of clothing lying on a chair was what looked like a well-worn nightgown.

The master bedroom had the same neat yet impersonal air as the rest of the house, with a huge bed draped in ivory silk sheets and duvet, and furniture made of carved ebony. It looked like a guest room in an extremely wealthy person's mansion.

As she walked through the room, she felt distinctly skeezy. Here John was being such a good friend by watching Landon for her, and she was sneaking around in his bedroom like a perv.

She pushed that feeling aside and refocused on her objective.

The master bathroom showed a few more signs of life, the usual toothbrush and toiletries. Her eyes slid right past the hairbrush before coming back to it, and she picked it up. There were quite a

ond hairs in it. But John wasn't blond, nor was his hair
was brunette. So, whose brush was this?

nd sorrow for the woman she'd only met once but rather
gged at her heart. Was that the explanation for the two
oms? Had Julia been right that she wasn't John's 'the one'?
eline imagined the scenario easily: Relationship problems
ween the two of them, but Julia unable to afford to move out on
er own and John too kind to kick her out. Julia moving into a
second bedroom to become a roommate even as... Even as John
brought a new girlfriend over? That last element didn't feel right. It
seemed a little too cruel to match what she knew of John. And
wouldn't he have mentioned anything about it if he and Julia had
broken up?

Why would he? Jacqueline chastised herself. *When was the last time
you asked him anything about his life? Isn't it always about you and your
own problems?* But she did mention Julia from time to time, and...
and he usually brushed past the topic as quickly as possible.

Once again, Jacqueline had to refocus on what she was doing.

Everything looked pretty normal in the bathroom otherwise.
Except for a few hand-labeled bottles whose labels seemed to be
written in some language she didn't know. But there were lots of
people who bought handmade hair and skin care products. Maybe
John even had a hobby of making them himself. Or Julia did.

This wasn't getting her anywhere. She left the master suite,
quickly checked the guest bathroom, and tried the one remaining
door in the hall. It was locked. Which meant that if there was
anything John was hiding, that was probably where it was hidden.
Jacqueline took out her lock-picking kit. It looked like she'd need it
after all.

She knelt by the door and carefully began to slide the tools into
the lock. A loud clattering, skittering sound from the skylight above
her head startled her into dropping the tools. Her head snapped up
to see what it was—and she saw the frantic flapping of a brown
wing at the edge of the skylight.

The hawk.

Jacqueline's pulse spiked in panic. If the hawk was back, then she was about to be caught out, if she wasn't already. And if John was the witch, when he came back... What would he do to her if he believed she'd discovered his secret?

She snatched up her tools and ran to the open window, scrambling outside just slowly enough that she didn't knock anything over on her way out, then dashed around the house to her car and drove away.

But as she headed back to her own home, she came back to her senses and chided herself for being a fool. It might not have been the hawk. It could have been any bird of approximately the same size and color, and the timing could have been entirely coincidental. She hadn't found any evidence at all that John was the witch, after all. If anything, she felt bad for prying into what seemed to be a delicate personal situation.

In the end, she'd panicked and wasted all the effort and planning she'd put into the incursion. What was even the point of breaking into the school if she was just going to botch her real mission?

"What's wrong?" Landon asked.

Kester realized he'd stopped stirring the cake batter, and his hands were shaking. He released the mixing bowl and forced his hands to his sides. "Nothing at all. Why do you ask?"

Landon raised a dubious eyebrow. If a six-year-old could see something was wrong, he must really be losing it.

Kester ruffled the boy's hair. "I'm fine, young one. I'm merely used to using a mixer, so when I stir for too long by hand, the muscles start to give out. It's perfectly normal for us elders. Do you want to keep stirring for me? I think it's nearly done."

Landon got up on the step stool and went about stirring the batter with an intense precision that was a bit uncanny in such a small child. Kester watched him in silent trepidation. Jacqueline had been about to break into his lab when Julia interrupted her, but how much had she seen before that? Enough to confirm her suspicions? And when had she started suspecting him? He hadn't gotten that impression at all. And if she suspected him of being the witch she hunted, why had she continued to allow him to watch her son?

Their son. His son. Who he would never see again if she'd seen enough at his house to make plain his true nature. The thought bothered him more than he ever would have expected it to.

Not that he couldn't outplay her or force his way into their lives again. He had a great deal of power and decades of practice in getting what he wanted. If he wanted to see his son, Jacqueline wouldn't ever really be able to keep him away. But she could make it a monstrous pain, and she'd always be on the lookout for him. And… he didn't really want to fight her on this. He didn't want to fight her at all.

There was nothing to do, then. If she called him out on his lies and demanded he leave her and her family alone, he would do so. He'd planned to leave when he got bored, anyway. It wouldn't be all that much different. Right now, all he could do was hope that she hadn't seen anything witchy at his house.

He gently guided his son through the rest of the recipe, savoring the moments in case they were the last he'd have. Two minutes after they put the cake in the oven, the front door opened and Jacqueline came in.

"You're just in time," he told her, offering his usual friendly smile.

She wasn't scowling, and she didn't fly into a rage at him or quietly tell Landon to leave the room. All she did was stroll closer to the kitchen, look at the mess and the two of them with wary curiosity, and say, "In time for what?"

"To help us clean up."

She rolled her eyes. "The one who makes the mess cleans the mess up. House rule."

Did that apply to kittens? he couldn't help but wonder. But he was too weak with relief at her breezy response to wonder too hard.

"You heard the woman," he told Landon. The two of them cleaned up everything they wouldn't need any longer. Jacqueline went back to her room, but she came back by the time they were finished cleaning up. "There's still a bit of time left on the cake, then it'll need to be frosted and finished," Kester told her.

"Thanks, John. I think I can manage that part. I have baked a few cakes before," she said with a wink. "I don't want to keep you any longer than I have to."

"Should I—" Despite himself, his throat closed around his words. He swallowed and tried again. "Should I expect to be needed tomorrow as well, or have you found the man you're searching for?"

She thought about it for long enough that Kester knew she wasn't as unsuspecting of him as she acted. "Better plan on it," she said at last. "If you're free."

The tightness that had begun to wind itself up in his chest released. "I am. I'll plan on being over in the morning, then."

———

After John left, Jacqueline checked the nanny-cam video. She watched the whole thing in real time, only stopping to help Landon finish with the cake. Although she watched with a mother's eagle eye for any sign of questionable intent or any hint of magic, she saw and heard nothing but her son enjoying wholesome quality time with a man he seemed to both like and respect.

Hopefully, she'd gotten lucky and John would find no evidence that someone had broken into his house. But if she continued pushing this, if she continued investigating him and he found out about it, he'd likely feel betrayed and offended. There was no way anyone would want to keep being friends with someone who behaved like she was behaving toward him. And while she was willing to risk losing a friend over it, she couldn't risk losing the positive influence that John was to Landon.

She didn't have any proof that John wasn't the witch, but she didn't have much evidence—let alone any actual proof—that he was. At this point, she had to choose whether to let her suspicion and protectiveness drive her to keep investigating John until she found evidence one way or the other, or to trust in the good man that she believed him to be and in the positive influence that he was having on Landon.

For her son's sake, she chose to trust.

———

Notice it. Notice it, Trick thought.

The familiar girl had come back to her room and was setting her things down. "So when I reminded them about my homework, my parents let me go home early," she was saying. She wasn't trying to be quiet, so her brother was probably back in his room with the door closed. "You're going to help me with it, right?"

What was she talking about? Trick wasn't really paying attention.

"Homework," she clarified. "You need to get yours done, too, so we'll do it together, okay?"

Trick didn't care about that. His eyes flicked to the mouse on her pillow, then back to her. When was she going to notice it?

"Trick?" she said slowly.

Oh, good.

"Is that... a dead mouse?"

"For you." He stood up from the desk chair and went over to stand beside it. "I caught it in the kitchen." *Praise me. Praise me!*

Her lips curled up in something that met all the requirements he could think of for a smile but still didn't look anything like one. "Um, that's... great, but..."

Why wasn't she praising him? Or thanking him?

"You... don't like my present?" he asked.

"Present?" she squeaked. Then she had another look at the mouse. "So that's what it is. Well, it's, um... it's very nice, Trick. But

—wait a minute. What do you mean you caught it in the k
When were you in the kitchen?"

"Your brother let me out during the day."

She jumped in surprise. "He did?"

"He let me explore, then I caught the mouse, then we cuddled c
the couch."

She snorted a laugh.

"What's funny?"

"Nothing. But you have to be careful. How long were you out?"

Trick shrugged.

"Hours?"

"I guess. He put me back in here a while before you got home."

The familiar girl rubbed her forehead like doing it helped her
think. "Has he let you out before when I wasn't here?"

"Yeah."

She kept thinking. "As long as he's keeping you secret from our
parents, I probably can't tell him not to. I didn't know he likes cats,
though. But what if Mom or Dad comes home without warning?"

Trick pointed at the mouse. "Are you not gonna eat that?"

"What? Ew, no!" she blurted.

He couldn't say that didn't hurt a little, but it was her loss. He
picked up the mouse and popped it into his mouth.

Then immediately spat it back out. "Ugh, that tastes gross!"

"YEAH, OF COURSE IT DOES!" She was gaping at him like he'd
gone absolutely insane.

Trick rubbed his tongue off with his hands. It didn't make any
sense. Mice usually tasted pretty good. That mouse had tasted fine
when he'd killed it earlier.

"You're not a cat right now, Trick!" the girl barked. "You can't eat
dead vermin! You'll get sick!"

"Sorry!" He backed away. Why was she yelling at him? Even if
she didn't like his present, she didn't have to yell at him.

With a sigh, the girl calmed down. When she stepped toward
him, he shied away, but she kept coming and he let her put a hand
on his shoulder. "I'm not mad at you. I'm worried for you. Cats and

can't eat the same things. You need to try to remember
body you're in."

e petted his head, and he felt better. "I'll... try." He really
n't known humans couldn't eat mice, though when he thought
out it, he'd never seen any of them do it. They ate other dead
nimals, though. How was it different? He didn't want to risk
asking her right now in case it upset her again.

"I appreciate the present," she said. "It was really sweet of you to
think of giving it to me, and it was really helpful that you caught it."

There was the praise, even though it didn't sound like she meant
it. It sounded like she was humoring him. He closed his eyes,
wishing he could purr as she petted his head.

"We can't really do anything with it, though," she said, "so I'm
gonna take it out and get rid of it, okay? If you catch any more mice
or anything, you don't have to show them to me. You can just tell
me you caught them, all right?"

That didn't sound nearly as satisfying, but he said, "Okay."

As the familiar girl moved around, taking the mouse out and
changing her pillow, Trick wondered if she thought he was useless.
He didn't want to be useless to her. But if he couldn't impress her
with his hunting, what would impress her? If he couldn't give her
his catches, what could he give her? If he couldn't offer her food,
what could he do for her? Trick knew it made her feel happy to pet
him and cuddle with him, but... that wasn't enough.

CHAPTER
TWENTY-THREE

Denneka had gotten used to the strange and invasive positions Trick got into when he slept, but this was too much. *Don't freak out*, she told herself, looking down her body at the situation she'd woken to find herself in.

She was on her back in a neutral enough position. It was Trick that was the problem. He was stretched out on his belly between her legs, with his feet hanging off the end of the bed and his face resting on her stomach. Which would have been awkward enough if the blanket between them weren't down at her hips and her pajama top hiked up to leave a couple inches of bare midriff.

"Trick," she whispered and lightly shook his shoulder.

His hands, which had been lying harmlessly at her sides, snaked down between her and the bed, his arms clutching her around the waist, his hands splaying out to hold her more tightly.

Adrenaline, panic, and something else shot through her whole body and made her jerk like she'd been shocked.

"Stay," Trick murmured without opening his eyes. "Sleep." When he said it, his lips moved against the bare skin of her belly, making her abs twitch uncontrollably.

"Trick!" she repeated, shoving his shoulders hard with both hands.

He released her and sat up with the aggrieved slowness of someone rudely awoken. "Hmm?"

"You're on top of me," she said, not able to meet those intense green eyes. "I need to get up."

He slid backward off the bed with a languid grace. The extensive stretching and yawning he then engaged in helped calm her down.

He's only a cat. Cats sleep between people's legs all the time. It doesn't mean anything.

But what about that hug? He'd never hugged her like that before. Then again, he'd been mostly asleep. Had he meant to do it? Did he remember doing it?

Was that the sort of thing Jacqueline had meant about treating her like a boy treats a girl?

She rubbed her head and got up. Things people did in their sleep didn't count. Pretending it did would only make her feel... things she didn't want to feel. Like groundless hope.

———

Kester's plans for Sunday abruptly changed when, at noon, he received a text from Marcus Parkes.

I'd like to meet, it said. *Lunch?*

The mystery of how the two phones were acquainted with each other was solved when Kester remembered that Parkes had called him to set up their earlier meeting in the park, and Kester hadn't thought to delete the record of that conversation before leaving. The fact that Parkes had neither used any salutation nor verified Kester's identity before asking to meet meant that he was certain whose number he had.

I'm growing abysmally sloppy, Kester thought with a grimace. Before replying, he called Jacqueline to see if she was available to come back home. She was. *Better see what he wants, then.*

They met half an hour later in a sandwich shop on Main Street.

"John McKenzie?" Parkes asked as Kester slid into the other side of the booth he occupied.

"Yes. And you're Officer Parkes, I presume. My cousin told me to expect to hear from you."

Parkes eyed him with suspicion. "Have we met before?"

"You and my cousin?"

"No." He waggled a finger between the two of them. "Us."

"You responded to my call about my student's disappearance, though I don't believe we talked then. And I was at Jacqueline's house when you and your partner came to interview her the next day."

Parkes shook his head. "I mean another time."

Kester pretended to think. "Not that I can recall."

Parkes held up his phone, which clearly displayed a contact listing with Kester's phone number and alias. "Then why is your number in my phone?"

"I assume you put it there when you were investigating the theft of my information from the school computer, though I can't imagine why you're asking me."

"No. It was in my phone before that."

Kester held up his hands. "It's your phone, Officer. I have no idea what you have in there or why."

"Yet you seemed to know who I was when I texted you. Which means you have my number in your phone."

"Lisa gave me your number in case I perceived a threat to Denneka, since she said you were concerned about her safety."

The other man's mouth tightened, unhappy to be losing this line of inquiry. "I really feel like we've met before. In a park, maybe."

This might be bad. Had Landon done such a poor job of erasing Parkes's memory, or were the memories coming back to him over time? Kester nodded amiably. "That might be possible. I do take a boy I babysit to the park sometimes. We may have bumped into each other there, though I don't recall."

Parkes's face twitched. "A boy. You mean Landon St. Andrew?"

Kester had to fight to keep his expression from slipping. "Yes, that's the one. You're familiar with him?"

"We've met, when I went back to talk to his brother after he came home."

"So we both became acquainted with the family because of that incident. What an amusing coincidence."

Parkes didn't appear at all amused. His deep brown eyes locked with Kester's and held him as if daring him to look away. To his extreme discomfort, Kester began to feel as if the man were looking straight through his magical disguise. "I'm gonna come right out and say it, McKenzie," Parkes said when the silence became uncomfortable. "There's something weird about you. I know I've met you before, and not just in passing."

"Oh?" Kester had to struggle not to falter under the policeman's stare. "I'd love to be enlightened as to when."

"I... I can't—remember." Parkes fought with the words. "But I'm sure of it. I'll figure it out one of these days. And when I do, if I find out you had something to do with Haug's murder—or if you're a threat to anyone else—this innocent act of yours won't stop me from bringing you in."

Kester didn't have to feign his confusion. "I assure you, Officer, I had nothing to do with the murder of my predecessor. I never met the man. I never even knew he existed until after I moved to this town."

"Then what are you hiding?"

"Hiding? You don't have any evidence that I'm hiding anything. Do you?"

Parkes gritted his teeth, then planted his hands on the table and stood. "Fine. But I'll get to the bottom of this, whether you cooperate or not. Count on it." He took a step away from the booth, but Kester stopped him.

"Aren't we having lunch? It's rude to take up a table like this and then leave without ordering anything."

The irritation on Parkes's face before he stormed out was amusing enough to make Kester feel better. When the waitress came, he ordered enough food to have a nice lunch with Jacqueline and Landon when he went back to their house. While he waited for it, he pondered the problem of Parkes. He was an interfering nuisance Kester hadn't anticipated, and he was becoming a real thorn in Kester's side.

———

"Did you get all your homework done last night?" Denneka's mom asked her.

Denneka looked up from sorting through a mixed-up shipment of pants. "Not quite."

Mom checked her watch. "It's two-thirty. Why don't you go ahead and go home? We can handle it from here."

Denneka hurried home, grateful to get off early. *There might be time to let Trick out for a while,* she hoped. *Maybe if Jonah's sleeping.* Her brother was still sick, which was why Denneka had had to work again today. And Trick didn't pay very close attention to how far from her he was when he was playing in the back yard. It wouldn't be good if Jonah looked out his window and saw him transform.

So when she opened the front door and stepped inside, she was a little disappointed to see the back of Jonah's head over the couch. The TV was on and loud, so he probably wasn't asleep.

"Hey," she said, going over to him, "how are you—"

In the same moment that Jonah turned his head to her, a sudden, large shape appeared right in front of him as if by magic.

Jonah shouted an expletive in surprise.

Denneka dashed to the front side of the couch.

And a very naked Trick tumbled from Jonah's lap onto the floor, banging himself hard against the coffee table on the way down.

Jonah scrambled up onto the couch, crouching there like the floor had suddenly become lava. He let out a few more shocked curses before falling into a coughing fit.

Trick moaned and clutched at his upper arm, curling his knees up to sit on the floor.

"What did I tell you?!" Denneka shouted at him. They'd talked about this *yesterday*. He was supposed to be careful. But it was her

417

fault, too, for forgetting that Jonah had let Trick out yesterday and might do it again today.

"You—know him?" Jonah asked between coughs.

"Uh, yeah?" she answered. This was bad. This was super bad. She had no idea what to do.

"Denneka, what the hell just happened? Who is this guy?"

"It's kind of complicated."

"Uncomplicate it! I was just sitting here petting your cat and then—" His head swiveled to Trick, his eyes going huge.

"This is Trick," Denneka told him. "He turns into a cat sometimes."

"My arm hurts," Trick complained.

"No way." Jonah's voice was hoarse.

"Yeah," Denneka said. "See?" She moved far enough away for Trick to turn back into a kitten. When she was sure Jonah had gotten the point, she moved back to Trick's side. Trick groaned on his hands and knees, then sat on his heels and rubbed the sore spot on his arm.

Jonah slid onto his butt on the couch and rubbed his temples with his palms.

"What's wrong with him?" Trick asked.

"He's just surprised," she told him, watching her brother carefully for how he might react next.

Trick crawled over to Jonah and offered his head. "You can still pet me."

Jonah jerked away so hard he rolled into it and came to his feet. But wheezing and more coughing stopped whatever he was going to say. Finally, he was able to rasp, "Who are you?"

Trick didn't respond, so Denneka did. "He's my friend."

This answer startled her brother, and he looked between the two of them several times. "You're naked," he said to Trick. Then he scowled at Denneka and asked, "Why is he naked?"

She felt herself blush. "That happens when he changes forms because his clothes don't change too."

"Why do you sound used to it?!" Jonah wheeze-yelled.

Denneka held out her hands. "Will you calm down and let us explain?"

Part of him seemed to want to punch Trick on general principle, but he sat down and nodded.

So Denneka explained the whole situation and finished with, "Will you please promise not to tell Mom and Dad?"

Trick was on the floor with a blanket in his lap, and he'd kept trying to get either Jonah or Denneka (it alternated) to pet his head while Denneka explained things.

Jonah was sitting with his arms crossed, frowning at the two of them. "I can't believe I'm saying this, but yes," he grunted. Before Denneka could breathe too big a sigh of relief, he added, "On one condition. He has to stay in my room at night."

"No!" Trick blurted.

"But he can't stay human if he's not with me," Denneka protested.

"All the better! Denneka, what kind of big brother would I be if I just let"—he waved a hand between the two of them—"*that* continue? You don't know how boys are."

"Look at him, Jonah. He's not really a boy. He's a cat."

Jonah laughed. "I can see he thinks that, and I trust what you just told me, which is why I'm not beating the crap out of him right now. But, I repeat, you don't know boys. That's my condition. Either take it, or if he's still here when Mom and Dad get home, I'll tell them you've been hiding a boy in your room."

How that would go over was too horrifying to imagine, but honestly, a small part of Denneka was relieved. "Okay."

Trick's head snapped to her, betrayal written all over his face.

"We don't have a choice, Trick," she told him calmly. "We can still hang out together at home before bedtime, as long as my parents aren't here. I'll still feed you and—" Her throat closed up on the words 'bathe you'. She hadn't gone into quite that level of detail in her explanation to Jonah. She doubted he'd allow them to keep up many aspects of the routine they'd gotten into. Which meant all of this probably wouldn't last much longer. She laid a hand on

Trick's head and rubbed it lightly. "It'll be fine," she told him. *Don't be sad that it's almost over*, she told herself. *Be happy that you got this chance at all*. Even if he forgot about her when he moved back to his normal life—whether that ended up being a normal life as a cat in his mom's house or a normal life as a boy going to school like a regular kid—she'd never forget him. How could she? Unlike her, he was unforgettable.

———

Trick was afraid his mom would yell at him for getting caught, but she took it pretty well.

"It was only a matter of time," she said. It was Monday morning, and she was driving them to school. "I'm surprised he even gave you any option for Trick to keep staying there."

"Yeah, he was… surprisingly cool about it, all things considered," the familiar girl said. "Trick, he didn't say anything weird or act mean to you last night, did he?"

"He kicked me off the bed."

Mom snorted.

"But I kept trying, and eventually he gave up and let me cuddle with him."

"He did?!" the familiar girl cried.

"Oh," Trick remembered, "but he said I wasn't supposed to tell you that."

Mom was giggling. "He must really love cats."

"Not that I ever knew of." The familiar girl sounded like she didn't know what emotion to feel.

They got to the school, but before Trick and the familiar girl got out, Mom said, "I'll bring you home tonight, Trick."

"What? No!" When Trick looked at the familiar girl for support, she didn't seem surprised at all. He begged his mom, "I want to stay with her!"

"It's too dangerous now," Mom said, "and things have gotten

too complicated. I'll be happy to have her come over and visit, and you'll still see each other at school."

"But I like sleeping with her. And I like how she washes my hair. And feeds me. And..." Trick trailed off, hating how needy he sounded. As if he was some pet who needed an owner and not... Not what?

Mom let out a breath. "Neither of you is moving out of town or anything. You can still be friends. We just have to adapt to the situation as it changes, and things are still changing a lot. Do you understand?"

Trick wasn't sure that he did, but he mumbled, "Okay."

When they got out and headed for the school building, the familiar girl said to him quietly, "Trick, remember what I said about not telling people we sleep together?"

"But she already knows."

"I know, but... still." She was staring at the ground as they walked. Was she sad again? Had his slip up made her sad?

"Sorry. I'll be more careful."

———

"Good afternoon, ma'am—I mean, Jacqueline." Marcus forced himself to relax. It wasn't easy. Every time he saw the woman, he was surprised by how strong his attraction to her was, as if when she wasn't around, his brain convinced itself that she couldn't possibly be as beautiful as he remembered. But he wasn't here for that.

She looked at him oddly, which was understandable. "Marcus?"

"Yeah. And *just* Marcus today." He waved vaguely at his jeans and t-shirt. "It's my day off."

Her eyebrows rose, her smooth forehead crinkling. "Oh?"

"What I mean is, I'm not here on official business, but-but I am here on business." Why was he tripping over his words like a teenager? *Get a grip, man.*

"Oh." Was there a hint of disappointment there?

"It's about... about... well, could we talk inside? I have several questions I'd like to ask you. They're not case-related, exactly, but sort of case-adjacent."

"Sure. Come on in."

He followed her into her house, taking a second to grab enough of his professionalism to see her as a potential source of information instead of as a hot, single woman. Mostly.

"It's nice to see you out of uniform," she said as she led him to the dining table.

He had to bite his tongue to stop from saying something so flirty it bordered on obscene. *Information*, he told himself. *Remember what you're here for.* As he took a seat at the table, he responded with, "My boss runs a tight ship, but he does allow us personal lives."

From the kitchen, she said, "And yet you're here, asking case-adjacent questions, on your day off. Doesn't sound like much of a personal life."

"I think most single men would consider visiting a gorgeous woman a good use of a day off." *Well, crap.*

Her bright laughter erased his immediate fear that she'd think he'd come into her house under false pretenses. "Do you like cream or sugar in your coffee?" she asked.

"Both," he answered, afraid to let himself say any more words.

She came to the table a few minutes later with two mugs of coffee, sat across from him, and slid him one.

"Most people usually offer tea," he said lamely.

"Yeah, but you look more like a coffee guy. Am I right?"

He nodded, sipped the coffee, and didn't mention that he'd have preferred about twice as much cream in it. "I need to make it clear that this is a personal thing I'm asking about, not something I'm asking as a police officer. You don't have to tell me anything."

She held her own mug in both hands and looked at him with an expression that was serious but not stern. "Then if I don't want to answer something, I won't. So shoot."

This was going to be awkward, but he had to start somewhere. "I hear you're friends with John McKenzie."

hy I v
d the face
e. I hadn't
t even known
I looked at my
hn McKenzie. I
s number in my

attention, so he

ed meeting with
." He decided to
s Landon for the
ll. It was like the
been driving me
is name, I get this
e I should know
oing on with him.
rrent case. I can't
s put me on leave
I have to."
rry or skepticism
ly sat back in her
houldn't tell you
mation from the

s you?"

I hadn't left any

he literal ones." At
he floor."

ve amused him so

him
hink a
ean to th
ery good w
when John's

would have used.
d possibly 'cunning

about himself. I don't
as a teacher when he
something else, then
f that were the reason

ange?"
anaged to choke the

o him. "Why? What's

one would think he
great look on a cop.
r days now, and he
ow for sure. But... I
an a feeling. About
I went to a park. I
ew, I was sitting on

idea w
emembere
drugged m
memory I hadn
gain. And when
phone call with J
g to him or putting hi

ssion was nothing but rapt

as I saw the call log, I remembe
here at the park. Just moments before
mention of the boy who he was sure w
eing. "I couldn't remember any details at a
ing had happened but hadn't happened. It's
uts ever since. Any time I see McKenzie or hear h
sense like there's part of my brain missing. Lik
something and I don't. I know there's something g
I don't know if it has anything to do with our cu
tell anyone at work about it because all they'll do
or something. But I've got to get to the bottom of i

Jacqueline was a study in non-reaction. No w
or pity about how he was losing his mind. She slo
chair and said in a soft, calm voice, "I probably
this, but I broke into the school to get his inf
computer."

Marcus's mouth fell open in surprise. "That w
"You knew about that?"

"Lisa reported it."

She nodded. "Lisa seems sharp. I'd though
tracks, though."

Her choice of word made him grin. "Except t
her questioning look, his grin widened. "Dirt on t

She winced.

Her confession of a crime really shouldn't ha

much. "It's too bad I left my work notepad at the office. Everyone knows how forgetful I can be without it."

She smirked back at him. "Well, I hope you're *really* forgetful, because I'm not finished. Last Saturday, while John was watching Landon, I broke into his house."

Marcus blinked in surprise. "You're a spunky one, aren't you?"

She laughed. "Spunky? I haven't been called that since I was five."

"So just a couple decades ago, then."

She winked in acknowledgment of his blatant flattery. "Closer to three."

So, she was only about one decade younger than him. *Workable,* he thought. *No. Focus.* He cleared his throat. "Did you, um, find anything?"

"No. But I... sorta got spooked and ran off before I got into all the rooms."

"Spooked by what?"

"A... bird."

"You're such a hardened criminal."

"The point I'm getting at is that I... had my suspicions about John, too. But I couldn't find out anything concrete, and he's so good with Landon, I decided not to risk the relationship they've built by continuing to investigate him."

Either McKenzie was fooling her well, or there was some part of him that was a decent person. And she didn't strike Marcus as the sort of woman to be easily fooled. "I understand. Does that mean you won't help me with my investigation of him?"

"No, it doesn't." She sighed. "I put it behind me. I decided to trust him. Then you come in and dig it all up again, making me think there really is something there after all. Now I *have* to know for sure. So I'll tell you what I know, as long as you promise to share what you find out with me."

That definitely wasn't the arrangement he'd planned on when he'd come here. But Marcus found he didn't mind the idea of partnering with this woman. "Agreed."

They didn't shake on it, but they nodded across the table on it.

"Would you tell me why you had your own suspicions?" he asked.

She chewed on her lower lip in thought. It was incredibly distracting. When she started speaking, his focus snapped to her lowered eyes. "There was an old woman I met once. She was a witch." She raised her hazel eyes to lock with his in some meaning he wasn't picking up on. "A literal witch."

He frowned. "What kind of literal witch?"

"The kind that uses magic. Spells, potions, all that."

"For real?"

"Very real. When I was pregnant with Landon, there was a problem. Doctors said he wouldn't survive. They wouldn't even try treating him, but I was desperate to save him. One day, I got a letter in the mail. No signature. No return address. But it told me to go to this place and talk to this woman. It said she was a witch and could use magic to help me in ways doctors couldn't."

"And you believed it?"

"Like I said, I was desperate. And I used to be very superstitious when I was young. I guess there was enough of that still in me to give it a try."

"So… the witch did magic to save your son."

She nodded. "A potion. All it took was some potion that tasted like pine needles, and my baby lived."

Is that what's strange about him? Marcus wondered. If magic really existed, could it be put into an unborn child?

"Fast forward to now," Jacqueline said. "Some strange things have been going on with Trick."

"What kinds of things?"

"That's… probably better left seen instead of explained. But definitely magical things. And he was sure they were caused by a male witch that he saw once."

"You mean here? In Agreste?"

"Yes. I'd just started trying to find this witch when I remembered

426

something John said when we first met. A small thing, almost nothing, but it was odd."

"What did he say?"

"We were joking around about something, and he said, 'What kind of witch do you take me for?' I brushed it off at the time, but now that I knew there was really a witch, it made me suspicious. But I didn't know much about him, and if he was going to be watching my son, I needed to know." She shrugged. "It wasn't much, and it still isn't, but if you think there's something strange about John too, I have to wonder if there isn't really something there."

"Don't underestimate the combined power of a mother's instinct and a cop's instinct."

"You believe me, then?"

"That there are witches and John McKenzie might be one?" He considered it. "I do. If it means I'm not going nuts in thinking that we had a conversation I can't remember having—but *can* remember *having had*—then I'm all for believing in witches."

"I don't think you're going nuts," she said. "You strike me as a very stable person. After some of the things I've seen, a little memory confusion is nothing."

I think I love this woman, Marcus thought melodramatically. "Hold on. You said Trick saw this male witch."

"Yes," she said like she already knew where he was going with this.

"John McKenzie is Trick's teacher. He'd recognize him if he saw him, so he would have known it if McKenzie was the witch."

She nodded. "But remember: magic. What if he doesn't always look the same?"

A shape-shifting witch? This was getting complicated. But there was one other element Marcus still needed to address. He hoped they'd established enough trust now that she wouldn't throw him out. "There's something else I haven't mentioned yet. In the memories—or non-memories—that I have of that meeting with McKenzie, he wasn't the only one there. A boy was with him."

Jacqueline's whole body stiffened.

"I… think it was Landon."

"What do you mean?" she asked in a dangerous voice.

"I'm not exactly sure. I remembered a boy, then when I saw him here the other day—"

"You went white," she breathed, remembering. Her tone wasn't dangerous anymore; it was afraid. "You looked like you'd seen a ghost."

"It wasn't a conscious thing. I was hit with this sudden terror like… like when a caveman hears a lion and his body tells him to run for it before his mind even knows why."

Jacqueline's eyes filled with pain. "Landon?" she whimpered. But the helplessness was gone in the next instant, and her face set in hard lines. "Come on." Her chair slid back with a screech, and then she strode to the living room and snatched up her purse.

Marcus had to hurry to catch up. "Where?"

"To get answers."

The point is

but does

The
nish
eka
ly

UR

on as Bobby pulled out a laser pointer, Denneka knew there
as going to be trouble.

They were in Spanish class, and Mr. Black had told them to pair
off and practice introducing themselves and making small talk with
the vocabulary they'd learned so far. Bobby Juarez, who was already
fully bilingual but still had to sit through the class because it was
required, got bored easily.

Denneka and Trick sat with their desks facing each other. She
was trying her best to get him to participate, but he wasn't coop-
erating.

"Hola," she said for the fifth time. "Me llamo Denneka."

Trick stared at her.

"Now you say your name."

"Trick."

"No, you have to say the whole sentence."

"Why?"

"Because that's what we're practicing."

"Why?"

"Because that's the class."

"But the words don't make sense."

they're in another language, Trick.

ney do make sense."

meet someone who doesn't speak English

sh, you can talk to them."

eka sighed and glanced over at Bobby and Jennife

girl seemed a bit dazed as Bobby rambled on in fluent Spa

beyond their beginner-level ability. Jennifer saw Denn

ching and gave her a *help me* look, but Denneka could o

rug and nod helplessly toward Trick.

"This is stupid," Trick said. "People should all speak the same."

"Maybe," Denneka allowed. "But they don't."

"Cats do."

"Cats don't speak at all."

He actually looked a little offended at that. "Yes, we do."

Denneka considered what he might mean. "Cats communicate, but they don't speak."

He didn't answer, which was probably his way of conceding the point.

"Cats don't communicate the same way dogs do, though, right?"

"Dogs are stupid. Why would we want to talk to them?"

This was going in an uncomfortable direction. Maybe a different approach. "You learned to get along with the hawk, right? You learned how to read it and make sense of what it's saying, even though it's not talking like a cat, right?"

After a few seconds, he said, "Yes…"

"And you had thought at first that it meant to hurt you, but now you can play with it, right."

"Yes…"

"It's like that."

Trick thought about this for a while. "I still don't like having to learn new words for things. It's hard enough remembering the rules for regular human language."

She decided not to correct him on his description of English as 'regular human language' when he appeared to have only just taken his first step in understanding languages as a concept.

It dawned on her that Bobby wasn't rambling anymore, so she looked over to see how Jennifer was getting on. But they still weren't doing the assigned exercise. Instead, Bobby was fiddling with something small and metallic in his hand. Denneka saw a red dot moving around his desk, and she got a very bad feeling.

From the corner of her eye, she saw Trick's head move to follow her gaze. "No, don't look," she hissed. But it was too late.

His body snapped to attention, his head twitching side to side as his sharp eyes followed the red dot around Bobby's desk, then across Jennifer's shirt. When it leapt to the floor, Trick jerked, rattling his chair, and Bobby noticed.

"Could you put that away?" Denneka asked Bobby. But he ignored her and grinned at how engrossed Trick was with the laser pointer.

The red dot shot off down the aisle between the chairs, and Trick was out of his seat and chasing after it in an instant. Bobby laughed. Other kids stopped what they were doing to watch Trick. The red dot leapt onto Ian, and Trick smacked him in the shoulder with both hands, trying to catch it.

"Dude!" Ian protested, slapping Trick away.

Trick had already followed the red dot to Wanda's desk and was smacking his hands down all over her papers.

Bobby was still laughing hysterically.

He's getting too far away from me, Denneka realized with a rush of panic. She got out of her chair and said, "Trick! Stop it!"

But he was too absorbed in the hunt to hear her. He chased the red dot all over the classroom, scrambling over or under desks, slapping his hands against whatever the dot landed on that he could reach—including people.

Mr. Black raised his voice. "Trick, stop disrupting the class and return to your seat."

All the kids were either laughing or annoyed. No one had any idea why he was acting this way, but Denneka picked out the words 'weirdo' and 'cat' from the general chatter. She tried to get closer to Trick, but he was moving so much and so quickly, she couldn't keep up, and her attempts only added to the chaos.

Then the red dot zipped over the floor, up the wall, and straight to an open window, where it vanished. Denneka was on the other side of the room when it happened, and she wasn't quick enough to follow Trick as he raced after the dot and dove through the window.

There was no loud thumping sound of a teen boy landing on the dirt outside. There was, however, a much smaller, lighter sound.

Oh, crap. Denneka froze in place, staring at the window. An eruption of shocked laughter burst out of several people. A few rushed to the window and looked out. Denneka held her breath.

"He's not there," said Wanda.

Peter tipped over the edge of the windowsill, his legs in the air as his upper body disappeared. When he came back up, he was holding Trick's shirt. "But his clothes are."

This is bad. This is bad. Denneka was still frozen with no idea what to do. She'd screwed up. She was supposed to stay close to Trick so this wouldn't happen. She should have tried harder to stop Bobby or Trick.

More people went to the window to see for themselves. Mr. Black pushed through to investigate, but when he saw what they were seeing, he didn't have any immediate answer.

"I'll go look for him," Denneka declared. "Can you give me his clothes?"

The boys had plucked all the pieces off the ground by then, so Peter wadded them all into a ball and handed it to her. "What happened to him?" he asked.

Since Denneka had no idea how to answer that, she grabbed the clothes and ran from the room without trying to explain.

———

"I called Landon's teacher, so he should be out in a moment," the school secretary told Jacqueline. "Oh, while I have you here, we need an updated pick-up release form for Landon's father."

Jacqueline, who had been watching the office door impatiently, snapped her head around to the secretary. "What?"

"I was certain we already had him in our system, but it doesn't seem to be there anymore. It must have been a computer glitch or something."

"What do you mean 'Landon's father'?" Jacqueline growled.

The woman didn't pick up on her tone. "When he was here the other day to pick Landon up, I was sure I saw the release in our system, but it's not there now." She pushed a form onto the front desk between them. "It's a short form, so it'll just take a second and we can get him back in the computer."

Jacqueline felt a hot weight settle in her chest. "You met him?"

"Yes." Finally, the secretary began to sound slightly confused.

"What did he look like?"

The secretary put her finger to her chin. "I can't really remember. Normal, I guess. It's been a couple weeks."

A couple weeks. Marcus had said it had been a couple weeks since whatever happened in the park. "Did he give his name?"

"Wasn't it... Mr. St. Andrew?"

"There is no 'Mr. St. Andrew.' Did he say it was?"

The woman's eyes glassed over for a moment. "I... don't remember."

"But he called himself Landon's father?"

"Well, no. He came by and said he wanted to take Landon to lunch, and when I checked the system, he was in there."

"If you didn't get his name, how did you check the system?"

The secretary stared into the middle distance. "I'm... not sure."

"What made you think he was Landon's father?"

"Landon told me, and he called the man 'Dad'. Is there a problem?"

Jacqueline's gut twisted. She'd feared Landon might have been used by John, if John was the witch. But why would Landon do something like that on his own?

The office door opened, and a young woman walked in with Landon beside her.

"Mom?" he asked, confused and innocent. Her little boy. He didn't look any different. Was there really something going on with him?

Jacqueline smiled. "Hi, sweetheart. We need to go out for a bit. Is that all right?" The last part was directed at the teacher.

The young woman nodded. "It's fine. He won't miss anything important." The woman was oddly standoffish toward Landon, cutting quick glances at him and keeping a deliberate distance. Almost as if she were afraid of him.

What is going on? Jacqueline thought desperately.

———

Landon didn't know why his mom had pulled him out of class, but he was glad he'd get a break from pretending not to notice the stares and whispers of the other kids. Last week, Cliff had been taken to the hospital, but it turned out he was fine. No one had any idea what had happened. At least, the adults didn't. Even Cliff couldn't remember. But the other kids, the ones who'd been there and had seen what Landon had done—they knew. They'd tried to tell the adults, but no one really believed them. Besides, almost all the adults liked Landon better than those other kids. So no one punished him for almost killing Cliff. None of the other boys tried to mess with him anymore, but no one really talked to him anymore either. Not even the girls.

He was so relieved to be out of the classroom that he didn't ask Mom where they were going. He only followed her out to the parking lot, trailing beside her without paying much attention. Until he looked up and saw a man sitting in the passenger seat of Mom's car.

Landon froze, his feet refusing to move. It was the policeman, Officer Parkes.

This was it. He'd been found out.

Landon looked up at his mom, startled and scared by what he saw. Her eyes got wet as he watched, and she turned her face away from him. She put a hand on his back, pushing him forward, and said, "Come on," like it was hard to get the words out.

No one said anything when they got to the car, not even Officer Parkes. Landon got in the back seat and buckled up without having to be told. Mom started driving, and she didn't say anything, but Landon could see her jaw clenching.

They were taking him to the police station. That had to be it. They'd found out what he'd done and were arresting him. This was even worse than Mom yelling at him. Her stiff silence scared him and made his insides feel like they were being eaten up by a black hole. He'd known she would be angry at him if she ever found out, but he hadn't known she'd be angry enough to skip punishing him and instead take him straight to jail.

But Landon stayed quiet because he knew he deserved it.

Except they didn't go to the police station. They went home. So, maybe they didn't know for sure. Or maybe Mom wanted to yell at him before taking him to jail. Or maybe Officer Parkes wanted to yell at him before taking him in.

When they were all standing in the living room, Mom said, "Tell me."

Landon didn't even know where to begin. "About what?"

"Are you—" she started, and then choked on the words. "Can you do—"

He'd definitely been caught. Landon didn't know how, but it didn't matter. He might have been able to not tell her certain things, but he couldn't bring himself to lie to her when she asked him directly. "I'm a witch," he said softly.

A sob and gasp burst out of her, one on top of the other, and her hand flew to her mouth. "How? When?"

"I don't know. Since forever, I think."

Mom fell to her knees. Officer Parkes gave a startled cry and rushed to her, laying a hand on her shoulder, but she waved him away. Landon felt like he'd been stabbed in the stomach, seeing how much his being a witch hurt her.

"I'm sorry, Mom," he said, beginning to cry. "I don't mean to be. I can't help it."

She shook her head, not able to talk through her tears, and then pulled him into a hug so tight that he lost some of his air. It wasn't the reaction he'd expected. "It's not your fault. I know it's not. But why didn't you ever tell me?"

"You don't like magic. I didn't want to worry you."

"I'm sorry. Landon, I'm so sorry I never noticed. I'm sorry you didn't think you could tell me."

She was apologizing to him? No, that was wrong! He hugged her back. "No, I'm sorry! It's my fault, Mom. Why are you crying?"

Mom sucked in deep breaths, trying to stop crying. "It's not your fault," she breathed, rubbing his back. "None of it's your fault. You're a good boy."

He stiffened, and his body jerked in her arms as he took tight breaths. She didn't know, then. She didn't know the worst parts. "I'm not a good boy."

"Landon, yes you—"

"I'm not," he whimpered.

She pushed him out to arm's length. "What do you mean?"

Landon rubbed at the tears in his eyes. He had to tell her everything. She had to know it was all his fault, not hers. Even if she yelled at him, even if she took him to jail, it couldn't be worse than seeing her hurting like this because of him. "I... I almost killed a boy at school with magic."

With her eyes so wide and her mouth opening and closing, she looked like a fish. Her crying had been horrible, but this was worse.

Officer Parkes grabbed Landon by the shoulder, turning him enough that Landon had to look at him. "Explain what you mean, Landon," he said gently but firmly.

"He... killed my lizard," Landon said. "I was angry, so... I told him to die, and he almost did."

Officer Parkes let go and stumbled back a step, looking at Landon like he had the other day when he was here. Landon really hated being looked at like that.

"But then I told him to live, and he did," Landon said, desperate to make sure they knew that part. Mom only kept staring at him like she couldn't believe it. But he needed to tell her everything. "And... I made him tell us things."

"Him?" Mom asked.

Landon pointed to Officer Parkes.

"Us?" the man repeated. "You mean you and John McKenzie?"

Landon nodded. "He told me how to control your brain so you'd answer questions. But he didn't like it when I did it to him."

Officer Parkes rubbed at his head. "That's both terrifying and a huge relief."

"Landon," Mom said carefully, "is Mr. McKenzie a witch?"

Landon nodded. He hated to tell Mr. McKenzie's secret, but it was Mom asking, so he had to. "I knew I should have told you. But I like him, and he was teaching me. I'm sorry, Mom." He sniffled. "I'm not a good boy anymore."

She hugged him, stroking his hair while he cried into her neck. "No, Landon, you are. Even if you did some bad things, you felt bad about them, and you tried to fix them if you could. And you're telling me about them now. It's good to feel bad when you do bad things. You're still my good boy."

He pulled back to look at her. "I—I am?"

"Yes, sweetheart. And now that I know about your magic, I can help you. We'll figure this out. I'll always be here for you." She wrapped one arm around him, and he clung to her side.

She still loved him, and she wasn't even angry. Landon didn't understand it.

"So, McKenzie's the witch you were trying to find," Officer Parkes said to her. "What does that mean for you?"

"I... I honestly have no idea. Landon, you said Mr. McKenzie was teaching you about magic?"

He nodded.

"Did he ever say why?"

"He's interested in me because I'm a witch."

"That's all? He didn't say anything else?"

Landon shook his head. "I... I made him talk. Like I did with Officer Parkes. But he stopped me before I could get him to say more."

"What do you think he's after?" asked Officer Parkes.

Landon didn't know what Mr. McKenzie *could* be after, but it was Mom who answered. "I don't know. Before I knew who the witch was, I assumed he was messing with my family because witches are selfish bastards who use others however they want. The old woman seemed relatively nice and reasonable for a witch, and she still demanded seven years of Trick's life to save Landon. But now that I know John is the witch... I just don't know. It's hard to believe that it was all an act."

"I know you said it's better seen," Officer Parkes said, "but maybe you could tell me what he was doing that made you want to hunt him down."

───────

Kester was in the middle of writing the English discussion questions on the board for the irrelevant eighth grade class (which is to say, the one Trick and Denneka weren't in) when he felt a spike of panic from Julia so intense that he dropped the dry erase pen.

Show me, he told her, tapping into her vision without bothering to leave the classroom.

He experienced a split second of vertigo when he switched to her perspective at least a hundred feet above the ground. She was flying above the school, looking down on an area in the back of the property. A girl was stumbling around in the grass alone. *Denneka? Why is she—?* He didn't even have to finish asking himself the question when he saw the bundle of fabric in her arms. *So, Trick got away from her after all. And they'd been doing so well.* But that didn't explain Julia's alarm.

Julia swooped closer and circled around to get a different angle. And then he saw what had her so spooked. A man was approaching from a side street that was overgrown with bushes. He was crouched low and heading straight for Denneka.

It's him. He really did come after her. The killer was stalking Denneka, and he was getting close. Even if she noticed him right now, it was possible she might not be able to outrun him, and she was too far from the school building to easily call for help.

Kester ripped his focus from his connection to Julia and spared only one moment to get his bearings. The students were looking at him as though he'd had a seizure, but that didn't matter. There was no time to waste making excuses.

I'm coming, Kester told Julia as he sprinted out of the room.

———

Maybe I really am stupid, Trick thought. He sure had acted like it, chasing that light around like he didn't have a brain in his head.

Oh, sure, it was obvious to him *now* that it had been a light. That was the only way to explain how it moved so fast and how it jumped to the back of his hand as soon as he caught it. But at the time, he hadn't been thinking enough to put that together. He hadn't been thinking at all. He'd let his instincts take over, and because of that, he'd almost gotten caught transforming and messed everything up.

The change back into a cat had jolted him to his senses, and he'd bolted away so fast that he left a trail in the dirt even a human could follow. And she did.

The familiar girl had made it through the dirt strip outside the school and onto the grass, where it was harder for her to track him. He knew it was hard because he was sitting high in a tree, watching her. She was calling for him, looking around in the grass and near bushes.

The tree he was in was still kinda far away from her, but she'd reach it soon if she kept heading this way. It was all the way at the edge of the grass, close to a back street and a concrete spot with some dumpsters.

He felt bad about letting her wander around, but he couldn't deal with facing her yet. She'd probably yell at him for making a scene, and he didn't know how he could explain getting fooled by something so simple except to say that he was a dummy.

But as he watched her searching the grass for him, movement a little way off caught his eye. It was a large shape, moving closer to her. A man. The big man from the graveyard.

Trick shot to his paws on the branch, but when he looked down, terror gripped him so hard, he almost fell. Not because of the height but because he knew he wouldn't be able to get down to warn her. He was too high in the tree, and he couldn't see any easy way to reach the ground.

He meowed as loud as he could, trying to get her attention. If she came close enough for him to transform, maybe he could use his bigger body to get down.

The familiar girl's head jerked up at his meow, and she started running toward him, shouting his name. But the big man started moving faster, too. He ran behind her, keeping near the bushes, until he came up to the concrete and ducked behind one of the dumpsters.

Trick meowed and meowed, trying to warn her.

"Trick, there you are," she said. "Are you stuck? How did you get up there?"

That doesn't matter! Look behind you! he thought at her, but the only sounds he could make were desperate, ear-splitting yowls.

"Hang on, I'm coming." But even when she got to the bottom of the tree, he didn't transform back. Why had he climbed this high?

Suddenly, the big man was right behind her. He grabbed her by the arm and pulled her away. She cried out in surprise and dropped the bundle of clothes she'd been holding, but she couldn't pull out of his grip.

"Finally got you." The big man's voice was just as rough as Trick remembered. He began dragging the famir away, and her struggling didn't even slow him down.

Trick ran out as far as he could on the branch. He had to something! He had to stop them!

A flash of brown shot toward the big man's head. He dodged away, and the hawk swooped around for another pass, screeching angrily. When it came down again, talons aiming for the man's neck, he crouched near the dumpster and picked up a metal pipe that had been lying there. But his body hid the pipe from the hawk, so it didn't see the danger until he snapped the pipe up and smacked the hawk out of the air. The hawk landed in the grass with a soft thud and didn't get up.

The man kept dragging the familiar girl away, ignoring her struggles and cries telling him to let her go. When she cried out too loudly, he turned and raised the pipe like he'd hit her with it, growling something to her that Trick couldn't quite hear, and she went silent but didn't stop trying to pull away.

He's taking her! He's taking her! Terror filled Trick's whole body with tremors, but he scrambled back and forth on the branch, desperate to find a way down. If he could get closer and become human again, maybe he could fight the man off and save her.

There. That other branch was a big jump down, and he wasn't sure he'd be able to grab it, but it was his best chance. He crouched, gauged the distance, and jumped. He nearly missed, but he caught the lower branch with his forepaws and scrambled up. It was still too far to the ground, though, and he had to find another branch lower down.

When he looked up, the man and the familiar girl were even further away.

But that was when he saw someone else running toward them. It was the teacher man. He was coming fast across the grass toward them, like he meant to slam right into the big man.

Facing the new threat, the big man threw the familiar girl hard

oncrete. She must have landed wrong, because she didn't
even when he turned away from her.

ey!" the teacher shouted when he saw the big man throw her.

What now?" the big man asked, going to meet the teacher.

The teacher said, "You've made a very big mistake," and reached
or something on his wrist. But before he could finish whatever he
was doing, the big man got to him, swung a huge fist, and the
teacher fell to the ground.

Trick stared in horror. He was so stunned, all he could do was
watch as the big man looked at the two bodies, grumbled something, then threw the teacher man over his shoulder and picked the
familiar girl up under his arm.

Where are you taking them?! Trick demanded—but, of course, he
couldn't say it aloud. He scrambled to find a lower branch, jumped,
caught it, and with a few more wild leaps landed on the ground in a
tumble. It banged him up a little, but he didn't even notice the pain.
He raced across the grass and concrete, struggling to keep sight of
the man, and watched helplessly as the man stuffed both humans
into the trunk of a car, then got in and drove off.

CHAPTER
TWENTY-FIVE

Julia shook herself awake, getting to her feet and ruffling her feathers back into the right positions. How long had she been stunned for? She thought about Kester and let her worry and fear fill her. It was enough that he would have stopped whatever he was doing to speak to her in her mind, to reassure her or tell her what to do.

She heard nothing.

Flapping her wings a few more times, she was sure she didn't have any broken bones. That pipe could have killed her, but she managed to turn at the last second just enough that it didn't strike her full-on. With two strong flaps, she took to the air.

When she got twenty feet up, she saw the killer hurrying toward a car... with two bodies.

Kester! she shrieked, but it only came out as a hawk's cry.

There was a small, black shape on the ground, darting through the grass after the kidnapper. So, the kitten boy had gotten himself out of the tree and was trying to save his girl. It was a nice thought, but there was nothing a kitten could do against a man like that.

When the man dumped Kester and Denneka into the trunk and started the car, Julia swooped down near the kitten boy. As soon as the car started to move, he was chasing it. As if he could catch it and stop it. He saw her flying near him but didn't spare her more than a glance.

Stop and think, she thought at him, but all she could do was cry out, and he couldn't understand that. They'd managed to communicate simple things between the two of them, the way any animals might, but it was impossible to communicate complex human thoughts with animal sounds or gestures.

He understood that she was trying to say something, though—maybe even that she was trying to stop him, given the defiant-sounding meow she got in return.

There was no use. He was going to keep chasing that car even if he got run over in the process, and she was too small to pick him up and carry him away. So she did the best thing she could think of and flew higher, trailing the car herself. She stayed high enough to keep a better view of it than Trick had from the ground, but low enough that Trick would be able to keep her in sight and use her as a guide if he lost track of the car.

In this way, the two of them followed the car to an abandoned building on the far south side of town. It was an older area—not vintage-old but dilapidated-old. The area was close to the river, far downstream from Kester's house. Based on the damage to the buildings, Julia guessed it may have flooded at one point, badly enough for the buildings to be ruined and abandoned as the people looked for less treacherous ground farther in.

The building had probably been a house originally, but now it was so covered in metal sheeting, it didn't look much like a house anymore. If this was where the killer had been hiding out all these weeks, he'd had plenty of time to shore the place up and make it uninviting to curious passersby.

The kitten couldn't move as fast as Julia could, so he was trailing behind. Julia perched on the roof of another building and watched the killer-turned-kidnapper haul Kester and Denneka out of the trunk and carry them into the house like two sacks of potatoes. Trick ran up the road, huffing and panting, just in time to see them disappear inside and a metal door clatter shut behind them.

Trick barely paused for breath but immediately started searching the house for a way in. As he covered the ground, Julia searched the roof. Old houses usually had plenty of broken slats or torn window screens that a bird could use to squeeze inside. But this one was nailed up tight, and she couldn't find an entrance.

It had been several minutes since her master had been kidnapped, and still she couldn't hear his voice. She'd seen him beginning to stir when the man carried him in, so she knew he had to be either awake or waking up. If so, surely he'd free himself and the girl and deal with the criminal at any moment.

But as Trick darted around the house on the ground below, minutes passed, and Julia heard nothing that sounded as if Kester had been able to free himself.

Finally, she heard his voice in her head. It sounded angry and hurt... and afraid. *My hands are tied. I can't get the watch off. Get help.*

———

Kester tugged at his bonds again. *All this power, and I'm foiled by duct tape.* He'd been arrogant and careless, in such a hurry to save the girl that he'd forgotten his power was locked away behind his disguise. When Julia had been hit, the sudden pain and silence from her had temporarily blinded him with rage and fear, driving the memory of his locked power even farther from his mind. By the time he remembered he needed to remove his watch, he'd been right on top of the killer—and had still allowed the killer to get too close before he was ready to fight. When a man isn't used to facing actual threats, he gets sloppy.

There was a fair chance Kester would die for it. Julia was all right, no thanks to him, and was on her way to find help, but there was still distance to cover and the human/bird language barrier to overcome. From the looks of their captor, Kester and Denneka might not have the sort of time Julia needed.

He was a large man, just as Parkes had said, and as he stomped around the house, his heavy steps caused vibrations in the floor.

"Mr. McKenzie," Denneka said in a terrified whisper, "what do we do?"

Their captor had put them in what was likely the largest bedroom, though there was no bed in it and holes in the walls gave them views into other rooms. The two of them were sitting on metal chairs in the center of the room, their hands bound behind them with that blasted tape, and their ankles taped to the chairs. The only light came from thin cracks in the metal sheeting that was covering the outside; there was only broken glass in the windows, and the original walls of the house had lost much of their structural integrity. Mold covered most of the external wall and the only piece of furniture besides the chairs—a dresser—looked and smelled like a haven for rats.

"Stay calm," Kester told Denneka because that seemed like the sort of thing an adult should tell a child in this situation. Easier said than done, though. Inside, Kester seethed with anger, fear, and wounded pride.

As their captor paced around the house, Kester could hear him muttering to himself but couldn't make out exact words. Not at first. The footsteps moved to the hall outside and the room behind them, and the mutters turned into, "I'm done for. I'm done for. This is it. Franco's gonna have me."

"What are you blathering on about?" Kester murmured.

"What's going on?" Denneka asked in a pleading whisper. The girl was already beginning to cry, though at least she did it quietly. "Why did he take us?"

Kester raised his eyebrows at her. "Us? It was you he was after. I'm only here because I got in his way and he didn't want to leave a body or witness behind." That was the conclusion Kester had come to since waking, at any rate. He'd already deduced after Jacqueline had broken into his house that the theft of his personal information had been perpetrated by her, so he had no reason to think *he* meant anything to their captor.

"Me?" Denneka squeaked. "Why?"

Maybe the man heard her, because the pacing footsteps stopped, then pounded in their direction until their captor thundered in through the open doorway of the bedroom. His head didn't actually touch the ceiling, but it came half an inch shy of brushing the door frame. A face only a boxer's mother could love glared at the girl so fiercely it could have made a grown man cower. Denneka froze in terror.

The man took two threatening steps toward her. "Do you have any idea what you've done to me?"

Now confused as well as terrified, Denneka could only shake her head.

"Siccing the cops on me. Spilling my secrets. What'd you think you'd get from that, huh? Think you were doing the right thing? That man was a worthless, good-for-nothing loser, and he was already dead. What good did you think you were doing narking about it?" He worked himself up more and more with each sentence so he was nearly shouting by the end.

"Excuse me," Kester said tightly. "She's only a girl. If you don't mind, kindly don't shout at her."

"And you!" The man punched Kester in the jaw so hard his head snapped around. "Why can't you just mind your own business?!"

Kester hadn't felt pain like that in a very long time. His face throbbed, and he could feel where the inside of his cheek had been cut on his teeth. Spitting blood on the floor, he said, "She is my business. Who are you, anyway?"

The man's eyes bulged in indignation. Then he shook his head and laughed hysterically. "You don't even know. You two have ended me, and you don't even know who I am."

"We do not. Why don't you tell us? You're going to kill us anyway, aren't you?" From the corner of his eye, Kester could see Denneka turn a terrified look on him.

"Oh, is that what you think?" said their captor. "I'm a murderer, so obviously I'm going to murder you? Is that it?"

"Isn't it?"

"It might be now!" The man let out a frustrated howl and paced back and forth in the room. "I don't like killing when I don't have to! It's messy. It complicates things. But that girl"—he thrust a finger toward Denneka—"saw me, so I had to do something about her."

"I didn't see you!" Denneka blurted.

The man scowled at her. "Lying's not gonna help you now. I don't know how, but I know you saw me bury Haug. I saw you come back to the grave when I was watching it, and you ran from me when I got closer, so I know you recognized me. Then you told the cops about the corpse. *Then* you gave them my description!"

"But I didn't! Except telling them about the body, but I wasn't the one—"

"Denneka," Kester said in soft warning. If the man didn't know about Trick, there was no reason to tell him.

Fortunately, their captor seemed to be on a roll and ignored her protest. But he wasn't looking at her anymore, having shifted somewhere between berating her and muttering to himself again. "Franco's gonna kill me. He said this was my last chance. It should have been easy. How hard could it be to scare a teacher into paying up? It wasn't my fault I killed him, and I tried to cover it up." His eyes shot to Denneka. "Then you had to go and screw everything up. I had it all nice and tidy, but no. You had to tell the cops. You had to blab about me to everyone. But you were still the only one who'd actually seen me, so I had to get you out of the way."

Denneka started hyperventilating.

"I wasn't gonna kill you! Just keep you here for a while. Get you out of the way. Who'd care about a dead nobody when a kid's missing? It would have worked! It would have given me time to clean things up so I could go back without Franco blowing my head off. But then you"—it was Kester's turn for the finger thrust—"had to get in the way. So I brought you both here. And what the hell am I supposed to do now?"

"You could let us go," Denneka cheeped. "We won't tell anyone."

The man eyed Kester. "Nah. I might have believed you, if you hadn't already blabbed so much. But your teacher here wants to kill me. I can see it in his eyes."

Kester couldn't deny it. His face throbbed, his wrists ached, and his head spun with the realization that this man could not let witnesses leave here alive.

But Julia was getting help. She would come back for him. All he had to do was stall for time and keep their captor from reaching for his gun. "Will you at least allow a condemned man his last confession? I promise it'll be interesting."

———

All things considered, Jacqueline thought Marcus had taken it all pretty well. Better than Jacqueline had taken the news that her own son had been a witch for apparently all his life and she'd been such a bad mother that she had never even noticed.

"You know, I thought there was something weird about him," Marcus said.

"Weird?" Jacqueline repeated. She couldn't help feeling a little defensive, even if 'weird' was an objectively accurate way to describe Trick.

Marcus held up his hands. "Not weird in a bad way. I really was glad when he got back safely. Though... I am a little annoyed now that he had us all worried just because he didn't want to tell you he was safe."

Jacqueline laughed. "Yeah. Welcome to my life."

Marcus shifted his attention to Landon. The fear in his eyes was gone now, or at least hidden by caution and concern. "Sounds like your brother causes your mom a lot of trouble."

Landon shrugged. He was sunken into the corner of the couch like he was trying to make himself look as small and non-threatening as possible. Which was ridiculous for a six-year-old boy. The fact that he saw himself as such a danger—and that Marcus saw or had seen him as such a danger—was something Jacqueline still couldn't quite wrap her head around.

To her surprise, Marcus got up from his chair and sat down beside Landon on the couch. "You love your mom a lot, don't you?"

Landon nodded.

"I bet you love your brother, too, even if he's a pain."

Landon nodded.

Marcus ruffled Landon's hair lightly. "You're a good kid, Landon."

Landon jumped in surprise and sat up out of his hole. "You're not mad at me?"

"I was never mad. Scared and confused, but not mad. Yeah, you did some things you shouldn't have, but you apologized and you're not going to do them anymore, right?"

"No. I mean, I... I don't want to."

Marcus nodded solemnly. "You're honest. I like that. It's good to ask for help when you're struggling, especially when you're struggling against yourself. That's what your family's here for."

Landon looked away with an expression Jacqueline couldn't quite interpret, but Marcus seemed to understand it.

"Even when they're dealing with their own problems," he told Landon firmly. "Family's got to be there for each other, even when they've got their own stuff going on." He rubbed the back of his head, suddenly looking much younger. "At least, that's what I figure." Looking at Jacqueline, he shrugged. "Been a while since I've really had any experience with that, but I don't think I'm wrong."

"You're not wrong." Jacqueline scooped Landon into a hug. "No matter what else is going on, you tell me if you need help, okay?"

Landon's small arms wrapped around her, and he nodded. "Okay, Mom."

The sweet moment was interrupted by a loud thump on the front door, quickly followed by the same sort of frantic flapping sound that had sent Jacqueline rushing out of John's house. A spike of irrational fear made her jump to her feet. Then reason kicked in a second later. This was her house, so she had no need to worry that she'd be caught doing anything.

"What is that?" Marcus asked.

Jacqueline said, "Landon, stay here," and went to open the door.

As expected, she found a red-tailed hawk on her front step. It stood there on the mat, looking up at her. "Are you finally going to talk to me?" she asked it.

The bird nodded once.

Jacqueline stepped aside, and the bird flew in. Marcus and Landon both jerked back from the hawk in surprise. It flew up to perch on Trick's cat tree and watched them all impatiently. How she knew the bird was impatient, Jacqueline wasn't quite sure. Maybe the way it kept ruffling its feathers every few seconds and stepping from side to side.

"You're the witch's familiar," Jacqueline asserted, sure enough in what the kids had told her that she didn't make it a question.

The hawk nodded.

"We know John is the witch."

If a bird could show surprise, the hawk did. Its head moved back in a way that was very birdish but also a close approximation of a human start of surprise. Then it looked directly at Landon.

"Yes, he told us," Jacqueline said, then gestured between herself and Marcus, "but we'd already basically figured it out ourselves."

The hawk's beak pointed toward Marcus, then its head cocked. Then cocked the other way. Then nodded.

"What does that mean?" Marcus muttered.

"I have no idea," Jacqueline admitted. But knowing that John was the witch and that the witch had a familiar, and based on the oddly human gestures coming from the hawk, Jacqueline had to assume that John's familiar was like Trick—a human transformed into an animal. And then it all made sense. "You're Julia, aren't you?"

The bird gave another, bigger start of surprise. Then it looked at Jacqueline for a long second and slowly nodded.

"Of course," Jacqueline breathed. Julia, the person with the closest direct connection to John, who Jacqueline had only met once and who never seemed to be available at any other time. The way Julia was always 'working' even on weekends. The wry smile John had worn when he'd agreed with Jacqueline that Julia's boss was a dick. "I'm sorry," she said softly, not quite sure why. Sorry that she hadn't noticed sooner. Or maybe only sorry for the other woman, who had struck her as smart and capable but was bound to a life of servitude to... Well, to the man she loved, wasn't it? If Julia had been honest with her about that, and Jacqueline thought she had been.

Still a life of servitude, though. One which Jacqueline had no intention of ever letting Trick get caught up in again. A thrill of fear ran through her body as a fresh idea occurred to her. Maybe John had found out there was a stray familiar—or former familiar—in town and wanted to add him to his collection? Do witches have more than one familiar? But why else would John be messing with Trick?

"He can't have Trick," Jacqueline told the hawk.

It—no, *she*—cocked her head, then shook it. Then ruffled her wings impatiently as if the very idea wasn't even worth discussing.

So, that wasn't what John wanted Trick for? "What does he want with him, then?"

Julia only flapped her wings and scratched at her perch with her talons.

"You think something's wrong?" Marcus asked. "She's acting pretty agitated."

The hawk nodded vigorously, then flew up to perch on Marcus's shoulder. He winced as her talons gripped him, but they didn't draw blood through his light shirt. Clearly, she had practice being gentle with soft human flesh.

"So, this bird's like Trick?" Marcus asked. "She's human?"

"Yes," Jacqueline answered. "John's girlfriend. Though that may have only been a cover story." If it was, she felt even worse for Julia. But she couldn't afford to spare much sympathy for this woman when she still didn't know what John meant to do with her family. "What's going on? Is there some kind of trouble?"

Julia nodded again and flapped her wings.

"Hey, careful with the claws," Marcus said, moving so that Julia was nearly shaken loose and had to hold on tighter, which made

ain. But the bird stopped .

ld loosen her grip.

turn human?" Jacqueline asked

er head.

That would make this difficult. "Then what's the

Trick?"

The bird shook her head.

"Is it John?"

The bird nodded and gave a quick flap.

This was going to take forever.

Landon's quiet voice interrupted her next question. "Can I try?

Jacqueline, Marcus, and Julia all turned to the little boy. "Did John teach you how to talk to animals?" Jacqueline asked.

"No..."

"Telepathy?" Marcus asked.

"No... But... sort of both? A little? I might be able to figure it out."

Jacqueline shared a concerned look with Marcus. "Do you think it's safe to let him do magic?"

Marcus shrugged.

But Julia was clearly worked up about something, and she wouldn't let up until they understood what. Jacqueline took a deep breath. "Okay, Landon. You can try. But if you feel like anything's wrong or... or anything"—she really wished she had the first clue how to guide him in this—"then stop, okay?"

"Okay."

Julia flapped from Marcus's shoulder to the arm of the couch. Landon gave Jacqueline a questioning glance, but when she nodded, he looked the bird in the eye. Their locked gaze was so intense, he didn't quite seem like a little boy at all.

"Is Mr. McKenzie in danger?" Landon asked Julia. She didn't nod, but he seemed to get some response from her, because he said, "The killer has him?"

"What?!" Marcus demanded, stepping toward them.

Jacqueline put a hand on his arm. "Don't interrupt."

Landon said.

id again, and Jacqueline had to tighten he

speak again right away, but he kept his gaze
's, nodding a few times as they—Jacqueline could
communicated telepathically.

d thought her life had been surreal before, when all
was a son who was a cat.

tually, Landon sat back and looked at her. "Mr. McKenzie
rick's friend were taken by the killer and are being held some-
ere. Trick's there, too, looking for a way in to save them."

"He's what?!" Jacqueline cried.

Marcus laid a hand on hers, which was still gripping his arm.
"It's okay. I'll deal with this."

"*We'll* deal with this!" she corrected, releasing him. "That's my
son out there!"

He held up his hands. "Okay. But let me call in backup, at least."

Julia flapped frantically.

"There's no time," Landon said. "She's afraid the man will kill
them soon."

Marcus let out a harsh breath. "And it would take days just to
convince someone I'm not crazy if I told them how I found out
about all this. McKenzie's a witch, right? How'd he get himself into
this mess?"

"He can't do magic right now," Landon explained. "I don't know
why. But when he was teaching me, I never saw him do any."

"Well, that's helpful," Marcus muttered.

Jacqueline turned to the bird. "Julia, can you lead us to where
they are?"

Julia leapt into the air and flew a few tight circles around them.

"Can I come?" Landon asked.

"No," Jacqueline and Marcus said in unison.

"But what if Ms. Julia needs to say something else?"

He had a point. Jacqueline hated that he had a point. If something changed and Julia needed to talk to them, she wouldn't be

able to without him. "All right." Once again, Jacqueline risk one son for the sake of the other. She hoped it wouldn'␣ to be a mistake.

———

The dirt was damp and sticky, and it got caked into Trick's fur mor and more the further in he dug. But he didn't stop. He'd finally found a way inside the house where the familiar girl was being kept by the big man, and he couldn't stop digging until he got to her.

He'd found a tight space between one of the metal sheets and the ground, and when he'd dug at it he'd found that the wood of the house had rotted away.

Even with the extra space, he had to dig for a while to reach a broad space under the house that was tall enough for him to stand up in. There were concrete blocks with posts sticking into them. The floor of the space was all dirt, and the ceiling was wood. Light came in through a bunch of holes, so he wouldn't have even needed cat vision to see his way around.

It was creepy under here, and he felt disgusting with all the mud matting up his fur, but the thrill of success was like lightning running through his body. He'd made it inside—or almost inside. Past the metal barrier the big man had put up around the house, anyway. He was here, and he was going to save the familiar girl. He knew he could do it. Maybe he'd failed to save her from the big man before, but he wouldn't this time.

I'm not useless, he thought fiercely. *I'll save you.*

The sound of the teacher man's voice made his ears perk up, and his head swiveled toward the right side of the house. The familiar girl was probably with the teacher. With all the stealth a cat could muster, Trick crept toward the sound.

———

worked through all his stories that were both interesting
hold a rough man's attention and relatively safe for a
ars (there weren't many) and was five anecdotes into 'don't
ur parents I said that in front of you' territory when he heard
skitter of claws on wood.

"What was that?" asked their captor. He'd been in a good mood
ly a moment ago, laughing at Kester's story, but if he was twitchy
enough for his mood to turn like that, things weren't going all that
well.

"Probably only a rat," Kester said. "I'm sure this place is full of
them. Now, as I was saying…" He continued with his story, but he
knew the claws hadn't been a rat. Having regained the other man's
attention, Kester glanced as carefully as he could toward the sound.

Through a large hole in the wall in front of him, Kester could see
a small, black shape moving silently across the wooden floor.
Directly toward an approximately five-inch hole at the bottom of the
wall between them. Which was just about ten feet from where
Denneka sat.

The idiot boy was going to kill himself.

"You know what?" Kester interrupted himself. "All this talking
has me quite parched. Do you have any water?"

The killer eyed him suspiciously.

"I know, I know, you're going to have to kill us anyway, but
don't pretend you're not enjoying my stories. And no one knows
we're here, so we're in no hurry. What could it hurt to get me a
drink?"

Their captor huffed and left the room.

"And some food, if you have any!" Kester called after him,
trying to buy as much time as he could.

As soon as the man's footsteps clomped down the hall, the black
shape of Trick darted toward the hole in the wall between the room
he'd entered the house through and the one Kester and Denneka
were held in.

"Trick, stop!" Kester commanded as loudly as he could without
his voice carrying to the killer a few rooms away.

It was the first time he'd said Trick's correct name directly him, which might have been the only reason the boy actual obeyed.

"Trick?" Denneka squeaked. She'd been silent the whole time Kester had told his stories, her only reaction being the changing pink tones of her face and the more or less widening of her eyes "What are you doing here?" she whispered shouted at the kitten.

He couldn't answer of course

Kester gave him another order, "If you don't want to cut yourself in half, back away from the hole."

Trick stayed frozen for another three seconds, then skittered backward away from the hole as if a snake had emerged from it.

Denneka gasped, watched with relief as Trick disappeared from their view to go another way around, and then gave Kester such a cartoonishly exaggerated look of shock that he knew she'd put it all together. "You're—you're ——"

"Yes," Kester murmured.

The pitter-patter of tiny feet preceded Trick's entrance into the room through the open doorway. He charged in at full speed, but one leap after he crossed the threshold, he transformed and landed ungracefully on his face. Without sparing even a glance at Kester, Trick scrambled to his hands and feet and crawled to Denneka.

"My wrists!" she whispered urgently, pulling at her hands. "Take the tape off!"

Trick scurried to the back of her chair and picked at the duct tape with his fingers and teeth. It didn't take him long to get it off, and then Denneka rubbed at her wrists and bent to pull the tape from her ankles. Seeing what she was about, Trick worked on one leg while she got the other. When she was free he stood and bent down to her, wrapping his arms around her shoulders in a hug so tight Kester could see the boy's arm and back muscles straining beneath his skin.

It would have been a shockingly human display from Trick, but it was somewhat ruined by the way he rubbed his head against Denneka's as fervently as a normal boy in a situation like this might

ve kissed her. But it was the urgent lick he ran from Denneka's
w to her temple that made her gasp, "Trick!" and push him away.

"Hurry and untie me," Kester told them. "He'll return soon."

The boy made no move toward him. Not even the dire situation
had done much to warm Trick toward the teacher he disliked.

"Trick," Denneka whispered. "He's the witch."

Surprise registered on Trick's face, but he said and did nothing,
possibly unsure how that information changed things.

"That's true," Kester said, beginning to lose his patience. "Now
untie me so I can get us all out of here."

Still, the children hesitated.

Kester directed his gaze to Denneka. "You're smarter than this."

The wheels turned in her head, and her mouth set in a firm line.
"Trick, get his ankles," she said as she knelt behind Kester's chair to
work on the tape at his wrists.

Kester didn't allow any fear to show on his face, but his heart
pounded harder and faster with every second that passed while the
children worked on his bonds. There was no more stalling. If their
captor returned before he was free, they were all dead. But
reminding the children of that would only make them panic, which
at best meant their fingers would become clumsier and freeing him
would take longer. At worst, it would make them do something
phenomenally stupid like try to run for the door and leave him
behind.

The faint clomp of boots from the other end of the house grew
more distinct. The man was coming back. Trick finished freeing
Kester's legs just as Denneka unwound the last of the tape to free
his hands.

Kester rose and tore the watch from his wrist, tossing it to the
floor. He ignored the shocked faces of the children as his disguise
vanished, instead reveling in the connection to his magic—his
power—that returned to him.

In the very next second, their captor entered the room with a
bottle of water in one hand and a microwaved sandwich in the
other. "Who the hell are you?" he asked Kester.

...k. She didn't
... in either form. But if
...osion went off...

...ating for him. "Trick! Trick!" Her feet
...through the debris with a dexterity she didn't
...still had. She could hear Marcus following behind her,
...casionally slipping on something with a surprised grunt, but she
couldn't wait for him. She had to know if her son was—

As she turned around the ragged edge of what remained of the house's exterior, she saw him. Past the splintered remains of two walls, he was huddled on the floor with Denneka, his arms around her protectively. There was shock and terror in their eyes, but that meant there was also life.

"Trick!" Jacqueline shouted, stepping into what was left of the house. But she stopped when she saw the man who was standing near Trick and Denneka. At first, she didn't recognize him, but... "It can't be," she breathed.

"Who is he?" Marcus asked beside her.

How could she answer that when the answer made no sense? She picked her way across the cluttered floor slowly, expecting the scene to change into something she could understand.

Julia flew down from above and landed on the man's shoulder.

SHAWNA CANON

haunted, eerie look that had been in his blue eyes melted into a
m smile. He reached up to stroke Julia's head, and the bird
ned into his touch. "Hello, beloved one," he said to her in a soft,
entle voice that Jacqueline could barely hear. "You came as I knew
you would, but I fear I grew impatient."

Marcus moved off to investigate something in the debris to their
right, but Jacqueline continued toward the three humans and one
hawk. "Trick," she called out. "Are you okay?"

At the sound of her voice, the man jerked, and his eyes met hers.
She knew those eyes. She'd seen them once before, as well as every
time she looked at her youngest son. *How?* she asked herself. *How?*

"We're okay," Denneka called back.

Jacqueline walked closer until she could speak to them without
shouting. "Kester?" Her voice was barely more than a croak.

He smiled sadly, wincing at the same time, and stroked Julia's
head. "It seems the game is up, my lovely."

"Who is he?" Landon asked.

Jacqueline spun to see that he'd followed her.

Landon pointed at his father. "Who is that man, Mom?" Something in his voice told her he already knew the answer.

Kester came to them, kneeling to look Landon in the eye. The
similarities between them were so striking, Jacqueline felt it in her
gut. The same blond hair. The same pale blue eyes. The same lines
and features.

The same sad, guilty smile.

"I'm no one," Kester told his son. "Only a troublemaker who
brings nothing but chaos and destruction. As your brother can attest
to." He stood and spoke to Jacqueline. "Don't worry; I'm leaving. I'll
make sure neither of you ever see me again." He took a step, as if to
move past her and walk out of their lives.

Jacqueline grabbed Kester's wrist, jerking it toward her. "Like
hell you will!"

...other slow breath. The boy

...n good.

...zie?" Landon didn't continue until Kester had
...ed his eyes and looked at him. "You're my dad, aren't you?"

All the strength in Kester's body and all his resolve seemed to leave him at once, and he dropped into a squat on the debris-strewn floor. He rubbed his head with his hands. He should have left days ago. Weeks, even. Now look at the mess he'd made, literally and figuratively.

"Are you really John?" Jacqueline asked.

He nodded without looking up at her. If he stayed down here, it would be easier for her to kick him.

"You're John and Kester and a witch."

He nodded.

She kicked him. Right in the kidney. Stars burst behind his eyes at the pain, but he managed not to fall over.

From his shoulder, Julia flapped in protest, and he could feel her desire to attack Jacqueline. It was only a fleeting desire, since she did like Jacqueline, but she always came to his defense even when e didn't deserve it. *It's all right, dear one,* he told her through their ond. *Let her do what she will.*

"You're a bastard," Jacqueline seethed. "How long have you known what Landon's been going through?"

That was not what he'd expected Jacqueline to be angry about. He looked up at her with a frown. She was waiting for an answer. "For… for years. Julia and I have been watching you all for a long time."

"And why did you only show up *now*?"

Maybe the blast of magic had done something to Kester's hearing, because it almost sounded like what she resented was not him showing up *at all* but the fact that he hadn't shown up *sooner*. He stood and said, "If you really must have the whole story, we should go somewhere more comfortable. It is not a short one."

"Tell me now," she insisted.

"He's right."

They both looked over to see Parkes stepping through the debris from where the living room used to be. Why on earth had she brought him?

"Sorry, Jac," Parkes said, "but I need you guys to put a hold on whatever drama this is, at least long enough for him to tell me about that corpse over there."

Was the man honestly going to try to arrest him? "You saw him for yourself, didn't you?"

"Corpse?" Jacqueline snapped. "What corpse?"

"It looks like the suspect we've been hunting," Parkes told her. "The one who drugged me and who I'm pretty sure killed Haug." His gaze shifted to Kester. "Am I right?"

Kester nodded. "He attacked Denneka at the school. I tried to intervene, but"—this was embarrassing—"I forgot I was still wearing the disguise which also kept my magic locked away. So he was able to knock me out. Denneka and I woke up here, and the man made it clear he would have to kill us because we were witnesses." As an afterthought, he asked Jacqueline, "I am to

...ate

...heard an

...down as our

...accident. At least his

...be able to run his prints."

..."...to it, then."

...you whatever recompense you desire,

...planation, I'll give it to you. You know where

...nna tonight at eight."

———

"Are we going to talk about it?" Julia asked. She'd waited hours for him to open up on his own, but he hadn't done it.

"About what?"

"About the sulking."

"I'm not sulking."

"You've barely said a word since we came home."

"I've been busy." Kester gestured toward the dining table, which was set and filled with food. Only moments ago, he'd added the last dish.

_"

.all me that."

. in surprise. "Why not?"

.ed, took her hand, and led her to the living room,
down beside him onto the couch. "I've decided to free

.e me?" What was there to free her from?

'm going to remove the spells I've placed on you."

.he spells? But the only spells were… "N-no!" she blurted, so
.sperate she could hardly get the word out right.

Her vehemence startled him. "Julia—"

"Don't you dare, Kester. You need me."

His eyes tightened. "That isn't the point. For once in my life, I
need to consider what's best for someone other than myself."

The earnestness of that admission warmed her heart and softened her tone. "Then tell me what the problem is and let me make
my own decision."

Shame crept across his features. "Your own decision. I suppose
that should have been obvious, but I couldn't even think of that
much."

"You're still moping. What's wrong?"

"I'm not a good man, Julia. Even though I love you more than
anything else in the world, I've expressed it only by keeping you
trapped and controlling your life. I've kept you away from schooling, from a career, from friends and lovers. I've kept you as a bird in
a cage, and you deserve to fly free."

Julia nearly rolled her eyes at his over-dramatic mixing of
metaphor and literalism. "First off, what makes you think you're not
a good man?"

His eyebrows rose. "I should think that was patently obvious. I
manipulate others and meddle in their lives for my own amusement. I use magic to outright control them when they don't
cooperate."

"You've been doing that for decades. Why does it bother you
now?"

. "You know, Kester, you're
taco made her laugh. "If magic is
g it,"

said you did, for weeks."

rowned in thought. "But I wasn't intentionally avoiding it."

"The 'how' can be worked through. The point is you did it, so you can do it again,"

"But I'm not—"

"Remember when I agreed you were changing but wouldn't tell you what into?

"You.

"Do you want to know now?"

His eyes narrowed, peering into hers like he was searching for the answer. "Please."

"You've become a better version of yourself, Kester. The man I always knew was in there." She laid her hand over his heart. "The man I love."

He winced like her words pained him. "Julia…"

you know it, but I want to finally say it. I love you,
ve for a long time."

nd wrapped gently around hers and pulled it away from
. "They call that Stockholm Syndrome, Julia."

scowled and pulled her hand out of his. "Give me some
, Kester. I'm not a child or some naïve teenager. I'm a grown
man. I know exactly who you are and what you've done and
nat I've missed out on by being tied to you. I love you anyway."

Kester stared at her with round eyes, leaning away from the
strength of her words, so she pressed her advantage.

"Love isn't out of your reach, Kester. It's right here. And maybe
it's not easy, and maybe there's risk, and maybe it means sacrificing
something else, but if you really want it, I'm offering." There. The
gauntlet was down. If he didn't want her, he really would break
their bond and set her free, and there would be nothing she could
do to stop him.

He stared at her for a long time, emotions flickering through his
sapphire eyes. Eventually, he said in a small voice, "If I say yes, will
you stay with me?"

Her heart danced. "For the rest of our lives."

"What would I have to do?"

The answer should have been obvious, but this was Kester.
"Marry me. Be mine and only mine. Not my master, but my
partner."

"Is that what you want?"

"You know it is. But is it what you want?" She knew he might do
it anyway, if he thought he owed her, but she didn't want it if it was
only out of obligation.

Kester's arms reached out to her, pulling her into a tight hug.
"Yes," he said into her neck. "I want that, Julia. I need your help. I
don't know how to make it happen. But I want it."

Then he kissed her. Gently, softly, as if she might break. Heat
flared through her whole body, but when she tried to return the kiss
with passion, he pulled away.

"No, Julia. If you do that, I won't be able to stop."

mistaking it for... He swam...
to finish the sentence. But she knew what he meant, and her love for him burned even hotter. She pulled away, putting space between them. He looked suddenly awkward, trying for a carefree grin, but too self-conscious to make it work. "So... when should we have the wedding? I want to give you something spectacular, so planning will—"

"Tomorrow," she said.

"Pardon?"

"Tomorrow. I don't want a big wedding. I just want to be married to you and start our new life as soon as possible."

He gave her a look of surprise, then shook his head and laughed. "As the lady wishes. But... Julia..."

"What is it?"

"I should still remove the spells on you. You can't have a life if you're a bird all day, and you're not my slave anymore."

"But does being your familiar have to mean being your slave?"

"Well... not technically..."

"I like our bond, Kester. I'd feel... lonely if it was gone. If you think it would be too much intimacy, I'll understand, but—"

"You really want to be my wife *and* my familiar?"

"Is that so strange?"

"I've never heard of it being done before. Not according to the more modern definition of 'wife', at any rate."

"Does that mean it can't?"

"No. But you would have to still be an animal at least part of the time."

"You can change the spell, can't you?"

He considered it, then shook his head at himself. "Of course I can. Not thinking selfishly is going to take some practice."

"What does that mean?"

"I could have given you full control over your transformation from the start. All witches could do it that way if we wanted to. But retaining control over your transformation is most of what makes us your masters. We control your humanity by saying when you get to be human. But I can make it so that you determine for yourself when you're human and when you're a hawk. I can even make it so you can partially transform if you wish to."

"Really?" Julia had never really considered what it would be like to transform at will. The thought thrilled her.

"Yes," he said. "But, once I do that... I think that should be the last magic I do. Ever. It... brings out parts of me I don't much like anymore."

"You believe now that you can do it?"

He took her hand. "Only with your help."

The doorbell rang.

Kester grimaced. "The invaders are at the gates."

Julia smoothed her dress and went to answer the door. "Don't be such a drama queen."

———

Jacqueline felt so nervous and irritated, she didn't know whether she wanted to kick the door down or make a run for it. But she tried not to show any of that on her face, for the kids' sake. She stood on the porch holding Landon's hand, with Denneka and Trick behind her. Bringing the girl had been a necessity, not only because Trick insisted but because he wouldn't be human without her here. Not until Jacqueline made Kester turn him human again. But the girl kept giving Landon strange looks.

... the

... this, whatever

... one believed Julia had been

... ing in love with John—with Kester—and

... was with Kester's son. She couldn't imagine how painful it must be for Julia to see the two of them.

But then Julia grinned and said, "Nice of you to ring the bell this time."

And Jacqueline said, "Nice of you to speak in English instead of meaningful head tilts."

And that was pretty much it.

Julia welcomed her with a hug as if they were old friends. "I really am glad to see you," she said into Jacqueline's ear. "And thank you for stopping him from running away."

"I like you, Julia," Jacqueline said because she meant it. "But him, I make no promises."

Julia held her hand out to Landon. "Nice to see you again, too, Landon."

Even though he was nervous and confused, Landon had manners. He shook her hand. "Hello, Ms. Julia."

Trick moved forward and sniffed Julia's shoulder, then eyed her suspiciously. "Hawk?"

Julia laughed. "Yes, it's me, Trick. I prefer 'Julia', though."

Trick stepped into Julia's personal space and sniffed her face, coming millimeters away from touching her without actually doing it. Most people would back off if someone got that close, but Julia stayed still.

"For the record, Trick," she said, "I was never trying to eat you. I was only ever watching over you. And," she added with a tone of full disclosure, "keeping tabs on you."

"You're like me," he said, which surprised Jacqueline. Trick hadn't been able to voice his thoughts for the past several years, but based on what she'd seen lately, she didn't think he ever really thought of himself as a familiar, only as a cat.

Julia nodded. "Yes, in a way, I am."

"Are you a hawk or a human?" he asked her.

Jacqueline was so stunned by his question, all she could do was wait to hear Julia's answer.

The other woman didn't hesitate for long. "I'm a human, Trick. You don't always have to have a human body to be a human."

Trick didn't look entirely satisfied with that answer, but when Julia reached up to give him a pet on the head, he didn't pull away from her.

"That's how I feel about it," Julia said. "But you're not me. You can come to your own conclusions."

Trick looked over his shoulder to Denneka but didn't say anything else.

Julia offered her hand to Denneka and introduced herself.

The girl shook it uncomfortably. "I guess you know who I am, since you've been watching in my window."

"I do," Julia said, unoffended and unashamed. "What do you think of all of this?"

"I don't know. It's weird. I'll... probably think it was all a dream by the time I'm an adult."

Julia raised her eyebrows, glanced at Trick, but made no response to her statement. "You should all come in. It's a chilly night."

"There isn't all that much to it, I'm afraid," Mr. McKenzie said. "So I'll keep it brief. Jacqueline, after we"—his eyes flicked to Landon for a second—"met, I kept an eye on you. Had Julia keep an eye on you, mostly. This wasn't... um... the first time this sort of thing had happened, and I like to stay informed of any... developments."

"You have other children?" Mom asked.

"I keep a spreadsheet."

Over in the love seat, Denneka squirmed, but Landon didn't know why.

Beside him, Mom made a huffing noise. "All right. Go on."

"That was how I learned of the troubles you had with your pregnancy."

Mom stiffened. "Let me guess. The anonymous note."

Mr. McKenzie nodded. "I couldn't do anything myself, of course, since that would have entailed getting involved in your life. But I knew that woman, and she had a reputation for being relatively reasonable."

"For a witch," said Mom.

"For a witch," Mr. McKenzie repeated. "The deal she made with you surprised me, as did her untimely death. You and your boys still held my interest at this point, and... well, to be honest, Trick has

proven highly entertaining. So, I kept an eye on him—on all of you
—over the years. When it became clear that Landon might have
inherited at least some of my magical ability, that only gave me
more reason to stay interested."

"When did you know?" Mom asked.

"When he was three," Mr. McKenzie said, "and he made a bowl
of dirt with his hands, then filled it with water without going to the
faucet. The two of you were in the back yard, but you were garden-
ing, so you didn't see."

Mom leaned forward. "But how did you—"

Ms. Julia raised her hand. "I was there, watching."

Mom gaped at her. Landon had a hard time imagining that Ms.
Julia had been there so long ago. The thought felt really weird.

Ms. Julia kept talking. "The familiar bond lets Kester see through
my eyes and hear through my ears."

"So, that night when you came for dinner..." said Mom.

Ms. Julia nodded. "He wanted me to ask you those things. He
was listening to everything. I'm sorry."

"No, *I'm* sorry," Mr. McKenzie said. "Jacqueline, truly. I'm sorry
for everything. Well... perhaps not everything. I can't really regret
helping you make Landon or pointing you to the help that saved
him, or even for what happened to Trick because of it."

"If *you'd* helped us, that wouldn't have had to happen," Mom
snapped.

"But Trick doesn't regret it," said Mr. McKenzie. "Do you,
Trick?"

"Regret what?" Trick asked.

"Being a cat."

"No."

"See there?"

Mom clenched her jaw at him. "He was six. Even now, he's too
young to know what he wants."

Trick turned toward her, and—being right between them—
Landon could see he was going to argue with her. But Mr. McKenzie

back and tried to teach you, you might never have realized how much power you have."

Landon thought of the scared looks on Officer Parkes's face and Miss Cutler's face and the faces of the other kids. Of how sure he'd been that he was a murderer until he'd brought Cliff back to life. Of how desperately he wanted to touch that kind of power again even though he hated how it had made people look at him and how it had made him feel. He couldn't answer Mr. McKenzie. All he could do was cry.

"Landon, it's okay." Mom wrapped an arm around his shoulders.

"What's wrong?" Trick asked.

"I—I—" Landon gasped. "I... hurt people. I almost killed someone."

A big, warm hand touched his cheek. "Oh, my little one," said Mr. McKenzie. When Landon looked into his eyes, they were wet. "What have I done to you?"

"Can you—keep teaching me?" Landon asked, his breathing too fast and hard.

"To use magic?" He shook his head. "I can't. First, because I'm giving it up myself. Second, because I don't believe your mother will let me. After what I've done—"

"Stop assuming what I will and won't do, if you don't mind," said Mom.

Mr. McKenzie looked up at her. "Do you mean you would?"

She breathed a big, loud breath. "Just tell me one thing, Kester. Was it all a lie? When you were 'John'. Why did you really do it?"

"At… at first, it was only to get a closer view of the entertainment I made of Trick. Then, I thought that while I was at it, while I was hidden and you wouldn't recognize me, I'd get a closer view of my son. But then… No, it wasn't all a lie."

"What did you mean that you're giving up magic?" Mom asked.

"I've realized… much, much too late… that it's not good for me. For any of us, I think. Witches have a reputation for being vain, arrogant, self-absorbed, and cruel. The reputation is well-deserved and entirely accurate. I don't think it's an accident or some cruel twist of fate that only people like us get such power. I now think… not that it's an excuse… but I believe the power itself makes us that way. That it brings out all the worst in us. I've dug myself in so deeply, I don't know if I can ever really make it out, but I'm going to try, and Julia is going to help me."

"If you can't teach him to use magic," Mom said softly, "can you teach him *not* to use it?"

"I'm hardly the best person to—"

"There's no one else. I'll do my best, but I won't know what he's struggling with. You will."

"Jacqueline—"

"Please, Kester. I don't want my son to become the type of person you just described."

Landon didn't want to be that type of person, either. And he knew—down to his bones—that he could be.

Mr. McKenzie looked at Landon and Mom like he didn't know what to say. "You would really let me?"

"He needs you, Kester," said Mom. "I hate that I didn't see it before, but after the time you two spent together, it's obvious to me. He needs you."

...ea what was going on. All he knew was his brother ...ying, the witch man who used to be the teacher man was crying and the familiar girl was sitting all the way over there on the love seat. Mom had made him sit with her and Brother at first, but now everyone was crying and hugging and it was getting weird, so he got up and went to sit beside the familiar girl.

What's going on?" he whispered to her.

"Have you not been paying attention?"

He shrugged.

"Mr. McKenzie is your brother's dad."

Yeah, Trick had heard that much. He'd never really thought about what it would mean to have a dad before. He'd gotten along fine without one so far. It was weird that his little brother was getting so sad about it. "Why is he sad?"

"He's not sad, Trick. They're crying because they're happy."

"If the teacher-witch man is Brother's dad, then that means he mated with Mom."

girl turned pink. "Yes."

thought of the witch man doing that to his mom made Trick
of angry, but the witch man wasn't trying to do it *now*, so Trick
ld probably get in trouble if he attacked him for it. "Why would
y mate if they're not mates?"

The familiar girl looked at him with raised eyebrows. "Why do
cats?"

"I don't know."

"Really?"

"I can smell when female cats are in heat, but I don't know why
it makes the males want to mate with them. *I* never do."

The familiar girl's face turned a different color now. It was close
to green. "Thank goodness for that."

The crying and hugging was finally over, and Mom and the
witch man were on their feet. "Now," said Mom, "just put Trick
back to normal and then we can have dinner."

Trick clawed at the cushion of the love seat, pressing himself
back into it. 'Normal' to his mom meant 'not a cat'. "No!" he
cried.

A soft hand pried one of his from the seat cushion and curled
around it. "It's okay," said the familiar girl. "It'll be fine."

"I want to be a cat!" he protested.

"See?" said the witch man to Mom. "I told you." Could the witch
man be his ally here? If he refused to change Trick, no one could
make him, right?

The familiar girl was still holding his hand. "You... you should
be human, Trick. I know you like being a cat, but I think you'll be
happier if you're human. You can make friends. Find... find other
people to hang out with."

What was she saying? He had thought she understood him.
What other people did she think he wanted to know?

Or... was she trying to get rid of him? He'd saved her from the
kidnapper. Hadn't that shown he wasn't useless?

The witch man came and stood in front of the love seat. "I'm
sorry to you two as well. Especially you, Denneka. You were never

…danger hadn't been Trick's fault. That was

The witch man ran a hand through his hair. "But I should prob ably admit that this whole ten-foot distance stipulation as the trigger of your transformation was because it was the most amusing thing I could think of. And it was. Positively delightful."

The familiar girl's hand clenched around Trick's. "I knew you weren't very nice," she muttered.

"No, I'm not," the witch man admitted. "But I'm going to work on it. For now, Trick, maybe I can offer a compromise between your mother and you. Jacqueline wants you to be human. You want to be a cat. None of you, I presume, want your transformation to continue to be tied to your proximity to Denneka."

"I want to be a cat," Trick said.

"All the time?" the witch man asked.

The word 'yes' was on the tip of Trick's tongue, but then he felt the warmth of the familiar girl's hand, and he hesitated.

The witch man smiled. "As I said before, I'm giving up magic. But before I do, I'm going to change the spell on Julia's transformation to give her total control over when and how much she changes. What if I did the same thing for you?"

"You can do that?" Mom asked.

"Of course. What do you think, Trick?"

Trick thought it over, looking for the catch. But if he could be a cat whenever he wanted and his mom couldn't stop him... He couldn't see a down side. And he didn't have to be a cat if he felt like being human sometimes, like when he was with the familiar girl.

He didn't really know why he would want to, but it seemed like a good thing to have the option. If nothing else, he could be better help for her if she got into trouble again.

"Okay," he said.

His mom argued that it would still be too dangerous since he'd have to be very careful and learn when not to transform and all sorts of other things that sounded a lot like rules. Trick didn't pay much attention. Instead, he looked at the familiar girl beside him, who was staring down at his hand in hers. He still wasn't at all sure he could read facial expressions right, but he thought she looked kind of sad.

The hawk lady knelt beside her. "What's the problem?" she asked softly, but not too softly for Trick to hear.

"I just can't believe it's over," said the familiar girl.

"With Kester, the crazy stuff is never over. Though it'll be different now."

"Not that," the girl said, still looking at Trick's hand. Did she know he was paying attention to her instead of his mom? "This."

The hawk lady's eyes met Trick's for a second, but even though he was confused, she didn't give him any answers. She asked the familiar girl, "What makes you think it is?"

"Trick won't need me anymore."

"He seems to like you, though."

Trick opened his mouth to say 'I do', but the hawk lady put a finger to her mouth in a gesture his mother had used enough times for him to understand as *be quiet*. The familiar girl was still staring at her hand instead of either of their faces, so she didn't see.

"He calls me 'the familiar girl'," said the familiar girl. "He only

beside Marcus's
...is old neighbor-
...es. "Does anyone
...king at the strange
...officially."
...nd Jacqueline turned
...the metal roof.
...he moved toward the

likes me becau...
plenty of o...
O... a blinding wave of light
...son, throwing him to the
...rcus dove on top of both of
...ething sharp and hot stung
...o sound but that of debris
...okay?"

drawing it in, pulling it t...

...nd
...ly know about

...awk lady, "because his animal
... perfectly normal human relationships
...an that."

...amiliar girl looked into the hawk lady's face,
...urprise.

...hawk lady winked, then came around the back of the love
...o talk softly in Trick's ear. "Do you know what humans do,
...ck, when they want to show someone they like them?"

Not that he could think of, no.

Mom and the witch man were still arguing. The hawk lady slipped around to the witch man's side, got his attention, and kissed him softly on the mouth. He smiled, took her hand, and kissed it, murmuring something.

Oh, right, Trick thought. Mom kissed him and Landon a lot, usually on the head or cheek. But he'd seen other humans kiss on the mouth sometimes. He'd never given it much thought.

The familiar girl still looked sad, and from what she'd told the hawk lady, she still didn't believe that Trick liked her. He'd told her in the strongest terms he could that he did, but maybe she hadn't understood him because he'd told her in cat language. [...] believe him if he told her like a human?

Still letting her hold his hand, he used his other hand [...] her chin and tilt her face toward him.

"Trick?" she said. Her face turned pink again, then kept brighter and brighter.

Trick pressed his lips to hers. They were soft. He... kind of [...] it. "I like you," he told her, adding words to make himself e[...] clear. "Please believe me."

Her face turned an even brighter red, and she whispered, "Oka[...] I do."

Someone laughed loudly. When Trick looked at the others, all the adults were smiling, the witch man was clapping, and Brother seemed as confused as Trick was about why everyone was excited.

But then Mom agreed that Trick could still be a cat, letting him take the offer the witch man made, and that was all Trick really wanted.

Well, maybe not *all*. Not anymore.

CHAPTER
TWENTY-SIX

"Are you sure this is it?" Jacqueline asked, standing beside Marcus's car. She hadn't seen anyone for a few miles, and this old neighborhood looked like it had been abandoned for decades. "Does anyone even live here?"

Marcus came around to her side of the car, looking at the strange house boarded up with metal sheeting. "No. Not officially."

"Ms. Julia's there," came Landon's voice, and Jacqueline turned to see him standing and pointing at the bird on the metal roof.

"Landon, stay in the car," she told him, but he moved toward the bird.

"This must be the place."

"Landon—"

The front half of the house exploded in a blinding wave of light and heat. Jacqueline dove on top of her son, throwing him to the ground to shield him with her body. Marcus dove on top of both of them. She heard him grunt just as something sharp and hot stung her arm.

A few seconds later, there was no sound but that of debris continuing to fall to the ground.

"Landon," she gasped. "Are you okay?"

"Think so."

Behind him, the children moved back, staying low. Good instincts.

"You never bothered to tell me your name," Kester told the man. "Why should I tell you mine?" An inferno of rage burned in Kester's chest. Pure, raw fury at this powerless, insignificant *nothing* who had threatened him. Who had taken and endangered what belonged to him. Who had made him—*him*—feel afraid.

Fear was for the weak. Fear was for victims. Fear was for prey. Fear was not for those like Kester McKenzie.

The worm who had dared to make him feel fear pulled a gun and pointed it at him.

Kester fed his rage with his magic, drawing it in, pulling it to him, preparing to aim it.

He would make this worm feel fear.

Very, very briefly.

likes me because I'm convenient. Once I'm not around, he'll find plenty of other friends and… girls."

Once she wasn't around? Was she planning to leave him?

The hawk lady leaned closer to the girl's ear, and Trick had to work to hear her over the argument his mom and the witch man were having about him. "Denneka, 'familiar' doesn't mean 'convenient'. It comes from the word 'family'."

The familiar girl didn't answer that, but a crease formed between her eyebrows.

"You forget I've been watching the two of you. He likes you, Denneka. And not just because you're the only girl around."

"He says he likes me, but when I asked him what he liked, all he could say was that I'm familiar." Her voice was getting tight and high, and tears pooled in her eyes. "What does he really know about me? What about me, myself, does he like?"

"Maybe he likes you," said the hawk lady, "because his animal instincts tell him to. A lot of perfectly normal human relationships are built on no more than that."

Finally, the familiar girl looked into the hawk lady's face, blinking in surprise.

The hawk lady winked, then came around the back of the love seat to talk softly in Trick's ear. "Do you know what humans do, Trick, when they want to show someone they like them?"

Not that he could think of, no.

Mom and the witch man were still arguing. The hawk lady slipped around to the witch man's side, got his attention, and kissed him softly on the mouth. He smiled, took her hand, and kissed it, murmuring something.

Oh, right, Trick thought. Mom kissed him and Landon a lot, usually on the head or cheek. But he'd seen other humans kiss on the mouth sometimes. He'd never given it much thought.

The familiar girl still looked sad, and from what she'd told the hawk lady, she still didn't believe that Trick liked her. He'd told her in the strongest terms he could that he did, but maybe she hadn't understood him because he'd told her in cat language. Would she believe him if he told her like a human?

Still letting her hold his hand, he used his other hand to touch her chin and tilt her face toward him.

"Trick?" she said. Her face turned pink again, then kept going brighter and brighter.

Trick pressed his lips to hers. They were soft. He... kind of liked it. "I like you," he told her, adding words to make himself extra clear. "Please believe me."

Her face turned an even brighter red, and she whispered, "Okay. I do."

Someone laughed loudly. When Trick looked at the others, all the adults were smiling, the witch man was clapping, and Brother seemed as confused as Trick was about why everyone was excited.

But then Mom agreed that Trick could still be a cat, letting him take the offer the witch man made, and that was all Trick really wanted.

Well, maybe not *all*. Not anymore.

EPILOGUE

Ten years later

"Hey, sis," Jonah said right into Denneka's ear.

"Aaah!" She jerked, her knees banging the bottom of the desk, and spun to see her brother standing behind her, laughing.

"Jumpy much?"

"I was distracted. What are you doing here?"

"Trick called and said his mom was making him help buy food and it was taking too long so they were going straight to the party."

"And since he has the car, he asked you to pick me up on your way," she guessed.

He nodded.

Crap. Now they wouldn't get a chance to talk for hours.

Jonah leaned against the other desk. "I'm surprised she got him to leave while you were still here."

"Yeah, she laid the guilt trip on pretty thick."

"And that worked?"

"Not until I told him he should go." Denneka regretted that now. The doctor had called right after he'd left.

"You ready?" Jonah checked the clock on the wall. "It's almost one."

She saved the copy she'd been working on as a new draft. "Yeah. Just let me close this out."

"How's the website coming?"

"Good. The new layout's nearly done, but there are all these places that need descriptions or calls to action, and it's hard to figure out how to be informative and enticing without being corny or annoying."

"Why didn't Mom and Dad just have Trick do it?" Jonah asked.

Denneka let out a bark of laughter.

Jonah took it a step further and did an impression of Trick. "'Shirt: this one is red. Shirt: this one is also red. Jacket: to go over shirt. Please buy them now.'"

"Pretty much." She shut the computer down and gathered her things.

"I still can't figure out why Mom and Dad hired him. Does he really make any sales?"

As they left the office, Denneka pondered how to answer. "Maybe not directly. But he does draw people in. Certain types of people, anyway. Kids think he's fun. Older women love him." When Jonah raised his eyebrows at that, she shrugged. "They think he's adorable."

"Mmm," Jonah said, nodding. "To be fair, he is. Though he's a lot cuter when he's"—he lowered his voice and made a cat-sized gesture with his hands—"smaller and furrier."

Denneka smacked her brother in the arm. They left through the front of the store, waving goodbye to Barb on their way out, and headed for Jonah's car.

As soon as they stopped chatting, Denneka's mind went back to the doctor's news, and it felt like moths were swarming in her stomach. It was hard to think of going the rest of the day pretending everything was normal. Everything wasn't normal, and it wouldn't ever be again. Every moment that passed when her brain wasn't engaged, it was thinking up new problems and worries. Each one brought brought up another one, and another, and soon her head was full of them. So while they drove down Main Street, she tried to distract herself with small talk. "How's Paul doing?"

"Better. It was pretty serious for a few days, but we put him on some antibiotics and other treatment, and he's nearly back to normal. I've switched him to a prescription food, though. Kyle, too, just to be safe."

"Isn't two cats a lot in your apartment?"

"Nah. We all get along, so it's fine." Jonah glanced sideways at her, a conspiratorial gleam in his eye. "Don't tell Mom, but I might get another soon."

Their mom still hated cats. It was part of the reason they still hadn't told either of their parents about Trick's... specialness. Mom didn't hide her hatred of cats, and although Trick didn't argue with her about it, it did make him act somewhat coldly toward her. Which her parents couldn't help but pick up on. Mom and Dad didn't *disapprove* of Trick, but the three of them didn't have the warmest relationship in the world.

Denneka rolled her eyes and said, "I won't. But why?"

He sighed. "Someone brought in a pregnant stray last week. The poor thing was tiny, barely eight months old, and... well, the kittens were too big. The sire must have been huge."

Denneka suddenly had trouble keeping her stomach settled.

Jonah was watching the road and didn't notice her discomfort. "She and three of the kittens didn't survive the birth, but two did. Someone's fostering them—it's not easy, fostering newborns—and has already said she'll take one of them, but the other needs a home."

A vision of a too-small, too-young mother cat lying dead on a table beside her three babies floated in front of Denneka's eyes, and she couldn't make it go away.

Somewhere out there a big tomcat was going about his life without a care in the world.

Denneka gripped the handle of the door, wondering if she

should ask Jonah to pull over or if she would manage to keep her lunch down.

"When I get her," Jonah said, oblivious to Denneka's queasiness, "I think I might call her Amy."

"Ugh," Denneka groaned. There was a name she didn't need to hear ever again.

"Okay, weirdly intense reaction. What do you think of 'Nicole'?"

"It's fine." Denneka didn't really care about her brother's odd tendency to give animals people names. She stared at the dashboard, focused on her breathing, and the nausea gradually passed.

Jonah didn't speak again, leaving Denneka to think up more worries as they drove the rest of the way to the McKenzies' house and parked next to three other cars on the brick turnaround. They didn't even bother going into the house but walked around the side to the back yard. The day was warm but not hot, and sunny but with plenty of fluffy clouds in the sky. Three kids chased each other on the elaborate play set—technically still in the back yard but well away from the riverbank—and the rest of the crowd was already clumped up in small groups.

As soon as they came around the corner of the house, Trick spotted them and ran over. He hugged her, rubbed the side of his head against hers, and purred loudly. She clung to him briefly, wondering if she should ask him to go inside to talk.

Satisfied with the amount of attention he'd gotten, Trick stepped back. "The food's almost cooked."

"Good," said Jonah. "I'm starving." He gave Trick a quick head rub and went over to put a wrapped present on the gift table.

Now was her chance to get Trick alone. But the thought of telling him the news made her stomach get fluttery again. And she really didn't want to hijack the party.

A seven-year-old so big he looked closer to ten took the decision out of her hands when he ran over from the play set, smacked Trick on the back, and yelled, "You're it!" He darted away, and Trick took off after him without a second glance at Denneka.

Kids really did love Trick. She was never entirely sure how he felt about them.

"Sorry about Vincent," Julia said, coming up to her. "I've tried to teach him not to interrupt people, but he loses his manners when he gets into a game."

"It's fine," Denneka told her. "I like watching them."

The two women did so together for a few minutes. Vincent did a good job of staying out of Trick's reach, despite having a height disadvantage. That likely wouldn't last forever, though. Trick was pretty average in height. Vincent, everyone said, was on track to be tall—probably several inches taller than Kester. And from the looks of him now, to probably outweigh his father by several dozen pounds of muscle as well. He took after his mom, for sure, all except for the color and striking prettiness of his eyes.

"Julia," Denneka began in a casual, conversational way, "you're sure Vincent's not a witch, right?"

Julia nodded. "He'd definitely have shown signs of it by now if he was."

"But what about… um, that is… he obviously takes after you…"

"What are you trying to ask, Denneka?"

"Does he have any… birdishness?"

Julia laughed. Then thought about it. "Well, his eyesight is pretty good. Not that that means anything. Really, I can't think of any reason why he should have inherited any of that. I was careful not to transform at all when we were trying to get pregnant. It seems like the sort of thing that could cause a miscarriage. Or worse."

Any follow-up questions Denneka might have asked were prevented by the approach of the two other women.

"Remind me again," Lisa said to Jacqueline, "which one is your oldest?"

"The one crouched in the grass," Jacqueline said with a tired sigh.

Trick was indeed on all fours, pressing himself into the grass as if it could camouflage him, while he slowly stalked toward Vincent, who was hiding behind a tree. The two other children did cart-wheels together nearby, but Trick was focused on the larger boy.

A little too focused. "Oh, no," Denneka murmured.

One second after Trick's butt started to wiggle, a long, black tail sprang out of the hidden hole in his pants and lashed about enthusi-astically. Jacqueline had had to modify all of Trick's pants to make room for such occurrences. When he managed to keep his rear end fully human, the hole was disguised with carefully overlapping fabric.

"Trick! Keep it in your pants!" Jacqueline barked at him, but he didn't listen. He was too busy sprinting toward Vincent.

Denneka eyed Lisa with concern, but her former principal only took another sip of the punch she was holding and turned casually away. "I see nothing. I know nothing." As far as Denneka knew, no one had ever told Lisa about the magic stuff, but since she was around them from time to time, she was bound to see it. Especially when Trick let his guard down because he thought of himself as being at home and among family. This was the most blatant strange-ness that Denneka knew of Lisa ever having witnessed, but her lack of shock made Denneka wonder how much she'd guessed.

Jacqueline rubbed her forehead. "I'm sorry about him."

"Sorry about what?" Lisa asked her. "I have no idea what you're referring to. My life is exactly as complicated as I want it already, thank you. By the way, Julia, how is your knitting business going?"

"Oh, I'm past that," Julia said with a wave. "It's photography now." Before knitting it had been eBay reselling, and before that, proofreading. She had a long list of jobs she'd tried and was always looking for one that would interest her for the long term. As long as she could do it from home on her own time and it didn't require any education that she couldn't get from the internet, she was willing to consider it.

Denneka quietly excused herself and made her way down the yard and around the gift table, toward the back deck. Since the stairs were on the side farthest from where she'd been standing, that

ᵻtuated at the

ve me, I would, but
e both know that."
ce where Denneka
e more awkward
be caught if she

as if physically
y say that in
've also been
easure we've
mentation if
"

think I'm

nto his
nding
een a

ut
a

men standing
done so when

, pointing a spatul
, and laughing together.
e only been with two of

ɔ was inspecting the cooked
the table beside the barbecue
g none of your lovers ever met

And they definitely didn't become

ɔot to foot, not sure how to interrupt at
do so.

d for me," Kester said, "I would endure all
world and never let her see it, for her to have
ed."

d the three women, the burgers on the grill in
ling away and tossing delicious smells into the air.
es, doesn't she? How is it not weird for *her*? Jac and
eir own histories, but Julia was never with anyone else,

r got strangely still and quiet for a moment. Now Denneka
to back away and give them more privacy, but she was sure
did, she'd make some sound, they'd notice her, and things
uld be as awkward as they could get. "Truth be told," Kester said
oftly enough that Denneka almost didn't hear him. She tried not to,
but she still couldn't help doing so. "I believe it is. Not often. But
there are times when we're together, and her happiness is interrupted by a sudden, intense... something. Disappointment, I think.
Longing. I'm not sure. I haven't asked her about it, and she doesn't

n it. If I could give her as much as she g

no point in wishing to change the past. W

here were several seconds of awkward silen

perately wanted to back away slowly, but th

silent it got, the more sure she was that she'

oved.

But then Kester grinned and shifted his posture

shrugging off the heavy moment. "You know, the

certain ways, when you've been with someone, you

with everyone they've ever been with. Since by that m

already been with each other, I'm up for some experi

you are."

Marcus pointed the spatula at him. "You are not funny

Kester's grin widened. "Are you certain? Because I

hilarious."

"Obviously."

Kester shifted to face Marcus, which brought Denneka i

line of sight. "Ah, Denneka. How long have you been sta

there? Never mind, I can see from your expression that it's b

while."

"S… sorry," she said.

Marcus glanced at her and looked slightly uncomfortable,

Kester only kept smiling and came over to her. "It's fine. You're

woman of discretion. I trust you. Rather, I should apologize fo

blathering on about my private life in front of you again."

Denneka had tried hard to forget the stories she'd heard Kester

tell the murderer who'd kidnapped them that one time, but they'd

been extremely memorable stories. In her youthful foolishness,

she'd even asked Kester later if they'd been true or if he'd been

inventing them on the spot. The answer had made it difficult for her

to look him in the eye for months. "It's fine! I should have made

more noise."

"Do you want some food?" Marcus asked, poking the spatula

toward the food table.

She waved off the suggestion. "I had a light lunch not hungry yet."

Kester cocked his head at her. "Do you have some want to talk about?"

"Um… just a quick question."

"All right." He held out a hand toward the back door followed her into the house. "What can I do for you?"

As they stood in the living room, Denneka fidgeted with her slee She hadn't meant to make such a big deal of this. It was supposed to b a casual question, not something she wanted to take someone aside for. "Well, since you're the one who knows the most about how magic works, I was just wondering… The, um, the transformations… Can that sort of thing be passed on? Um, genetically, I mean?"

Kester's pale blue eyes narrowed at her, and they were so intense that they made her squirm even more. "To children?"

What else could 'genetically' mean? "Yeah."

A knowing, foxy grin spread across his face. "Not that I'm aware of," he said. "But there has not been sufficient opportunity for study on that topic. I suppose it might depend on whether the parent in question was at all transformed when the conception took place."

Denneka could feel her face heat, betraying her.

Kester chuckled.

"Just the ears and tail!" she blurted defensively. "And the eyes, if it's dark. And"—she waved a hand around her chest—"whatever it is that lets him purr."

Kester laughed.

Denneka tried to scowl at him, but the furious blushing she couldn't help was probably ruining the effect. "He's like that all the time at home! It's how he's most comfortable!"

The outrageous man actually rubbed his hands together in glee. "This is going to be fun. I can't wait to see what you two have concocted."

"'Concocted'?" she repeated, hardly able to believe he'd used that word. "This isn't a scheme! They're children!"

idened. "They?"

Denneka grabbed her head in her hands and squatted
ng room floor. "I—I just assumed. Because cats have

atted her shoulder. "There, there, young one. Think about it
ally. Nothing about what Trick is would make your body
se more eggs, would it?"

That made sense. Yes, okay, that made sense. She took some deep
eaths, calmed herself, and stood back up. "I haven't had the
chance to tell him yet," she said glumly. She really hadn't meant to
tell anyone else before him. She should have found the time to talk
to him first before going around asking other people about any of
the stuff she was worrying over.

"My lips are sealed," Kester assured her. "And I'm sorry I
couldn't give you more definite answers. But it is quite thrilling,
isn't it?"

Thrilling? More like terrifying.

When they went back outside, they found the deck much more
crowded than when they'd left it. Half the group was getting food
or standing around eating food they'd just gotten. She went over to
where Trick stood with Jonah and Julia, scarfing down a burger
while the other two chatted. He still had his tail out, and it was
swaying contentedly as he ate.

"Where's the birthday boy?" Julia asked.

Jonah raised his chin to look around the yard.

Trick answered with his mouth full and without withdrawing
his attention from his food. "Brother's in the gazebo with Boy Twin
and Girl Twin. The smiley boy went to look for him."

Julia snickered.

"Trick," Denneka reminded him gently. "Names." He'd gotten
much better at calling people by their names, but whenever he was
stressed, emotional, or distracted, he still tended to fall back on
whatever he called people in his head.

Trick met her eyes, looked at Julia and Jonah, and then swallowed his food. "Landon's in the gazebo with Jace and Maris, and I saw Sawyer running that way, too."

"I'll go make sure they all know everyone's eating," Denneka volunteered. It would be hard to get Trick alone right now without attracting attention, and there was no point trying to talk to him while he was hungry, anyway.

She walked out to the elegant, white gazebo that Kester had erected on the far side of the back yard, past where the tree line started. It was in a cozy little spot near the river's edge. She found Landon sitting inside, silently reading a book on a bench while his two younger siblings sat on the floor, playing one of those collectible card games. Even without their unusual eyes, they'd have been striking. Both had Jacqueline's red hair, and even though they were different genders, the eight-year-olds looked so similar in every aspect that they were frequently thought to be identical.

"The food's ready, and everyone's eating," Denneka announced.

The twins gathered their cards, arguing over which of them had claim to what Denneka assumed was a particularly good one. They seemed in most ways to be pretty typical kids. It was only their odd looks that made them stick out.

Maris had been born with brown eyes and Jace with hazel eyes. When the twins had been infants, Landon had only been eight and still hadn't had very good control of his powers. In looking at them in the cradle, he'd commented that they would look even more similar if their eyes matched.

And then... they did. Sort of. Now, Jace and Maris each had one hazel eye and one brown eye, though on opposite sides. Remembering which had the hazel eye on the left and which had it on the right was the easiest—and sometimes only—way for most people to tell them apart.

The eye switch hadn't caused the twins any real damage. Landon, though, had been so horrified by what he'd accidentally done that he'd refused to try to fix it in case he made it worse. Since it wasn't life-threatening, Julia refused to allow Kester to break his magical sobriety by fixing it himself. And even though Kester knew other witches who could do it, it wasn't worth the price any of them would ask.

Maris ran over and tugged on one of Landon's hands. "Are you coming, big brother?"

"In a moment," Landon said without looking up from his book.

"Maris, come on, I'm hungry," ordered Jace, grabbing his sister's other hand and pulling her away from Landon. The twins ran off together toward the rest of the family.

Landon didn't make any move to get up. Denneka sat beside him on the bench. Neither of them said anything for a minute or two.

"Are you gonna go eat?" she asked after he turned a page and kept reading.

"Yeah," he said. "In a bit."

"The food smells really good."

"Yeah. Stepdad's not much of a cook, but his barbecue's good."

They sat there for a few more minutes. Landon turned another page.

"They're gonna want to do the cake and presents soon," she said.

"I know. I'm almost done."

"Happy birthday, by the way."

"Thanks."

Another few minutes of silence. The river was sure pretty, and the sound of it was soothing.

"Denneka," Landon said, "what are you hiding from?"

"What are *you* hiding from?" she countered.

He closed the book and looked at her with complete dispassion. "The same thing I'm always hiding from. The same thing I'll be hiding from until my hormones stop driving me crazy. Everything."

"You're seventeen now. That's one more year down," she said encouragingly. "Only four or so more to go."

"Why does it take so long?"

"I hear most people enjoy their teenage years."

"Most people aren't liable to become monsters if they give in to temptation even once."

"Landon, you're not going to become a monster."

He shook his head. "You don't know. I can't even let myself *think* about wanting anything from anyone else. You have no idea how easy it would be for me to get it. And if I used magic for that, I wouldn't be able to stop using it for everything. I don't want to be the person that would make me."

"There are no scantily clad teen girls at your birthday party," Denneka told him. The truth was, there were no unrelated kids his age to even invite. He'd been homeschooled for years now, and he avoided being in social situations with other kids. That was why everyone in the family had made a particular effort to show up today.

"I know. But I can't risk getting annoyed or angry or..." He shook his head again.

"It's your birthday party, Landon. You're supposed to be happy. It's okay to be happy."

He took in a deep breath, held it, and let it out. "I know. I just don't want to bring everyone down."

"You won't bring anyone down. We all understand. Well, the kids don't understand. And most of us only understand in theory. But it's okay. We support you."

"I appreciate it."

"Landon... do you really think you'd be as bad as that? Just because your dad got that way?"

"It's not just because of him. Mostly, it's because of me. I nearly killed someone when I was *six*. Without even really trying. What could I do now if I tried? I'm really not afraid I'll become like Dad was. I'm afraid I'll become much, much worse."

The calm way he said that made Denneka's heart hurt for him. She wanted to put her arm around him and comfort him, but he'd told them all years ago that he didn't want to be touched by any females other than his mom or his little sister. Even his stepmom wasn't allowed to touch him unless she was in hawk form. It must have been hard for a teen boy to lay out his struggles so openly to his whole family like that. Denneka admired him more than she could figure out how to say.

"Don't worry, Landon," said a cheerful voice. "We won't let you become Voldemort." A lean sixteen-year-old boy slightly taller than Landon bounded into the gazebo and perched atop the back of the bench on the opposite side of Landon from Denneka.

"Where did you run off to?" When Landon spoke to his nearest brother, his expression visibly relaxed in a way it hadn't when he'd been talking to Denneka, the corner of his mouth even curling up a little.

"I saw these"—the boy flourished a bouquet of yellow flowers—"and thought I'd get some for everybody. Here's one for you, and one for you." He handed a flower each to Landon and Denneka.

For some absurd reason, the flower made Denneka's mood brighten a little. "Thanks, Sawyer."

"Aren't they pretty?" he enthused.

"You know Julia will kill you if you picked these from her garden," Landon warned him, sniffing the flower.

Sawyer seemed to be counting the remaining flowers in his bouquet. "Nah, Mom won't mind. These were wild. Took me a little while to gather enough because I had to search around."

"You probably didn't have to get one for everybody," Landon suggested, but Sawyer only cocked his head like the comment didn't make sense.

Sitting beside Landon on the bench back like he was, Sawyer reminded Denneka even more than usual of the 'angel on the shoulder' from those old cartoons—the ones where a character is being tempted to do something bad and miniature versions of themself appear on their shoulders dressed as an angel and a devil. Only usually it was Kester whose shoulder she pictured Sawyer sitting on.

Not long after they'd gotten married, Julia had encouraged Kester to make contact with the other kids he had by other women. Among them was Sawyer, who'd been in the foster system since he was a baby. It had been a pretty obvious move at that point for Kester and Julia to adopt him.

Much like Landon, Sawyer took after Kester almost entirely in his looks. He had sunshine blond hair and sky blue eyes, and a face similar enough to Landon's—in the rare moments when he wasn't smiling—that the two could pass as at least fraternal twins. But Sawyer wasn't a witch. Maybe for that reason, Sawyer seemed to have all the playful good cheer that Kester did but without the underlying selfishness and arrogance which Kester still struggled with. He was like a smaller (or younger, anyway, not so much smaller these days), pure and wholesome version of Kester. Just like that little cartoon shoulder angel.

Denneka hoped that didn't make Landon the devil.

Sawyer jumped up. "Come on, let's go eat."

And when Sawyer said it, Landon got up and followed him out of the gazebo.

As Denneka followed behind them, a stray thought crossed her mind. *'Familiar' comes from 'family'.*

Between one thing and another, she didn't get a chance to talk to Trick alone until later that night in their apartment. The party had gone late, so by the time they got home, it was time for the nightly wind-down.

Denneka was at the computer checking her e-mail when Trick came in, fully naked, took her hand, and pulled her behind him to the bathroom. He did this sort of thing more nights than not, so she went along with it without arguing, taking off her clothes and getting into the shower with him. He didn't even touch her that much; it was mostly about having her near. And, even though he was now perfectly capable of washing his own hair, he still liked her to do it sometimes. Tonight was one of those times.

He sat on the floor of the tub, the easier for her to reach his head as she stood behind him. His purring was so loud, she could hear it even over the thrumming of the water—and the pounding of her heart.

When it was time to rinse the soap out, he stood up, facing her with the back of his head to the flow of water. He was taller than her, but not so much that it was awkward for her to reach up and wash the soap out for him.

"Trick," she said, knowing she was a coward for waiting until his eyes were closed against the soap, "I have something to tell you."

"Mmm?" he hummed, waiting.

There didn't seem to be a best way to ease into this. "I'm pregnant."

His eyes shot open. Soapy water immediately trickled into them. With a noise of pain, he spun toward the water and frantically rinsed off his face and head. When he was done, he slammed off the faucet. In the sudden silence of their small bathroom, he turned back to her, his eyes still wide. "Kittens?"

She almost laughed. She might have, if it weren't so close to her own worries. "I hope not."

"Kitten humans," he corrected. Then corrected himself again. "Babies?"

"Probably only one." She hoped. She wasn't sure she was ready for more than one. Especially if...

He was staring at her in shock, his eyes going from her face to her belly and back like he was trying to put the ideas of 'Denneka' and 'pregnant' together in his mind. It was not the face of a man who was happy to hear about his impending fatherhood.

She stepped out of the tub, grabbed a towel, and dried herself off on the way to the bedroom. Trick took so long following after her that by the time he did, she was in her pajamas, under the covers, and well into imagining the worst case scenario.

"A baby," he said from the doorway. He was still naked, but he was dry and in his usual partially-transformed at-home state. His black cat ears were perked forward, and his tail had gone bushy.

"Yes."

He walked over to her and sat on the bed. The lamps on the nightstands made the slits in his green eyes narrow. "Why did you run away?"

There was no point avoiding the issue. She needed to just say it. "Because... I was afraid you would. I'm... afraid you will."

One of his ears twitched, and his tail thumped against the bed. "Explain."

"We weren't planning to have kids. Not yet, anyway. You've never even said you want any. So I was afraid to tell you. I was afraid when you found out, you'd... you'd want to leave."

Both of his ears laid flat in anger for a second before going neutral again. His tail thumped a few more times. None of the emotion displayed with his cat parts showed in his face or voice.

He braced his hands on the bed either side of her hips and leaned in so his face was close to hers. "Denneka. I said I won't leave you. I'd been telling you for years that I won't leave you, but you didn't believe me until I said it in front of a bunch of people and signed a piece of paper. Why are you doubting me again?"

She suddenly remembered promising him after their wedding that she wouldn't doubt him on that point again, and now she was. No wonder he was irritated at her. This *shouldn't* be bothering her, but suddenly it did. It had been all afternoon. Why? She fingered the blanket on her lap, not able to meet his penetrating gaze. "Your dad left. When he found out about you. And... and tomcats aren't exactly known for their stellar parenting skills."

Trick stared at her, unmoving, for so long that she had to look at him to try to figure out what he was thinking. Once their eyes met, she saw nearly no expression on his face, but he said softly, "I am a tomcat. And I am my father's son. But I'm also me. And *I* say that I will never leave you, Denneka St. Andrew. Not if you have a dozen babies. Not for anything. Not ever."

The tightness that she'd felt in her chest for the past several hours relaxed. She smiled and reached up to rub behind his ears. He groaned in pleasure, then pressed his forehead to hers, purring.

"I really hope I don't have a dozen babies," she said.

"Me, too," he confessed. "I don't even know what to do with one."

"We'll have lots of help," she said, thinking of their very strange but supportive family.

"Yeah." He kissed her. When he pulled back, she saw that his feline pupils were huge and round, despite the light not having changed. Lifting the blankets, he got into bed with her. He rubbed his head against hers, licked her, bit her, kissed her.

"I love you, Trick," she told him.

He didn't repeat the words back to her. He was too far gone for that. When he did speak, his voice was an insistent whisper. "Mate." It was both an endearment and a request, simultaneously calling to her and beseeching her.

She bit his neck and purred her answer into his ear. "Mate."

AUTHOR LINKS

Thank you for reading *Seven Years Awesome Luck* by Shawna Canon. To find more of my books or sign up to get an e-mail when I publish a new book, visit shawnacanon.com

instagram.com/shawnacanon

goodreads.com/shawnacanon

amazon.com/author/shawnacanon

facebook.com/shawnacanon

bookbub.com/authors/shawna-canon

patreon.com/shawnacanon